Hormones and Cancer: Breast and Prostate

Guest Editor

ALICE C. LEVINE, MD

ENDOCRINOLOGY AND METABOLISM CLINICS OF NORTH AMERICA

www.endo.theclinics.com

Consulting Editor

DEREK LEROITH, MD, PhD

September 2011 • Volume 40 • Number 3

SAUNDERS an imprint of ELSEVIER, Inc.

W.B. SAUNDERS COMPANY
A Division of Elsevier Inc.

1600 John F. Kennedy Boulevard ● Suite 1800 ● Philadelphia, Pennsylvania 19103-2899

http://www.theclinics.com

ENDOCRINOLOGY AND METABOLISM CLINICS OF NORTH AMERICA Volume 40, Number 3
September 2011 ISSN 0889-8529, ISBN-13: 978-1-4557-1029-4

Editor: Rachel Glover
Developmental Editor: Donald Mumford

Endocrinology and Metabolism Clinics of North America (ISSN 0889-8529) is published quarterly by Elsevier Inc., 360 Park Avenue South, New York, NY 10010-1710. Months of issue are March, June, September, and December. Periodicals postage paid at New York, NY and additional mailing offices. Subscription prices are USD 290.00 per year for US individuals, USD 503.00 per year for US institutions, USD 146.00 per year for US students and residents, USD 364.00 per year for Canadian individuals, USD 616.00 per year for Canadian institutions, USD 422.00 per year for international individuals, USD 616.00 per year for international institutions, and USD 216.00 per year for international and Canadian and foreign students/residents. To receive student/resident rate, orders must be accompanied by name of affiliated institution, date of term, and the signature of program/ residency coordinator on institution letterhead. Orders will be billed at individual rate until proof of status is received. Foreign air speed delivery is included in all *Clinics* subscription prices. All prices are subject to change without notice. **POSTMASTER:** Send address changes to *Endocrinology and Metabolism Clinics of North America*, Elsevier Health Sciences Division, Subscription Customer Service, 3251 Riverport Lane, Maryland Heights, MO 63043. **Customer Service: Telephone: 1-800-654-2452** (U.S. and Canada); **1-314-447-8871** (outside U.S. and Canada). **Fax: 1-314-447-8029. E-mail: journalscustomerservice-usa@elsevier.com** (for print support); **journalsonlinesupport-usa@elsevier.com** (for online support).

Reprints. For copies of 100 or more, of articles in this publication, please contact the Commercial Rights Department, Elsevier Inc., 360 Park Avenue South, New York, NY 10010-1710; phone: (+1) 212-633-3813; fax: (+1) 212-462-1935; e-mail: reprints@elsevier.com.

Endocrinology and Metabolism Clinics of North America is covered in *MEDLINE/PubMed (Index Medicus), EMBASE/Excerpta Medica, Current Contents/Clinical Medicine, Current Contents/Life Sciences, Science Citation Index, ISI/BIOMED, BIOSIS,* and *Chemical Abstracts.*

Printed and bound by CPI Group (UK) Ltd, Croydon, CR0 4YY

Transferred to Digital Print 2011

Contributors

CONSULTING EDITOR

DEREK LEROITH, MD, PhD
Chief, Division of Endocrinology, Metabolism, and Bone Diseases, Department
of Medicine, Mount Sinai School of Medicine, New York, New York

GUEST EDITOR

ALICE C. LEVINE, MD
Associate Professor of Medicine and Oncological Sciences, Division of Endocrinology,
Diabetes and Bone Disease, Mount Sinai School of Medicine, New York, New York

AUTHORS

KERIN ADELSON, MD
Assistant Professor of Medicine, Division of Hematology and Medical Oncology, Mount
Sinai School of Medicine, New York, New York

OLUYEMI AKIN-OLUGBADE, MD
Resident, Department of Urology, Mount Sinai School of Medicine, New York, New York

PETER C. ALBERTSEN, MD, MS
Professor and Chief, Division of Urology, University of Connecticut Health Center,
Farmington, Connecticut

MARY HELEN BARCELLOS-HOFF, PhD
Professor of Radiation Oncology and Cell Biology, Departments of Radiation Oncology
and Cell Biology, New York University School of Medicine, New York, New York

NOA BIRAN, MD
Resident Physician, Samuel Bronfman Department of Medicine, Mount Sinai Medical
Center, New York, New York

WENDY Y. CHEN, MD, MPH
Assistant Professor in Medicine, Channing Laboratory, Brigham and Women's Hospital;
Department of Medical Oncology, Dana Farber Cancer Institute, Harvard Medical School,
Boston, Massachusetts

CONSTANTINE DIMITRAKAKIS, MD
Developmental Endocrinology Branch, National Institute of Child Health and Human
Development, National Institutes of Health, CRC, Bethesda, Maryland; 1st Department
of Obstetrics/Gynecology, Athens University Medical School, Alexandra Hospital,
Athens, Greece

DORIS GERMAIN, PhD
Associate Professor, Division of Hematology/Oncology, Department of Medicine, Tisch
Cancer Institute, Mount Sinai School of Medicine, New York, New York

SERGE GINZBURG, MD
Chief Resident, Division of Urology, University of Connecticut Health Center, Farmington,
Connecticut

MATHIS GROSSMANN, MD, PhD, FRACP
Senior Research Fellow, Department of Medicine, Austin Health/Northern Health,
University of Melbourne; Endocrinologist, Department of Endocrinology, Austin Health,
Heidelberg, Victoria, Australia

SHUK-MEI HO, PhD
Jacob G. Schmidlapp Professor and Chair, Department of Environmental Health,
Center for Environmental Genetics, Cancer Institute, College of Medicine, University
of Cincinnati; Cincinnati Veterans Affairs Medical Center, Cincinnati, Ohio

JEFF M.P. HOLLY, PhD
Professor, School of Clinical Sciences, University of Bristol, Southmead Hospital, Bristol,
United Kingdom

ALEXANDER KIRSCHENBAUM, MD
Associate Clinical Professor of Oncological Sciences; Associate Clinical Professor
of Urology, Department of Urology, Mount Sinai School of Medicine, New York, New York

DAVID L. KLEINBERG, MD
Professor of Medicine, Department of Medicine (Endocrinology); Director,
Neuroendocrine Unit, New York University School of Medicine; Consultant, Veterans
Affairs Medical Center, New York, New York

HUNG-MING LAM, PhD
Research Associate, Department of Environmental Health, College of Medicine,
University of Cincinnati; Cincinnati Veterans Affairs Medical Center, Cincinnati, Ohio

CHRISTINE H. LEE, BA
Assistant Researcher, Department of Genetics and Genomic Sciences, Mount Sinai
School of Medicine, New York, New York

MING-TSUNG LEE, MPhil
Graduate Student, Department of Environmental Health, College of Medicine, University
of Cincinnati, Cincinnati, Ohio

YUET-KIN LEUNG, PhD
Research Assistant Professor, Department of Environmental Health, Center for
Environmental Genetics, Cancer Institute, College of Medicine, University of Cincinnati,
Cincinnati, Ohio

ALICE C. LEVINE, MD
Associate Professor of Medicine and Oncological Sciences, Division of Endocrinology,
Diabetes and Bone Disease, Mount Sinai School of Medicine, New York, New York

FARYAL SARDAR ALI MIRZA, MD
Assistant Professor of Medicine, Division of Endocrinology, University of Connecticut
Health Center, Farmington, Connecticut

ELAHE A. MOSTAGHEL, MD, PhD
Assistant Member, Clinical Research Division, Fred Hutchinson Cancer Research Center, Seattle, Washington

CLAIRE M. PERKS, PhD
School of Clinical Sciences, University of Bristol, Southmead Hospital, Bristol, United Kingdom

STEPHEN PLYMATE, MD
Professor, Department of Medicine, School of Medicine, University of Washington and VAPSHCS/GRECC, Seattle, Washington

GEORGE RAPTIS, MD, MBA
Associate Professor, Division of Hematology and Medical Oncology, Mount Sinai School of Medicine, New York, New York

JEAN D. WILSON, MD
Emeritus Professor of Internal Medicine, Department of Internal Medicine, University of Texas Southwestern Medical Center, Dallas, Texas

WEI YANG, BA
Division of Endocrinology, Diabetes and Bone Diseases, Department of Medicine, Mount Sinai School of Medicine, New York, New York

JEFFREY D. ZAJAC, MBBS, PhD, FRACP
Professor of Medicine, Department of Medicine, Austin Health/Northern Health, University of Melbourne; Director, Department of Endocrinology, Austin Health, Heidelberg, Victoria, Australia

Contents

> Mammary development begins in puberty in response to an estrogen (E_2)
> surge. E_2 does not act alone. It relies on pituitary growth hormone (GH)
> to induce insulin-like growth factor I (IGF-I) production in the mammary
> stromal compartment. In turn, IGF-I permits E_2 (and progesterone) action.
> During puberty, E_2 and IGF-I synergize for ductal morphogenesis. During
> pregnancy, progesterone joins IGF-I and E_2 to stimulate secretory differen-
> tiation necessary to produce milk. Prolactin stimulates milk production,
> while transforming growth factor-β inhibits proliferation. The orchestrated
> action of hormones, growth factors, and receptors necessary for mam-
> mary development and function are also critical in breast cancer.

> Many studies have reported a correlation between elevated estrogen
> blood levels and breast cancer and this observation has raised contro-
> versy concerning the long-term use of hormonal replacement therapy.
> This review will not address further this controversial topic; but rather,
> this review focuses on the role of estrogen signaling in first, the normal
> development of the breast and second, how alterations of this signaling
> pathway contribute to breast cancer.

> Given the worldwide epidemic of obesity, it is inevitably an increasingly
> common comorbidity for women who develop breast cancer; therefore,
> it is critical to understand its impact on this disease. This review focuses
> on the influence of obesity on breast cancer development and progression
> and describes the hormonal factors that may underlie the observations,
> with particular emphasis on the roles of estrogen, insulin/insulin-like
> growth factor axis, and adipokines.

> Many women take hormone therapy (HT) for menopausal symptom relief. Studies have tried to clarify whether various factors can modify the risk of HT, such as the age at initiation, dose, duration, or type of HT, or characteristics of the individual, such as family history or body mass index. The relative risks of breast cancer associated with HT across various subgroups of women should be considered similar, but absolute risks can vary significantly among women and this may inform individual decision making. For breast cancer survivors, systemic HT should be discouraged.

> This article explores the history of endocrine therapy for the treatment of breast cancer, the clinical evidence behind the current standards of care, and controversies that may change these standards in the future.

> Abundant clinical evidence suggests that androgens normally inhibit mammary epithelial proliferation and breast growth. Clinical and nonhuman primate studies support the notion that androgens inhibit mammary proliferation and, thus, may protect from breast cancer. On the other hand, administration of conventional estrogen treatment suppresses endogenous androgens and may, thus, enhance estrogenic breast stimulation and possibly breast cancer risk. Addition of testosterone to the usual hormone therapy regimen may diminish the estrogen/progestin increase in breast cancer risk, but the impact of this combined use on mammary gland homeostasis still needs evaluation.

> Estrogen deficiency at menopause is associated with increased risk of bone loss and osteoporosis. Aromatase inhibitors (AIs) are increasingly being used for the treatment of postmenopausal hormone-sensitive breast cancer because of better disease-free survival compared with tamoxifen seen in clinical trials with AIs. This article reviews the effect of endocrine therapies of breast cancer on bone and the management of bone disease with these endocrine therapies. The effect of these therapies on bone mineral density and bone turnover along with possible interventions is discussed. AIs are also associated with skeletal-related events, which are not discussed.

> The human prostate is heterogeneous with regard to its embryologic origin. The two most prevalent diseases of aging males, benign prostatic

hyperplasia and prostate cancer (PCa), arise from different zones within the prostate. The biology of PCa is also heterogeneous and even within a single individual there often exist prostate cancers with varying potential to progress and metastasize. Through careful study of the histology and molecular signatures of both the human and mouse-modeled disease, treatment decisions can be tailored to individual cases so as to optimize efficacy and minimize side effects from therapy.

Androgens are involved in every aspect of prostate development, growth, and function from early in male embryogenesis to prostatic hyperplasia in aging men and dogs. Likewise, androgen deprivation at any phase of life causes a decrease in prostate cell number and DNA content. The process by which the circulating androgen testosterone is converted to dihydrotestosterone in the tissue and dihydrotestosterone in turn gains access to the nucleus where it regulates gene expression, largely via interaction with a receptor protein, is understood, but the downstream control mechanisms by which hormonal signals are translated into differentiation, growth, and function are being unraveled.

The mainstay targets for hormonal prostate cancer (PCa) therapies are based on negating androgen action. Recent epidemiologic and experimental data have pinpointed the key roles of estrogens in PCa development and progression. Racial and geographic differences, as well as age-associated changes, in estrogen synthesis and metabolism contribute significantly to the etiology. This article summarizes how different estrogens/antiestrogens/estrogen mimics contribute to prostate carcinogenesis, the roles of the different mediators of estrogen in the process, and the potentials of new estrogenic/antiestrogenic compounds for prevention and treatment of PCa.

Androgen deprivation therapy (ADT) is an effective means of palliating symptoms of prostate cancer but is associated with significant toxicities that increase with treatment duration. Primary ADT in men with localized disease provides no survival advantage. Neoadjuvant ADT, when combined with external beam radiation, improves survival for men with locally advanced disease. Immediate adjuvant androgen deprivation does not seem to benefit most men undergoing radical prostatectomy. No evidence supports combined androgen blockade or monotherapy with nonsteroidal antiandrogens for locally advanced prostate cancer. ADT with orchiectomy or gonadotropin-releasing hormone agonists or antagonists is standard care for men with metastatic prostate cancer.

VISIT US ONLINE!
Access your subscription at:
www.theclinics.com

FORTHCOMING ISSUES

December 2011
Endocrine Disorders During Pregnancy
Rachel P. Pollack, MD, and
Lois Jovanovič, MD, Guest editors

March 2012
Insulin-Like Growth Factors in Health and Disease
Jeff M.P. Holly, MD, and
Claire M. Perks, MD, Guest Editors

RECENT ISSUES

June 2011
Endocrine Hypertension
Lawrence R. Krakoff, MD,
Guest editor

March 2011
Gastroenteropancreatic System and its Tumors: Part 2
Aaron I. Vinik, MD, PhD, Guest Editor

December 2010
Gastroenteropancreatic System and its Tumors: Part 1
Aaron I. Vinik, MD, PhD, Guest Editor

RELATED INTEREST

Urologic Clinics Volume 37, Issue 1 (February 2010)
Advances and Controversies in Prostate Cancer
William K. Oh, MD, and Jim C. Hu, MD, MPH, Guest Editors

VISIT US ONLINE!

Access your subscription at
www.theclinics.com

Foreword

Hormones and Cancer: Breast and Prostate

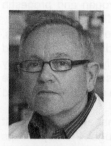

Derek LeRoith, MD, PhD
Consulting Editor

This current issue of *Endocrinology and Metabolism Clinics of North America* compiled by Dr Alice Levine covers the important topic of hormones and cancer and focuses on two hormone-dependent cancers, breast and prostate. The first seven articles cover the mammary gland and breast cancer and the second seven articles cover the prostate gland and prostate cancer.

In the opening article, Dr Kleinberg discusses the development of the adult mammary gland that is seen at puberty and is the result of multiple hormonal interactions. Both estrogen and progesterone are critical, estrogen for mammary ductal morphogenesis, while the combination of both is required for lobulo-alveolar development. On the other hand, growth hormone is also needed for ductal morphogenesis and GH plus prolactin are required for lobulo-alveolar development. Importantly, IGF-1 apparently mediates all the effects of GH on mammary development.

Estrogens are well known to be important for breast development, but also play a role in breast cancer. In her article, Dr Germain describes the emerging studies that show that in addition to estrogen and estrogen receptor's nuclear effects on gene transcription, the ER also has significant nongenomic effects that emanate from the plasma membrane and cytosolic compartment. The nuclear events involve activation or suppression of co-activators or co-repressors, whereas the extranuclear effects of ER activation involve intracellular signaling pathways.

Epidemiological studies have established an increased risk for developing breast cancer in obese individuals. A number of factors have been identified that may be causative. These include sex hormones, the insulin/IGF-1 axis, leptin, and inflammatory cytokines such as IL-6. Furthermore, Drs Perks and Holly describe how lifestyle changes have been shown to affect the prevalence of breast cancer in obesity.

Endocrinol Metab Clin N Am 40 (2011) xiii–xvi
doi:10.1016/j.ecl.2011.05.015
0889-8529/11/$ – see front matter © 2011 Elsevier Inc. All rights reserved.

Following publication of the results from the Women's Health Initiative, the use of hormonal replacement therapy (HRT) has decreased significantly. However, as estrogens remain the most effective therapy for hormonal symptoms, many questions still remain. Dr Chen's article reviews the literature data on postemenopausal HRT and breast cancer risk. It seems clear that women who have had breast cancer or have other associated risk factors should refrain from HRT. However, it is apparent that estrogen therapy is less harmful than the combination of estrogen and progestin and is still commonly used by women with postmenopausal (PMP) symptoms.

In their article on the use of hormonal modulation, Drs Adelson, Germain, Raptis, and Biran describe its use as primary cancer prevention, as adjuvant therapy, and even as palliative therapy, in cases of breast cancer. Traditionally tamoxifen therapy is used in cases of premenopausal cancer, whereas aromatase inhibitors are the mainstay for PMP cases. However, as the authors discuss, more research is required to determine if these are the optimal approaches.

Dr Dimitrakakis discusses an interesting concept, namely, that androgens inhibit mammary epithelial proliferation. Furthermore, conventional estrogen therapy inhibits endogenous androgen production and the balance favors mammary epithelial proliferation. Thus the possibility that needs to be tested is the addition of androgens to estrogen/progestin (E2/P) therapies to decrease the impact of E2/P on breast cancer risk.

In PMP women with breast cancer, tamoxifen has been used as an anti-estrogen for the cancer and pro-estrogen protecting, to some degree, against bone loss. Aromatase inhibitors decrease circulating and possibly local estrogen levels and when used to treat breast cancer generally cause a reduction in BMD. As discussed by Dr Mirza in her article, bisphosphonates have been successful in preventing the PMP bone loss associated with aromatase inhibitors. The recent addition of the RANKL as a therapy for bone loss may prove to be another important way to prevent bone loss in these patients.

Drs Lee, Akin-Olugbade, and Kirschenbaum describe many aspects of the prostate gland, including its anatomy, histology and pathology with particular relevance to two common disorders, benign prostatic hyperplasia, and prostate cancer. They underscore the marked heterogeneity of the gland, which is particularly relevant in prostate cancer. In addition, they review the current understanding of the location and characterization of prostate epithelial stem cells. As they discuss, while there is a large body of information on all these aspects, further research on molecular aspects may help in our understanding of the normal and abnormal gland and in the development of both biological markers that predict disease progression and more efficacious, targeted therapies for both hyperplasia and cancer.

Dr Wilson describes the critical role of androgens in prostate differentiation, early development, and hyperplasia later in life. A complex interplay between prostate stromal and epithelial cells, under the influences of androgens, dictates fetal, pubertal, and adult growth of the gland. Androgen deprivation, conversely, results in apoptosis and a reduction in prostate cell number. The relative roles of testosterone and its metabolite, dihydrotestosterone, have been dissected at both the biologic and the molecular levels. Despite these well-known effects, Dr Wilson reports that downstream events of androgen action, particularly gene expression, is not well defined and awaits further research.

While androgens are traditionally considered to play important roles in prostate cancer (PCa) and anti-androgen therapy is often used especially in metastatic PCa, there is accumulating evidence that estrogens may also play a role. As discussed by Drs Ho, Lee, Lam, and Leung, both genomic and noncanonical effects of the ER maybe involved. For example, alterations in the estrogen/androgen ratios, changes in sex hormone binding globulin, and the potential genotoxic carcinogenic effects may all be involved. Thus, estrogen and anti-estrogens may be important in the etiology as well as potential therapeutics for PCa.

In their article Drs Ginzburg and Albertsen discuss the history, clinical trials, and current indications for androgen ablation therapy for PCa. Although castration therapy has long been the mainstay of treatment for bone-metastatic, symptomatic disease, it is not indicated for localized disease as it has serious side effects and has no proven long-term benefit in that setting. Neo-adjuvant androgen deprivation when combined with external beam radiation does improve survival for men with locally advanced disease. Androgen deprivation therapy, with orchiectomy or with GnRH agonists or antagonists, is the current standard of care. They underscore that more randomized clinical trials are needed to guide clinicians as to the proper use of androgen deprivation therapy in men with prostate cancer at various stages of the disease.

Although most patients with advanced, metastatic prostate cancer will respond to androgen deprivation, the majority of cancers inevitably relapse and progress. The majority of castrate-resistant prostate cancers still express androgen receptors (AR) and depend on AR-signaling for their survival and continued proliferation. Recent studies have demonstrated that prostate cancer cells are capable of de novo synthesis of androgens under castrate conditions, reviving the interest in targeting the androgen/AR pathway even in so-called castrate-resistant disease. Therapeutic strategies designed to more effectively ablate tumoral androgen activity are required to improve clinical efficacy and prevent disease progression. Thus newer forms of anti-androgen therapy are constantly being pursued. Drs Mostaghel and Plymate in their article discuss these new hormonal therapies that target the androgen/AR signaling pathway that are currently being translated into the clinic.

Drs Yang and Levine explain the conundrum regarding androgen deprivation therapy (ADT) that is used in cases of prostate cancer and bone metastases. The proven value of ADT as neoadjuvant therapy in high-risk advanced localized disease receiving external beam radiotherapy may be attributed to castration-induced reduction in tumor angiogenesis, invasion, and suppression of androgen-induced osteoblast-derived paracrine growth factors that stimulate PCa growth in the bone microenvironment. However, most clinical studies have not shown any beneficial effect of ADT in terms of prevention of bone metastases or survival in patients with localized PCa and this may be due to the increase in osteoclastogenesis that ensues following ADT. Increased bone resorption with the subsequent release of stored growth factors in the bone matrix promotes PCa bone-targeting and growth in bone. The combination of ADT with anti-resorptive therapy could overcome this effect and be used as a strategy to prevent bone metastases in patients with early-stage disease.

As ADT becomes more commonplace, so do the side effects. In their article Drs Grossmann and Zajac describe these effects that include bone and muscle loss, increased fat mass with the consequent metabolic syndrome, and sexual dysfunction. As discussed, some of these unwanted effects can be managed, such as prevention of fractures with bisphosphonates and prevention of the metabolic syndrome with diet, lifestyle, and metabolic therapies. Other important considerations that need to be explored include intermittent therapy that may reduce the impact of ADT.

This is undoubtedly a very important issue. The articles cover both basic and clinical aspects and are therefore a great resource for many subspecialties, including primary care, oncologists, urologists, and endocrinologists. Dr Levine has certainly brought together experts in this field!

Derek LeRoith, MD, PhD
Division of Endocrinology, Metabolism, and Bone Diseases
Department of Medicine
Mount Sinai School of Medicine
One Gustave L. Levy Place
Box 1055, Altran 4-36
New York, NY 10029, USA

E-mail address:
derek.leroith@mssm.edu

Preface

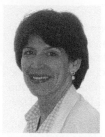

Alice C. Levine, MD
Guest Editor

In order to understand the pathogenesis of breast and prostate cancer and to design newer, more effective treatments for these common and sometimes deadly disorders, it is essential to dissect the processes involved in the normal growth and differentiation of these organs. This issue of *Endocrinology and Metabolism Clinics of North America* focuses on the profound role that hormones play in the normal development of the breast and prostate and the influence of these same hormones on the development and progression of breast and prostate cancer. It has become clear that even in the most advanced, so-called castrate-resistant breast and prostate cancers, hormones and their receptors still play a pivotal role in cancer progression. In advanced prostate cancer, for example, de novo synthesis of androgens from cholesterol has been reported. This realization has led to newer hormonal therapies that attempt to disable the hormone-receptor system to an even greater extent than previously deemed possible or even desirable.

The most well-studied hormonal effects are those of estrogens on the breast and androgens on the prostate. Herein, authors uncover less obvious but equally critical relationships between hormones and cancer including the influence of IGF-1 and androgens on the breast and estrogens on the prostate. In our aging population, hypogonadism in both sexes has adverse effects on quality of life as well as on metabolism and bone health. Dissecting the risks of hormone replacement therapy as it relates to breast and prostate cancer risk is difficult, as there are many confounding factors that may modulate risk such as family history, lifestyle, diet, and obesity. Hormone-ablative therapy has been the mainstay of treatment for both breast and prostate cancer for over 60 years, but the timing and extent of these treatments remain controversial. Finally, as patients with both disorders are highly likely to live with these diseases for many years, the potential benefits of castration therapy must be weighed against the known risks and all efforts made to preserve a good quality of life and prevent the side effects.

I am grateful to the panel of authors from diverse fields, including basic science, urology, epidemiology, oncology, and endocrinology, who have contributed to create

---

Endocrinol Metab Clin N Am 40 (2011) xvii–xviii
doi:10.1016/j.ecl.2011.05.014
0889-8529/11/$ – see front matter © 2011 Elsevier Inc. All rights reserved. **endo.theclinics.com**

this comprehensive and up-to-date issue. I hope that it illustrates the value of collaborative and translational science. If we are to conquer breast and prostate cancer, it will most certainly take a village.

Alice C. Levine, MD
Division of Endocrinology, Diabetes and Bone Disease
Department of Medicine
Mount Sinai School of Medicine
One Gustave L. Levy Place, Box 1055
New York, NY 10029, USA

E-mail address:
alice.levine@mountsinai.org

PART 1:
Hormones and Breast Cancer

The Pivotal Role of Insulin-Like Growth Factor I in Normal Mammary Development

David L. Kleinberg, MD[a,c,*], Mary Helen Barcellos-Hoff, PhD[b]

KEYWORDS

- IGF-I • Estradiol • Ductal morphogenesis
- Progesterone • TGF-β

Adult mammary development begins at puberty. A surge of estradiol (E₂) begins the process before menarche. In humans, breast development is referred to as thelarche. The early contributions of the various hormones important in mammary development have largely been studied in mice. The identification and isolation of estrogen,[1] prolactin (PRL),[2] and growth hormone (GH)[3] together with improved surgical techniques in mice permitted investigators to begin to understand the hormonal control of mammary development. The work began in the 1920s and continues today.

Turner and Frank[4] showed that although estrogen alone stimulated mammary ductal morphogenesis, the combination of estrogen and progesterone caused lobuloalveolar development similar to that seen during pregnancy.[5] Several investigators in the 1930s determined that the pituitary gland was essential for mammary development because mammary development did not occur in hypophysectomized animals even if estrogen was administered in high concentration.[6,7] Several years elapsed before pituitary hormones were sufficiently purified to help determine which of the pituitary hormones played a role in mammary development.[8-10] The laboratories of Lyons and colleagues[11] and Nandi[12] provided evidence that GH, together with estrogen, was responsible for ductal morphogenesis, whereas estrogen,

a Department of Medicine (Endocrinology), New York University School of Medicine, 550 First Avenue, New York, NY 10016, USA
b Departments of Radiation Oncology and Cell Biology, New York University School of Medicine, 566 First Avenue, New York, NY 10016, USA
c Veterans Affairs Medical Center, 423 East 23rd Street, New York, NY 10010, USA
* Corresponding author. Department of Medicine (Endocrinology), New York University School of Medicine, 550 First Avenue, New York, NY 10016.
E-mail address: David.Kleinberg@nyumc.org

Endocrinol Metab Clin N Am 40 (2011) 461–471
doi:10.1016/j.ecl.2011.06.001
0889-8529/11/$ – see front matter © 2011 Published by Elsevier Inc.

progesterone, GH, and PRL interacted to stimulate lobuloalveolar development in preparation for lactation.

MAMMARY DEVELOPMENT
Ductal Morphogenesis

At birth, the mammary gland is made up of a fat pad, with a small area of rudimentary ductal structures called ductal anlagen arising at the nipple.[13,14] An increase in circulating E_2 levels starts the process of ductal morphogenesis. GH-stimulated insulin-like growth factor (IGF) I, together with E_2, stimulates formation of terminal end buds (TEBs). These are club-shaped multilayered organelles that bifurcate, and perhaps trifurcate. Eventually, the entire mammary fat pad is filled with a network of branching ducts.[15–18] As the TEBs proliferate and extend, programmed cell death causes lumen formation within the ducts behind the TEBs.[19] As the network extends to the limits of the mammary fat pad, TEB formation stops and further extension is halted. Transforming growth factor β is an inhibitory factor that prevents proliferation of the mammary epithelium.[20] Except for transient proliferative response to each estrous cycle,[21–23] the mammary gland is quiescent until pregnancy. Although estrogen and progesterone are critical for proliferation, it is clear that mammary epithelial cells differ in their ability to respond to these signals. During both ductal and lobuloalveolar mammary growth, the distribution of proliferating cells is heterogeneous, suggesting the involvement of local factors in dictating the specific response to systemic hormones.[24–26]

PARTICIPATION OF INDIVIDUAL HORMONES
GH

Purer preparations of GH and PRL and the ability to make these or mutant forms of PRL and GH by recombinant techniques allowed further insights into the relative roles of these hormones in normal development. Ductal morphogenesis requires binding of GH to the GH receptor in the stromal tissue.[23,27] Both lactogenic and nonlactogenic GHs are capable of stimulating IGF-I messenger RNA (mRNA) in the mammary fat pad.[28] Some GHs are lactogens, but PRLs are not somatotropic. IGF-I is formed in the stromal compartment and presumably affects TEB formation by paracrine means.[29] There is also evidence that IGF-I can be produced within the TEBs, but little is known regarding the role of that pool of IGF-I in mammary development (estrogen receptor [ER]).

IGF-I

Studies in mice suggest that all known actions of GH in mammary development are mediated by IGF-I. IGF-I has been shown to substitute for GH in mammary development in hypophysectomized animals.[30] GH has no direct effect on TEB development, aside from stimulation of IGF-I. This finding was noted in oophorectomized IGF-I$^{-/-}$ female mice.[31,32] Neither E_2 nor GH had any effect on ductal morphogenesis unless animals were also treated with IGF-I. In contrast, IGF-I alone was capable of stimulating some degree of ductal branching in the complete absence of GH, E_2, and progesterone.[32] IGF-I binds to the IGF-I receptor as shown by stimulation of phosphorylated insulin receptor substrate 1 (IRS-1). Most of the known effects of IGF-I are mediated through the IGF-I pathway, which results in cell proliferation and inhibition of apoptosis. Animals deficient in either GH or IGF-I fail to develop pubertal mammary glands when treated with estrogen, GH-deficient dwarf animals and IGF-I–deficient animals, including IGF-I$^{-/-}$ female animals, follow this pattern A schema for hormonally induced mammary development is presented in **Fig. 1**.[23]

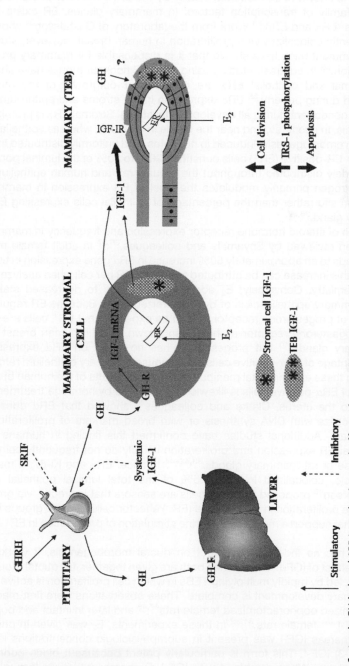

Fig. 1. Systemic GH-induced IGF-I production and effect of GH on mammary development. GH-R, GH receptor; GHRH, GH-releasing hormone; SRIF, somatotropin release–inhibiting factor. (*Reprinted from Wood TL, Furth PA, Lee AV. Growth hormone and insulin-like growth factor-I in the transition from normal mammary development to preneoplastic mammary lesions. Endocr Rev 2009;30:51–74; with permission.*)

E_2

E_2 plays a crucial role in mammary gland development and carcinogenesis. The estrogen signal is known to be mediated initially by the ER, a member of the nuclear receptor superfamily of transcription factors. In mammary glands, ER exists in 2 molecular forms: ERα and ERβ.[33] Work from the laboratory of Gustafsson[34] showed that ERβ frequently colocalizes with proliferation in human breast; however, studies using ERβ null mutant mice have shown that it is dispensable for mammary growth and differentiation.[33] In contrast, studies using the ER knockout mouse have shown that both stromal and epithelial ERα are required for outgrowth of the mouse mammary gland during puberty.[35] ERα expression in the stroma and epithelium are not necessarily concurrent during all developmental states. Stromal ERα is prominent in embryogenesis, in neonates, and near the nipple in the adult, whereas epithelial ER is absent during embryogenesis, induced in neonates, and uniformly distributed in the adult gland.[36,37] ER-positive (ER^+) cells constitute 20% to 30% of the luminal population and are widely distributed throughout the mouse, rat, and human epithelium.[38] Importantly, estrogen primarily modulates the level of ER expression in mammary epithelial cells in situ rather than the percentage of epithelial cells expressing ER in adult mammary gland.[36,37]

The regulation of steroid hormone receptor expression and frequency in mammary glands has been reviewed by Shyamala and colleagues.[36,37] In adult female mice, ovariectomy leads to an approximately 50% increase in ERα gene expression in tissue extracts,[39] but this increase can be attributed to greater ER per cell when analyzed by immunocytochemistry. Conversely, E_2 administration leads to decreased staining intensity in mammary epithelial cells of ovariectomized mice. Because ER regulates the expression of progesterone receptor, it is to be expected that ER^+ cells are also positive for progesterone receptor as has been shown in adult human breast and rodent mammary glands,[40] but progesterone has no effect on ERα expression. Thus, the percentage of ERα-positive cells in the mouse mammary epithelium remains constant during these experimental manipulations. In xenografts of the human breast, the frequency of ERα-positive cells is likewise not affected by hormone treatment.[41]

In contrast to the uterus, Clarke and colleagues[40] showed that ERα does not frequently colocalize with DNA synthesis or with broad markers of proliferation in the human breast. Additional studies have confirmed this finding in humans and have shown that ER expression and proliferation usually do not frequently coincide in normal mouse or rat mammary glands.[33,42–44] In mice, ERα and Ki-67, a marker of cells in cycle, colocalized in only 1.5% of the total luminal epithelial cells (**Fig. 2**).[45] Anderson[46] proposed that ER^+ cells are sensors that indirectly, via growth factors, regulate proliferation in ER-negative (ER^-) effector cells. Several groups have reported data that support a model of paracrine stimulation of proliferation in ER^- cells by ER^+ cells.

Although E_2 has no independent effect on ductal morphogenesis, it works by enhancing the effect of IGF-I.[30,32,47] When both are given together, full ductal morphogenesis occurs, led by rapidly multiplying TEBs in which cell proliferation is active until pubertal mammary development is complete. These observations were first made in hypophysectomized oophorectomized female rats[47,48] and later in intact and oophorectomized IGF-I$^{-/-}$ female rats.[31,32] In those experiments, E_2 was given in physiologic doses, whereas IGF-I was present in supraphysiologic concentrations in the form of des (1-3) IGF-I. This form is particularly potent because it binds poorly to IGF binding proteins. When combined with IGF-I, E_2 increases activity through the IGF-I pathway to increase cell proliferation and phosphorylation of IRS-1. E_2 had no

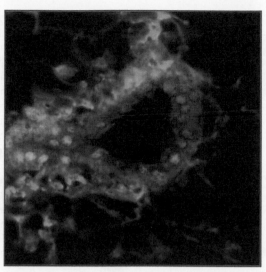

Fig. 2. Immunolocalization of nuclear ER (*green*) and Ki-67 (*red*) in the mouse mammary gland at estrous.[45] Nuclei are counterstained blue. Nonnuclear green staining is nonspecific staining. Note that ER and Ki-67 do not colocalize in the mammary epithelium.

independent effect on stimulation of IGF-I mRNA, but the level IGF-I mRNA was increased when E_2 was given along with human GH (**Fig. 3**).[49] Thus, it seems that the major action of E_2 is to enhance the effect of IGF-I at and downstream of its receptor. In addition, IGF-I has been shown to activate ERα,[50] and there are other known mechanisms through which IGF-I and E_2 cross talk.

IGF-I mediation of the entire effect of GH in mammary development is shown in **Fig. 4**. Neither E_2 alone nor E_2 together with human GH stimulated ductal morphogenesis in mammary glands of IGF-I$^{-/-}$ female mice. In contrast, IGF-I together with E_2 induced substantial ductal branching and following areas of TEB formation.

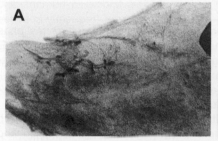
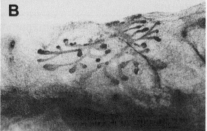

Fig. 3. (*A*) A mammary gland from an IGF-I$^{-/-}$ mouse treated for days with E_2 (note the lack of development). (*B*) A mammary gland from a representative animal having been exposed to E_2 + human GH. Note the degree of ductal morphogenesis after 5 days of treatment with des (1-3) IGF-I + E_2. (*Reprinted from* Ruan W, Kleinberg DL. Insulin-like growth factor I is essential for terminal end bud formation and ductal morphogenesis during mammary development. Endocrinology 1999;140:5078; with permission; and *Data from* Ruan W, Catanese V, Wieczorek R, et al. Estradiol enhances the stimulatory effect of insulin-like growth factor-I (IGF-I) on mammary development and growth hormone-induced IGF-I messenger ribonucleic acid. Endocrinology 1995;136:1296–302.)

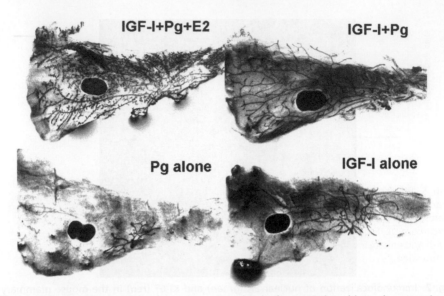

Fig. 4. Whole mounts of lumbar mammary glands from 98-day-old oophorectomized IGF-I$^{-/-}$ female mice treated for 28 days with progesterone alone (*bottom left* ×12). The area of the fat pad occupied by ducts is slightly but significantly increased compared with control. When IGF-I was given along with progesterone (*top right* ×12), the entire fat pad is filled with a network of narrow elongated branching ducts and side branches, in contrast to IGF-I alone, which increased ductal branching to a lesser extent (*lower right*). Only when E_2 was given together with IGF-I and progesterone was there a profusion of formation of alveoli as seen during midpregnancy (*top left* ×12). Pg, progesterone. (*Reprinted from* Ruan W, Monaco ME, Kleinberg DL. Progesterone stimulates mammary gland ductal morphogenesis by synergizing with and enhancing insulin-like growth factor-I action. Endocrinology 2005;146:1170–8; with permission.)

The relative effects of IGF-I and E_2 on ductal morphogenesis are shown in **Fig. 3** (2005).

Progesterone

The major effect of progesterone in mammary development is during the luteal phase or pregnancy when progesterone decorates the mammary ducts or interacts with E_2, PRL, and IGF-I to prepare the mammary gland for lactation. Progesterone receptor knockouts seem to develop normally during early puberty but fail to participate in differentiation of the mammary gland when lobuloalveolar development is to take place.[51] The authors differentiated between the effects of E_2 and progesterone in oophorectomized IGF-I$^{-/-}$ female mice. Although progesterone had no effect on the mammary gland during 28 days of treatment, progesterone was found to enhance the effect of IGF-I when the 2 were given together. They led to a form of ductal morphogenesis in which TEBs extended and bifurcated into a treelike pattern of wispy thin branching ducts that filled the entire mammary fat pad. The appearance was different from that of E_2 plus IGF-I induction of ductal morphogenesis, as shown in **Fig. 4**.

Thus, it is a different form of ductal morphogenesis, but progesterone also acts by increasing the action of IGF-I through its receptor,[32] which leads to increased cell proliferation and decreased apoptosis. The effects of progesterone with or without IGF-I in cell proliferation and apoptosis is shown in **Fig. 5** in comparison with the

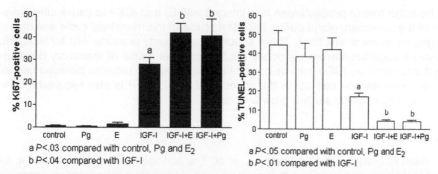

a P<.03 compared with control, Pg and E₂

b P<.04 compared with IGF-I

a P<.05 compared with control, Pg and E₂

b P<.01 compared with IGF-I

Fig. 5. Effect of different combinations of E_2, progesterone, and IGF-I on cell proliferation (*left panel*) and apoptosis (*right panel*). Pg, progesterone; TUNEL, terminal deoxynucleotidyl transferase deoxyuridine triphosphate nick end labeling. (*Reprinted from* Ruan W, Monaco ME, Kleinberg DL. Progesterone stimulates mammary gland ductal morphogenesis by synergizing with and enhancing insulin-like growth factor-I action. Endocrinology 2005;146:1170–8; with permission.)

relative effects of E_2 and IGF-I. It is not clear whether progesterone serves a physiologic role in pubertal ductal morphogenesis.

Only when E_2 is present with progesterone and IGF-I is alveolar differentiation suggestive of pregnancy. IGF-I is also essential for the combination of E_2 and progesterone to permit lobuloalveolar differentiation.

POSTPUBERTAL EFFECTS OF GH AND IGF-I

In addition to IGF-I playing a crucial role in normal mammary development, administration of supraphysiologic concentrations of GH or IGF-I or overexpression can lead to hyperplasia during or after puberty. GH can and does cause hyperplasia in rodents[32,52] and in primates.[53] Overexpression of des (1-3) IGF-I or des (1-3) IGF-I that interacts with mutant p53 leads to accelerated mammary tumorigenesis,[54,55] as does transgenic expression of a constitutively active IGF-IR.[56]

SUMMARY

In contrast to many other organs, including the prostate, mammary development occurs almost entirely at the time of puberty. Development involves several hormones and growth factors that are produced either in distant endocrine glands or locally in the mammary gland. Although development starts with a surge of E_2 levels, the participation by other hormones and growth factors is essential.

GH is one of the essential contributors. Although GH is produced in the pituitary gland, it works in the stromal compartment of the mammary gland to induce production of IGF-I. IGF-I works by paracrine means in the glandular compartment of the mammary gland. IGF-I activates the IGF-IR pathway that leads to proliferation of the ductal tree of the mammary gland through increased proliferation and decreased apoptosis.

E_2 acts by enhancing the action of IGF-I on ductal morphogenesis. The 2 hormones synergize so that ductal morphogenesis can be complete. E_2 may act through ERα in the glandular compartment by causing an effect in the stromal compartment that allows synergy of the 2 hormones in the developing gland. The number of mammary gland cells that express ERα is fixed, but E_2 increases expression in these cells. ERβ does not seem to be necessary for growth and development of the mammary gland.

The major role of progesterone is to interact with E_2 and IGF-I to cause differentiation of the mammary gland during the luteal phase of the menstrual cycle and during pregnancy when alveoli form. These structures eventually produce milk for lactation.

Even though the steroid hormones are the proximal cause of mammary development and function, IGF-I may be considered central to the process because neither E_2 nor progesterone can act in the absence of IGF-I. IGF-I is also required for the action of other hormones and growth factors.

REFERENCES

1. Allen E, Francis BF, Robertson LL, et al. The hormone of the ovarian follicle; its localization and action in test animals, and additional points bearing upon the internal secretion of the ovary. Am J Anat 1924;34:133–81.
2. Stricker S, Grueter F. Action du lobe anterieur de l'hypophyse sur la montee laiteuse. Compt Rend Soc Biol 1928;99:1978–80 [in French].
3. Wilhelmi AE. Comparative biochemistry of growth hormone from ox, pig, horse and sheep pituitaries. In: Smith RW, Gaebler OH, Long CN, editors. Henry Ford Hospital International Symposium on the Hypophyseal Growth Hormone: nature and actions. New York: McGraw-Hill; 1955. p. 59–69.
4. Turner CW, Frank AH. The effect of the ovarian hormones theelin and corporin upon the growth of the mammary gland of the rabbit, vol. 174. Research Bulletin Missouri Agricultural Experiment Station; 1932. p. 1–28.
5. Kleinberg DL, Ruan W. IGF-I, GH, and sex steroid effects in normal mammary gland development. J Mammary Gland Biol Neoplasia 2008;13:353–60.
6. Reece RP, Turner CW, Hill RT. Mammary gland development in the hypophysectomized albino rat. Proc Soc Exp Biol Med 1936;34:204–17.
7. Gardner WU. Growth of the mammary gland in hypophysectomized mice. Proc Soc Exp Biol Med 1940;45:835–7.
8. Li CH, Evans HM, Simpson ME. Isolation and properties of the anterior hypophyseal growth hormone. J Biol Chem 1945;159:353–66.
9. Li CH. Growth and adrenocorticotropic hormones of anterior pituitary. Harvey Lect Series 1950;46:181–217.
10. Li CH, Moskowitz M. Ultracentrifugation of hypophyseal growth hormone. J Biol Chem 1949;178:203–5.
11. Lyons WR, Li CH, Johnson RE. The hormonal control of mammary growth and lactation. Recent Prog Horm Res 1958;14:219–54.
12. Nandi S. Hormonal control of mammogenesis and lactogenesis in the C3H/He Crgl mouse. Berkeley (CA) and Los Angeles: University of California Press; 1959.
13. Daniel CW, Silberstein GB. Postnatal development of the rodent mammary gland. In: Neville MC, Daniel CW, editors. The mammary gland: development, regulation, and function. New York: Plenum Press; 1987. p. 1–36.
14. Richert MM, Schwertfeger KL, Ryder JW, et al. An atlas of mouse mammary gland development. J Mammary Gland Biol Neoplasia 2000;5:227–41.
15. Hinck L, Silberstein GB. Key stages in mammary gland development: the mammary end bud as a motile organ. Breast Cancer Res 2005;7:245–51.
16. Silberstein GB. Postnatal mammary gland morphogenesis. Microsc Res Tech 2001;52:155–62.
17. Howlin J, McBryan J, Martin F. Pubertal mammary gland development: insights from mouse models. J Mammary Gland Biol Neoplasia 2006;11:283–97.
18. Sternlicht MD. Key stages in mammary gland development: the cues that regulate ductal branching morphogenesis. Breast Cancer Res 2006;8:201.

19. Humphreys RC. Programmed cell death in the terminal endbud. J Mammary Gland Biol Neoplasia 1999;4:213–20.
20. Daniel CW, Robinson S, Silberstein GB. The role of TGF-beta in patterning and growth of the mammary ductal tree. J Mammary Gland Biol Neoplasia 1996;1: 331–41.
21. Silberstein GB, Van Horn K, Hrabeta-Robinson E, et al. Estrogen-triggered delays in mammary gland gene expression during the estrous cycle: evidence for a novel timing system. J Endocrinol 2006;190:225–39.
22. Anderson TJ, Battersby S, King RJB, et al. Oral contraceptive use influences resting breast proliferation. Hum Pathol 1989;20:1139–44.
23. Kleinberg DL, Wood TL, Furth PA, et al. Growth hormone and insulin-like growth factor-I in the transition from normal mammary development to preneoplastic mammary lesions. Endocr Rev 2009;30:51–74.
24. Bresciani F. Topography of DNA synthesis in the mammary gland of the C3H mouse and its control by ovarian hormones: an autoradiographic study. Cell Tissue Kinet 1968;1:51–63.
25. Daniel CW, Silberstein GB, Strickland P. Direct action of 17 beta-estradiol on mouse mammary ducts analyzed by sustained release implants and steroid auto-radiography. Cancer Res 1987;47:6052–7.
26. Christov K, Swanson SM, Guzman RC, et al. Kinetics of mammary epithelial cell proliferation in pituitary isografted BALB/c mice. Carcinogenesis 1993;14: 2019–25.
27. Feldman M, Ruan W, Cunningham BC, et al. Evidence that the growth hormone receptor mediates differentiation and development of the mammary gland. Endocrinology 1993;133:1602–8.
28. Walden PD, Ruan W, Feldman M, et al. Evidence that the mammary fat pad mediates the action of growth hormone in mammary gland development. Endocrinology 1998;139:659–62.
29. Wood TL, Richert MM, Stull MA, et al. The insulin-like growth factors (IGFs) and IGF binding proteins in postnatal development of murine mammary glands. J Mammary Gland Biol Neoplasia 2000;5:31–42.
30. Ruan W, Newman CB, Kleinberg DL. Intact and aminoterminally shortened forms of insulin-like growth factor I induce mammary gland differentiation and development. Proc Natl Acad Sci U S A 1992;89:10872–6.
31. Ruan W, Kleinberg DL. Insulin-like growth factor I is essential for terminal end bud formation and ductal morphogenesis during mammary development. Endocrinology 1999;140:5075–81.
32. Ruan W, Monaco ME, Kleinberg DL. Progesterone stimulates mammary gland ductal morphogenesis by synergizing with and enhancing insulin-like growth factor-I action. Endocrinology 2005;146:1170–8.
33. Saji S, Jensen EV, Nilsson S, et al. Estrogen receptors alpha and beta in the rodent mammary gland. Proc Natl Acad Sci U S A 2000;97:337–42.
34. Jensen FV, Chong Q, Palmieri C, et al. Estrogen receptors and proliferation markers in primary and recurrent breast cancer. Proc Natl Acad Sci U S A 2001;98:15197–202.
35. Mueller SO, Clark JA, Myers PH, et al. Mammary gland development in adult mice requires epithelial and stromal estrogen receptor alpha. Endocrinology 2002;143:2357–65.
36. Shyamala G, Chou YC, Louie SG, et al. Cellular expression of estrogen and progesterone receptors in mammary glands: regulation by hormones, development and aging. J Steroid Biochem Mol Biol 2002;1655:1–12.

37. Shyamala G, Chou YC, Louie SG, et al. Cellular expression of estrogen and progesterone receptors in mammary glands: regulation by hormones, development and aging. J Steroid Biochem Mol Biol 2002;80:137–48.
38. Petersen O, Hoyer P, van Deurs B. Frequency and distribution of estrogen receptor-positive cells in normal, nonlactating human breast tissue. Cancer Res 1987;47:5748–51.
39. Shyamala G, Schneider W, Guiot MC. Estrogen dependent regulation of estrogen receptor gene expression in normal mammary gland and its relationship to estrogenic sensitivity. Receptor 1992;2:121–8.
40. Clarke RB, Howell A, Potten CS, et al. Dissociation between steroid receptor expression and cell proliferation in the human breast. Cancer Res 1997;57: 4987–91.
41. Laidlaw IJ, Clarke RB, Howell A, et al. The proliferation of normal human breast tissue implanted into athymic nude mice is stimulated by estrogen but not progesterone [see comments]. Endocrinology 1995;136:164–71.
42. Russo IH, Russo J. Role of hormones in mammary cancer initiation and progression. J Mammary Gland Biol Neoplasia 1998;3:49–61.
43. Zeps N, Bentel JM, Papadimitriou JM, et al. Estrogen receptor-negative epithelial cells in mouse mammary gland development and growth. Differentiation 1998;62: 221–6.
44. Turgeon JL, Shyamala G, Waring DW. PR localization and anterior pituitary cell populations in vitro in ovariectomized wild-type and pr-knockout mice. Endocrinology 2001;142:4479–85.
45. Ewan KB, Oketch-Rabah HA, Ravani SA, et al. Proliferation of estrogen receptor-alpha-positive mammary epithelial cells is restrained by transforming growth factor-beta 1 in adult mice. Am J Pathol 2005;167:409–17.
46. Anderson E. Progesterone receptors—animal models and cell signaling in breast cancer: the role of oestrogen and progesterone receptors in human mammary development and tumorigenesis. Breast Cancer Res 2002;4:197–201.
47. Ruan W, Catanese V, Wieczorek R, et al. Estradiol enhances the stimulatory effect of insulin-like growth factor-I (IGF-I) on mammary development and growth hormone-induced IGF-I messenger ribonucleic acid. Endocrinology 1995;136: 1296–302.
48. Kleinberg DL, Ruan W, Catanese V, et al. Non-lactogenic effects of growth hormone on growth and insulin-like growth factor-I messenger ribonucleic acid of rat mammary gland. Endocrinology 1990;126:3274–6.
49. Kleinberg DL. Endocrinology of lactation. In: DeGroot LJ, Jameson JL, editors. Endocrinology. Philadelphia: Elsevier; 2006. p. 3461–73.
50. Yee D, Chavez JB, Ruan WF, et al. Inhibition of normal mammary gland development and breast cancer growth by IGFBP1. Proc Am Soc Clin Oncol. Annual Meeting, 2000 [abstract].
51. Lydon JP, DeMayo FJ, Funk CR, et al. Mice lacking progesterone receptor exhibit pleiotropic reproductive abnormalities. Genes Dev 1995;9:2266–78.
52. Kleinberg DL, Ameri P, Singh B. Pasireotide, an IGF-I action inhibitor, prevents growth hormone and estradiol-induced mammary hyperplasia. Pituitary 2011; 14(1):44–52.
53. Ng ST, Zhou J, Adesanya OO, et al. Growth hormone treatment induces mammary gland hyperplasia in aging primates. Nat Med 1997;3:1141–4.
54. Hadsell DL, Bonnette SG. IGF and insulin action in the mammary gland: lessons from transgenic and knockout models. J Mammary Gland Biol Neoplasia 2000;5: 19–30.

55. Bonnette SG, Hadsell DL. Targeted disruption of the IGF-I receptor gene decreases cellular proliferation in mammary terminal end buds. Endocrinology 2001;142:4937–45.

56. Carboni JM, Lee AV, Hadsell DL, et al. Tumor development by transgenic expression of a constitutively active insulin-like growth factor I receptor. Cancer Res 2005;65:3781–7.

Estrogen Carcinogenesis in Breast Cancer

Doris Germain, PhD

KEYWORDS

- Estrogen receptor • Breast cancer • Transcription factor
- Knockout mice • Mammary gland development

Many studies have reported a correlation between elevated estrogen blood levels and breast cancer, and this observation has raised controversy concerning the long-term use of hormonal replacement therapy. Analysis of the catechol metabolites of estrogen revealed that they can act as carcinogens by causing genotoxic stress and mutations. However, because the formation of these metabolites required specific conditions, and several pathways exist to repair DNA damage, the contribution of these metabolites to breast cancer remains unclear. This review does not address this controversial topic, but interested readers are invited to read the review of Dr Chen in this issue and other recent reviews on the topic.[1,2] Rather, this review focuses on the role of estrogen signaling in the normal development of the breast and how alterations of this signaling pathway contribute to breast cancer.

DEVELOPMENT OF BREAST FROM BIRTH TO ADULTHOOD IN MICE

Mice have been the most useful experimental models to dissect the role of estrogen in breast development. The breasts of mice are called mammary glands and, like the breast in humans, they are composed of 2 main compartments: the ductal tree and the stroma. Female mice have a total of 10 mammary glands, 5 on each side of the body, and are distributed in a line from the neck to the lower body. As for the development of breasts in human, the majority of the development of mammary glands takes place after birth, with the onset of puberty. Before birth the mammary glands are composed of a fat pad or stroma, which is duct-free with the exception of a short rudimentary ductal tree around the nipple. At birth these ducts remain short and underdeveloped until approximately 3 weeks of age when the ovaries begin to produce hormones. At this time, the ducts start to elongate and are characterized by a structure

The author has nothing to disclose.

Division of Hematology/Oncology, Department of Medicine, Tisch Cancer Insitute, Mount Sinai School of Medicine, One Gustave L. Levy Place, Box 1079, New York, NY 10029, USA

E-mail address: doris.germain@mssm.edu

Endocrinol Metab Clin N Am 40 (2011) 473–484
doi:10.1016/j.ecl.2011.05.009
0889-8529/11/$ – see front matter © 2011 Elsevier Inc. All rights reserved.

called the terminal end bud at the tip of each elongating duct. The terminal end bud is composed of a mass of cells of different types, including stem cells that respond to growth signals from the stroma and are responsible for the formation of the newly forming ducts. Remarkably, each duct grows in a very precise direction and distance from other ducts. Ductal elongation continues until 10 to 12 weeks of age when the terminal end buds reach the edge of the fat pad. At this point, the terminal end buds disappear, leaving the mammary gland as a fat pad invaded by a perfectly organized ductal tree. In addition to the formation of the ductal tree, during puberty the mammary gland begins a second important transformation. At this time, the ducts start branching into decreasingly smaller ducts, which terminate in more specialized structures called lobules. Each lobule is composed of underdeveloped alveoli, which remain underdeveloped unless pregnancy occurs. During pregnancy, the alveoli develop fully and will be responsible for milk production upon delivery of the newborn. In mice, once the mother is separated from her pups, the mammary gland begins yet another important transformation that involves the elimination of the alveoli. This process is referred to as involution, and, upon completion of this process, the mammary glands return to a state that resembles the mammary gland of a virgin mouse. For more extensive reviews of the development of the mammary gland the reader is invited to consult the referenced reviews.[3,4] Therefore, the development of mammary glands in mice mimics the development of breast in humans and has, therefore, been extensively used to understand the role of estrogen and the estrogen receptor in the development of the breast.

One of the first indications that estrogen plays a critical role in the development of the breast came from the observation that ovariectomized mice fail to develop mammary glands, and the rudimentary ductal near the nipple fails to proliferate at puberty. However, if a source of estrogen is inserted surgically into the fat pad of ovariectomized mice, the mammary glands resume development.[5,6] This observation demonstrates the importance of estrogen in mammary gland development.

CLONING OF THE ESTROGEN RECEPTOR

The crucial role of estrogen in breast cancer was recognized as early as the late 1800s, following the observation that in premenopausal women with metastatic breast cancer, oophorectomy led to tumor regression in one-third of patients. This observation was followed by a now famous experiment by Jensen and Jacobson in 1950. Using tritium-labeled estrogen, they demonstrated that estrogen is retained in specific tissues, including the breast.[7] This finding led to the hypothesis that a receptor for estrogen is present in these tissues. However, it took nearly 30 years to prove this hypothesis because the result of the cloning of the first estrogen receptor (ER), now referred as ERα.[8–11] Nearly 10 years later, a second estrogen receptor, ERβ, was identified.[12,13] The identification of the second receptor raised important issues because clinically only the ERα is targeted for treatment of breast cancer. The following sections describe the role of both the ERα and the ERβ in mammary gland development.

THE ERα IS ESSENTIAL FOR THE DEVELOPMENT OF THE MAMMARY GLAND

Advances in molecular genetics have led to the establishment of techniques that allow the elimination of specific genes. Mice that have been manipulated genetically to delete a specific gene are referred as knockout mice. Several different knockout mice have been created to investigate the role of specific genes on the development of the mammary gland. Such analysis has lead to an immense amount of information on what drives the growth and development of mammary glands, and, not surprisingly, this process is highly complex, involves several genes, and is not yet fully understood. The next section focuses on the analysis of the mammary gland in ERα knockout mice.

Generation of ERα Mice

ERα knockout mice are mice that have been genetically manipulated such that the estrogen receptor gene has been eliminated. The analysis of these mice revealed that the ducts in the mammary glands of the ERα knockout mice fail to develop and they resemble the mammary glands of ovariectomized mice.[14,15] However, these ducts remain short and underdeveloped even when the ovaries begin to produce hormones, indicating that in the absence of the estrogen receptor, estrogen alone is not sufficient to promote ductal elongation.[14]

Although the ERα is required for normal mammary gland function, not all cell types of the mammary gland express the estrogen receptor gene and the same observation is also true in humans. This point is best illustrated by the fact that at any time only a fraction of cells in a duct expresses the ERα.[16–18] During development, for instance, the cells at the tip of the growing ducts do not express the ERα; however, the cells in the fat pad do suggest that the role of the ERα in mammary gland development is mediated via the cells in the fat pad. In agreement with the role of cells in the fat pad in the development of mammary glands when the rudimentary ducts of an ERα knockout mouse are surgically removed and place into the fat pad of a normal mouse, the transplanted ducts are then able to grow.[19–21] Therefore, this observation indicates that the presence of the ERα in cells of the fat pad from the normal mouse is sufficient to promote the development of the ducts even if these ductal cells do not themselves have the ER.

In addition to the expression of the ERα in the cells in the fat pad, the ERα is also expressed in a small fraction of cells in the duct. In an adult breast, approximately 20% of cells have the ERα, and from experiments in mice, it is also known that this percentage varies depending on the stage of mammary gland development. What exactly regulates the expression of the ERα gene in one ductal cell and not the other is still not clearly understood.

ESTROGEN RECEPTOR BETA KNOCKOUT

Although the importance of the ERα in the development and function of the breast has reached a consensus, the role of ERβ remains much more unclear. To clarify the potential contribution of ERβ, the ERβ gene was knocked out in mice using various approaches. As a result, 3 different ERβ knockout mice were generated and each were reported to have different phenotypes.[22] Namely, Course and Korach[23,24] reported that the ductal tree and differentiation of the mammary glands were normal, whereas Forster and colleagues[25] reported normal development but impaired branching, and Palmieri and colleagues[26] found an age-related severe cyst breast disease. The inconsistency of the phenotypes was finally resolved by the discovery that the approaches used to generated these knockout mice led to the expression of aberrant forms of the ERβ. As a result, an additional knockout was generated in which a complete elimination of the expression of the ERβ gene was created. This study revealed that the mammary glands of these mice are entirely normal, suggesting that ERβ has no role in the normal development of the breast.[27] The remaining sections of this review, therefore, concentrate uniquely on the ERα and are referred to thereafter as ER.

MECHANISM OF ACTION OF THE ESTROGEN RECEPTOR

The best-characterized function of the ER is as a transcription factor. The structure of the ER can be divided into 6 functional domains: the activation functions (AF) 1 and 2, the DNA binding domain, the estrogen binding domain, the hinge, and the nuclear localization domain.[28] When functioning as a transcription factor, the DNA binding domain of the ER binds to specific DNA sequences in the promoter of target genes, whereas the AF domain serves to bind to the transcription machinery. AF-1 of the ER is the estrogen-independent domain that can lead to the activation of the ER as a result of its phosphorylation in response to various growth factors. The AF-2 function of the ER is estrogen dependent.

The classical view of the ER is that, in absence of estrogen, the ER is inactive and resides in the cytoplasm. When estrogen binds to the ER, it forms a dimer, which results in a conformational change that exposes the nuclear localization signal and promotes the translocation of the ER into the nucleus. Once in the nucleus, the DNA binding domain targets the ER to the estrogen receptor response element, a specific DNA sequence motif that is present in the promoters of several genes. The ER is, however, unable to promote transcription alone and requires the formation of a complex. The cellular response generated by the binding of ER is dependent on the composition of the ER complex.[28] Several different ER complexes exist and their formation is a reversible process. Any given complex may contain several corepressors and coactivators.[29] For example, a complex containing several corepressors but few coactivators could inhibit transcription of a estrogen responsive gene.[29] Therefore, the ER complex can activate the transcription of some genes and repress the transcription of others, leading to a complex genomic landscape. In terms of specificity between the ERα and ERβ, a recent study has shown that there is a high degree of overlap between the DNA binding regions bound by ERα and ERβ, but that there are also regions that are specific to either receptor.[30] This study also revealed that ERβ might act to recruit ERα to some regions because these genes were bound to ERα but only if ERβ was present. Therefore, the genomic landscape of ERα and ERβ is complex and includes genes that are regulated only by one receptor and not the other, genes that can be regulated by either receptors, whereas other genes require both receptors to be expressed.[30] However, because the deletion of the ERβ has no effect on the development of the mammary gland, presumably the genes regulated by ERβ are not essential for this process.

NONGENOMIC ACTION OF THE ER AT THE PLASMA MEMBRANE

Although the classical view of the mode of action of the ER is as a transcription factor, it is now well accepted that the ER also localizes to the plasma membrane. The rapid effect of estrogen was first reported more than 30 years ago.[31,32] Treatment of breast cancer cells with estrogen leads to the phosphorylation of proteins within 10 minutes after the addition of estrogen.[31,32] Such a rapid event is inconsistent with the transcriptional effect of the ER because activation of the expression of genes, followed by the translation of the mRNA into proteins, which then mediate their action, is a process that requires hours to take place. Rather, the rapid effect of estrogen acts by activating the ER at the plasma membrane where the ER associated with several growth factor receptors, such as EGFR, neu-2, and IGFR-1.[33–35] How the ER associates with the membrane remains a question of debate, but palmitoylation of the ER, a post-translational modification, has been reported to allow the association of the ER with membranes.[36] The complex of the ER with these growth factors receptors acts as large signalosomes, which allow the activation of signaling pathways leading to cellular proliferation.

In addition, the ER is also found in the mitochondria,[37,38] an organelle that is central in the control of cell death by apoptosis. The ER found in the mitochondria is identical to the nuclear form, so how the ER is imported into the mitochondria remains entirely unknown. However, it is well known that mitochondria are highly sensitive to estrogen, and it has been suggested that ER in the mitochondria is linked to resistance to radiation-induced cell death.

In summary, the ER is essential for normal breast development. The ER is best known as a transcription factor in the nucleus, but the nongenomic action of the ER at the plasma membrane and possibly in the mitochondria are rapidly gaining interest because alteration in these mechanisms are likely to be equally important in estrogen-mediated carcinogenesis.

MECHANISMS OF ESTROGEN CARCINOGENESIS

There are several mechanisms by which the activity of the ER becomes abnormally hyperactivated and contribute to the breast cancer formation, including (1) amplification of the coactivator of the ER; (2) repression of the expression of corepressor; (3) overexpression of proteins that act as the adaptor to facilitate the recruitment of the coactivator to the ER; (4) mutations in the ER itself, which allow its activation at a lower concentration of estrogen; and (5) localization of the ER at the plasma membrane and the activation of the signaling cascade. These 5 mechanisms are discussed in the following sections.

Amplification of Coactivators

Ultimately, the activity of the ER is determined by the delicate balance between coactivators and corepressors in the ER complex. Overexpression of the coactivator represents a powerful mechanism to promote the ER-dependent growth of breast cancer cells.

Gene amplification is a frequent mechanism of elevated gene expression in cancer, and in breast cancers, amplification of chromosome 20q is frequent. The identification of genes within this amplicon led to the discovery of the gene that was termed amplified in breast cancer-1 (AIB1)[39] because it is expressed at high levels in 64% of primary breast cancers. Further, AIB1 is associated with poor prognosis and tamoxifen resistance in cell lines that coexpress erbB2,[39] suggesting a crosstalk between AIB1 and erbB2. AIB1 binds directly to the ER and acts as a coactivator of the ER, therefore, enhancing the transcriptional activity of the ER. Thus far, AIB1 is the only coactivator of the ER that has been linked to breast cancer. This result raised the possibility that AIB1 is an oncogene, but whether the action of A1B1 is dependent on the binding of estrogen to the ER formally remains to be determined experimentally.

A demonstration of a role of AIB1 in breast cancer was confirmed using a mouse model where AIB1 was abnormally overexpressed in the mammary gland of mice to mimic the overexpression of AIB1 in primary breast cancer in humans.

Amplification of AIB1 in mice leads to the formation of mammary gland carcinoma

To determine the effects of AIB1 overexpression on mammary carcinogenesis, the AIB1 gene was expressed in the mammary gland using the mouse mammary tumor virus (MMTV) promoter, which leads to the expression of genes in the mammary glands.[40] The MMTV-AIB1 mice showed an increased size of the mammary gland starting at 4 weeks of age; hyperplasia and accelerated differentiation of the mammary gland; delayed involution following lactation; and adenocarcinoma of various pathologies as early as 9 months, with an average latency of 16 months.[40] Further, the adenocarcinoma of the MMTV-AIB1 mice were highly metastatic, showing tumor formation in lung and bones, indicating that AIB1-positive tumors are highly aggressive.

Of interest was the observation that the level of progesterone receptor (PR) is low in these tumors.[40] Because activation of the insulin growth factor (IGF) receptor-mediated signaling has been linked to a decrease in the expression of the PR, the investigators analyzed the IGF signaling pathway in these mice and found that it is highly activated[40]; additionally, 85% of all adenocarcinoma were positive for the ER.

Although a link between the ER and AIB1 was established in both humans and mice, 2 additional models tested whether the AIB1-mediated tumors in transgenic mice are, in fact, dependent on the activity of the ER.[41] In the first model, AIB1 transgenic mice were ovariectomized, and such ablation of estrogen blocked the ability of AIB1 transgenic mice to form invasive adenocarcinoma.[41] However, ovariectomization of mice after tumors were formed led to a 4-fold increase in the rate metastases.[41] This observation indicates that the timing of estrogen depletion impacts the outcome, with the early depletion of estrogen capable of preventing AIB1 carcinogenesis, whereas late depletion, after tumors are formed, aggravates metastasis, suggesting a protective role of estrogen against metastasis in this setting. The clinical implication of such a finding is that the treatment of patients suffering from AIB1-positive tumors with aromatase inhibitors should be restricted to early stage disease, whereas other antiestrogen drugs should be used in the metastatic setting.

The second model that was used to test the dependency of AIB1 tumor formation on the ER is more elaborate and consists of crossing the AIB1 transgenic to the ER knockout mice, leading to mice with overexpressed AIB1, but absent ER.[41] In this second model, the formation of carcinogenesis was entirely abolished and metastasis was also abolished.[41] Therefore, the results of these experiments strongly support that the formation of AIB1-mediated mammary carcinoma is highly dependent on the activity of the ER.

Loss of Expression of Corepressor

The repressor of estrogen receptor activity (REA) was originally identified using a screen for protein that was able to bind to the ER in the presence of the ligand. When bound to the ER, REA potentiates the action of antiestrogen drugs.[42] The level of REA varies widely in primary breast cancers,[43,44] and REA expression correlates directly with the ER level. As such, high REA and ER expression is prognostically favorable, but conversely low expression of REA is associated with worse prognosis.[43,44] In mice, the inhibition of REA expression leads to mammary gland hyperproliferation and an acceleration of the mammary development during pregnancy.[45] This finding suggests that REA is normally required to limit the action of the proliferative action of ER.

Abnormal Expression of Proteins that Act to Recruit Coactivators

Another mechanism by which the composition of the ER complex is altered is the abnormal expression of proteins that gain the ability to bind to the ER when their levels are elevated. Although these proteins have specific cellular function in normal tissues, they aberrantly interact with the ER when overexpressed. One of the best-characterized examples of this mechanism is the overexpression of cyclin D1, a protein that normally acts as a regulator of the cell cycle.

Cyclins act as the regulatory subunits of the cyclin-dependent kinases (cdk). Binding of D-type cyclins to cdk4 and cdk6 leads to the phosphorylation of the retinoblastoma protein (Rb) and the release of the E2F family of transcription factors for Rb. This action in turn activates downstream targets of E2F required for the G1-to-S phase transition and results in cellular proliferation.[46,47] In addition to its original role as a cdk-dependent regulator of the cell cycle, cyclin D1 also affects the activity of various transcription factors in a cdk-independent manner, including the ER.[48–51] Importantly, cyclin D1 not only interacts with the ER but also with steroid receptor coactivators.[50,52] Therefore, by binding to both the ER and its coactivators, cyclin D1 acts as a bridging factor to recruit ER coactivators, even in the absence of estrogen. The affect of cyclin D1 on the ER is independent of the interaction of cyclin D1 and cdk4. Cyclin D1 mutant proteins that are unable to bind to cdk4 can still regulate ER coactivators.[51] Cyclin D1 is overexpressed in 35% of breast cancers, and cyclin D1 positivity is tightly linked to ER positivity. This observation has led to the hypothesis that cyclin D1 overexpressing tumors may have hyperactive ER even in the absence of estrogen, and, therefore, cyclin D1 may help identify the subset of patients that do not benefit from tamoxifen treatment.

Cyclin D1 knockout mice

A specific role of cyclin D1 in breast cancer is supported by the observation that mice, where the cyclin D1 gene has been deleted, are remarkably viable and show limited defects, including a defect in the development of the mammary glands. These mice have normal development of the mammary gland during puberty but fail to proliferate during pregnancy.[53,54] This finding suggested that cyclin D1 plays a critical role in the pregnancy-associated proliferation of the mammary gland. This possibility was subsequently confirmed by the observation that the mammary gland of the cyclin D1 knockout fails to respond to prolactin, a major signaling cascade responsible for the proliferation and differentiation of the mammary gland during pregnancy.[55]

Another important finding is that the formation of the neu2-mediated mammary gland carcinoma in mice is entirely blocked by the deletion of the cyclin D1 gene.[56] Whether this observation is linked to the role of cyclin D1 in the activation of the ER remains to be determined.

Cyclin D1 transgenic mice

Although the frequent overexpression of cyclin D1 in human breast cancer and its role in the cell cycle and the activation of the ER suggest an important functional role of cyclin D1 in breast cancer, the demonstration that cyclin D1 is in fact an oncogene was demonstrated experimentally using cyclin D1 transgenic mice, where the cyclin D1 gene was overexpressed in the mammary gland in mice using the MMTV promoter. The analysis of these mice showed that, indeed, cyclin D1 is an oncogene because these mice develop adenocarcinoma.[57]

Cyclin D1 and tamoxifen

A further link between cyclin D1 and the activation of the ER was established by 2 recent clinical studies that have found a strong link between cyclin D1 overexpression and the resistance to tamoxifen.[58,59] First, in postmenopausal women, high levels of cyclin D1 protein were found to promote resistance to tamoxifen.[58] Second, in premenopausal women, elevated levels of cyclin D1 protein also abolished the beneficial effect of tamoxifen on recurrence-free survival. In this study, elevated levels of cyclin D1 gene correlated with a 6.38-fold increase in the relative risk of breast cancer recurrence and a 5.34-fold increase in the relative risk of death following tamoxifen treatment.[59]

The author and colleagues published a study suggesting a mechanism by which cyclin D1 overexpression confers tamoxifen resistance.[60] In that study, the author and colleagues characterized the interactions between cyclin D1, the ER, and the anti-apoptotic transcription factor STAT3 in response to tamoxifen treatment. The author and colleagues showed that repression of STAT3 by cyclin D1 inhibits tumor growth in vivo; however, treatment with tamoxifen abolishes cyclin D1-mediated repression of STAT3 and growth suppression. The author and colleagues demonstrated that tamoxifen induces a redistribution of cyclin D1 from STAT3 to the ER, which results in the activation of both STAT3 and the ER. Their data recapitulates and fully supports the clinical observation of an adverse effect of cyclin D1 gene amplification in premenopausal women treated with tamoxifen.[59]

Mutations of the ERα

Reversible post-translational modification to the ER protein, such as phosphorylation and acetylation, determines the binding of coactivators and corepressors and, thus, dictates the composition of the ER complex.

The somatic mutation K303R was found in 34% of hyperplastic breast lesions and in the majority of primary breast cancers.[61] Lysine 303 resides at the border of the hinge and ligand-binding domain of the ERα. Lysine 303 is a major site of ER acetylation, and although the K303R mutation does not affect the ability of estrogen or tamoxifen to bind to the pocket, cells expressing the mutated receptor had a doubling time of 1.3 days in the presence of 10^{-12} molar estrogen, whereas cells expressing the wild type receptor required 2.2 days to proliferate under these conditions.[61] It is hypothesized that in the presence of this mutation, there was an increased affinity for the binding of the coactivator. Because this mutation confers hypersensitivity to estrogen, the implication is that it may also be associated with resistance to antiestrogens, raising the possibility that it could be used as a biomarker to predict resistance to tamoxifen.[62] Ultimately, the creation of a knockin mice, where the ER gene is replaced by the ER gene expressing the K303R mutation, would be useful to test the effect of this mutation in vivo. However, there is currently no report of such mice.

Tyrosine 537 of the ER is an important phosphorylation site regulating ligand binding, homodimerization, and activation of the ER.[63] The Y537S mutation was shown to promote the transcription of 4 different ER target genes (vitellogenin, pS2, cathepsin D, and lactoferrin) to a 5- to 20-fold higher level than the wild type promoter.[63] These findings indicate that this mutation allows the phosphorylation-independent activation of the ER.[62]

Activation of the ER at the Plasma Membrane

The association of the ER with the receptors, such as EGFR, neu-2, and IGFR-1, is reported to increase with breast cancer progression and to contribute to the emergence of estrogen-independent tumors because these associations allow for the activation of the ER in minimal concentrations of estrogen.[64] Because the biologic outcome of these associations is the activation of signaling cascades, such as the MAP kinases and ERK, the overall regulation of these pathways impacts on the proliferation and survival of cancer cells and represents a considerable mechanism of estrogen-mediated carcinogenesis.[64]

The biologic consequence is resistance to antiestrogen drugs. For instance, laboratory models show that long-term estrogen deprivation, such as that created by the treatment with aromatase inhibitors, force the selection of adaptive changes in the localization of the ER and the acquired overexpression of growth factors. These changes then allow cells to proliferate in such estrogen-depleted conditions. Because neu-2 is the target of Herceptin, it has been proposed that combining fulvestrant, which leads to the degradation of the ER, and Herceptin, which blocks the action of neu-2, may represent a viable option to overcome such mechanisms of carcinogenesis. Several groups confirmed this possibility.[65–67]

Finally, because drugs are being developed to target the IGF receptor and several MAP kinases, combining fulvestrant to these new drugs also represents an important rationale for future clinical trials.

CONCLUDING REMARKS

Although only a few specific mechanisms of estrogen carcinogenesis are discussed in this review, several others exist. Although ERβ knockout mice do not show a defect in the development of the mammary gland, it remains possible that in breast cancers, ERβ may bind to and form heterodimers with the ERβ and are likely to affect its activity. Further, estrogen receptors-related (ERR) α, β, and γ also interact with the ER and may modulate its function.[68] In addition to competing with ERα for coactivators and corepressors, ERR attract an entirely new set of coactivators and repressors.[28] In light of the complexity of this pathway and the variety of mechanisms by which the transcriptional activity of the ER can be modulated, the classical strategy of endocrine therapy aimed at blocking the transcriptional activity of the ERα solely may be far too simplistic.

SUMMARY

The importance of estrogen in the etiology of breast cancer has long been recognized, but a definitive scientific demonstration of the link between estrogen and breast cancer has required the cloning of its receptor and the discovery of its function as a transcription factor and, more recently, as a partner of several growth factors at the plasma membrane, explaining some of the observed rapid effects of estrogen. The development of transgenic and knockout mice for isoforms of ER and ER coregulators has further elucidated the function of the ER in both normal breast development and in breast cancers. Research aimed at understanding all levels of the complexity of this signaling pathway has allowed the identification of mechanisms by which various genetic alterations contribute to estrogen carcinogenesis. These mechanisms include amplification of the coactivator AIB1; loss of expression of the corepressor REA; overexpression of cyclin D1, which acts as a adaptor between the ER and its coactivators; mutations in the ER itself that bypass mechanisms that restrict the activation of the ER; and, finally, the localization of the ER to the plasma membrane. Although much more remains to be discovered about estrogen-mediated carcinogenesis, it is now up to the scientists and clinicians to come together and design clinical trials based on strong scientific rationales that have emerged from this research.

REFERENCES

1. Yager JD, Davidson NE. Estrogen carcinogenesis in breast cancer. N Engl J Med 2006;354(3):270–82.
2. Mueck AO, Seeger H. Breast cancer: are oestrogen metabolites carcinogenic? Maturitas 2007;57(1):42–6.
3. Hennighausen L, Robinson GW. Information networks in the mammary gland. Nat Rev Mol Cell Biol 2005;6(9):715–25.
4. Silberstein GB. Postnatal mammary gland morphogenesis. Microsc Res Tech 2001;52(2):155–62.
5. Kumaresan P, Turner CW. Effect of various hormones on mammary gland growth of ovariectomized rats. Proc Soc Exp Biol Med 1967;125(2):556–8.

6. Flux DS. The effect of adrenal steroids on the growth of the mammary glands, uteri, thymus and adrenal glands of intact ovariectomized and oestrone-treated ovariectomized mice. J Endocrinol 1954;11(3):238–54.
7. Jensen EV. On the mechanism of estrogen action. Perspect Biol Med 1962;6:47–59.
8. Walter P, Green S, Greene G, et al. Cloning of the human estrogen receptor cDNA. Proc Natl Acad Sci U S A 1985;82(23):7889–93.
9. Greene GL, Gilna P, Waterfield M, et al. Sequence and expression of human estrogen receptor complementary DNA. Science 1986;231(4742):1150–4.
10. Greene GL, Press MF. Structure and dynamics of the estrogen receptor. J Steroid Biochem 1986;24(1):1–7.
11. Green S, Kumar V, Krust A, et al. Structural and functional domains of the estrogen receptor. Cold Spring Harb Symp Quant Biol 1986;51(Pt 2):751–8.
12. Tremblay GB, Tremblay A, Copeland NG, et al. Cloning, chromosomal localization, and functional analysis of the murine estrogen receptor beta. Mol Endocrinol 1997;11(3):353–65.
13. Mosselman S, Polman J, Dijkema R. ER beta: identification and characterization of a novel human estrogen receptor. FEBS Lett 1996;392(1):49–53.
14. Lubahn DB, Moyer JS, Golding TS, et al. Alteration of reproductive function but not prenatal sexual development after insertional disruption of the mouse estrogen receptor gene. Proc Natl Acad Sci U S A 1993;90(23):11162–6.
15. Bocchinfuso WP, Korach KS. Mammary gland development and tumorigenesis in estrogen receptor knockout mice. J Mammary Gland Biol Neoplasia 1997;2(4):323–34.
16. Clarke RB, Howell A, Potten CS, et al. Dissociation between steroid receptor expression and cell proliferation in the human breast. Cancer Res 1997;57(22):4987–91.
17. Zeps N, Bentel JM, Papadimitriou JM, et al. Estrogen receptor-negative epithelial cells in mouse mammary gland development and growth. Differentiation 1998;62(5):221–6.
18. Smith GH. Label-retaining epithelial cells in mouse mammary gland divide asymmetrically and retain their template DNA strands. Development 2005;132(4):681–7.
19. Curtis Hewitt S, Couse JF, Korach KS. Estrogen receptor transcription and transactivation: estrogen receptor knockout mice: what their phenotypes reveal about mechanisms of estrogen action. Breast Cancer Res 2000;2(5):345–52.
20. Bocchinfuso WP, Lindzey JK, Hewitt SC, et al. Induction of mammary gland development in estrogen receptor-alpha knockout mice. Endocrinology 2000;141(8):2982–94.
21. Korach KS. Estrogen receptor knock-out mice: molecular and endocrine phenotypes. J Soc Gynecol Investig 2000;7(Suppl 1):S16–7.
22. Harris HA. Estrogen receptor-beta: recent lessons from in vivo studies. Mol Endocrinol 2007;21(1):1–13.
23. Krege JH, Hodgin JB, Couse JF, et al. Generation and reproductive phenotypes of mice lacking estrogen receptor beta. Proc Natl Acad Sci U S A 1998;95(26):15677–82.
24. Couse JF, Korach KS. Estrogen receptor null mice: what have we learned and where will they lead us? Endocr Rev 1999;20(3):358–417.
25. Forster C, Makela S, Warri A, et al. Involvement of estrogen receptor beta in terminal differentiation of mammary gland epithelium. Proc Natl Acad Sci U S A 2002;99(24):15578–83.
26. Palmieri C, Cheng GJ, Saji S, et al. Estrogen receptor beta in breast cancer. Endocr Relat Cancer 2002;9(1):1–13.

27. Antal MC, Krust A, Chambon P, et al. Sterility and absence of histopathological defects in nonreproductive organs of a mouse ERbeta-null mutant. Proc Natl Acad Sci U S A 2008;105(7):2433–8.
28. Pearce ST, Jordan VC. The biological role of estrogen receptors alpha and beta in cancer. Crit Rev Oncol Hematol 2004;50(1):3–22.
29. Ariazi EA, Leitao A, Oprea TI, et al. Exemestane's 17-hydroxylated metabolite exerts biological effects as an androgen. Mol Cancer Ther 2007;6(11):2817–27.
30. Liu Y, Gao H, Marstrand TT, et al. The genome landscape of ERalpha- and ERbeta-binding DNA regions. Proc Natl Acad Sci U S A 2008;105(7):2604–9.
31. Pietras RJ, Szego CM. Endometrial cell calcium and oestrogen action. Nature 1975;253(5490):357–9.
32. Pietras RJ, Szego CM. Specific binding sites for oestrogen at the outer surfaces of isolated endometrial cells. Nature 1977;265(5589):69–72.
33. Migliaccio A, Di Domenico M, Castoria G, et al. Tyrosine kinase/p21ras/MAP-kinase pathway activation by estradiol-receptor complex in MCF-7 cells. EMBO J 1996; 15(6):1292–300.
34. Nemere I, Farach-Carson MC. Membrane receptors for steroid hormones: a case for specific cell surface binding sites for vitamin D metabolites and estrogens. Biochem Biophys Res Commun 1998;248(3):443–9.
35. Kelly MJ, Levin ER. Rapid actions of plasma membrane estrogen receptors. Trends Endocrinol Metab 2001;12(4):152–6.
36. Li L, Haynes MP, Bender JR. Plasma membrane localization and function of the estrogen receptor alpha variant (ER46) in human endothelial cells. Proc Natl Acad Sci U S A 2003;100(8):4807–12.
37. Yang SH, Liu R, Perez EJ, et al. Mitochondrial localization of estrogen receptor beta. Proc Natl Acad Sci U S A 2004;101(12):4130–5.
38. Pedram A, Razandi M, Wallace DC, et al. Functional estrogen receptors in the mitochondria of breast cancer cells. Mol Biol Cell 2006;17(5):2125–37.
39. Anzick SL, Kononen J, Walker RL, et al. AIB1, a steroid receptor coactivator amplified in breast and ovarian cancer. Science 1997;277(5328):965–8.
40. Torres-Arzayus MI, Font de Mora J, Yuan J, et al. High tumor incidence and activation of the PI3K/AKT pathway in transgenic mice define AIB1 as an oncogene. Cancer Cell 2004;6(3):263–74.
41. Torres-Arzayus MI, Zhao J, Bronson R, et al. Estrogen-dependent and estrogen-independent mechanisms contribute to AIB1-mediated tumor formation. Cancer Res 2010;70(10):4102–11.
42. Montano MM, Ekena K, Delage-Mourroux R, et al. An estrogen receptor-selective coregulator that potentiates the effectiveness of antiestrogens and represses the activity of estrogens. Proc Natl Acad Sci U S A 1999;96(12):6947–52.
43. Murphy LC, Simon SL, Parkes A, et al. Altered expression of estrogen receptor coregulators during human breast tumorigenesis. Cancer Res 2000;60(22): 6266–71.
44. Simon SL, Parkes A, Leygue E, et al. Expression of a repressor of estrogen receptor activity in human breast tumors: relationship to some known prognostic markers. Cancer Res 2000;60(11):2796–9.
45. Mussi P, Liao L, Park SE, et al. Haploinsufficiency of the corepressor of estrogen receptor activity (REA) enhances estrogen receptor function in the mammary gland. Proc Natl Acad Sci U S A 2006;103(45):16716–21.
46. Sherr CJ. D-type cyclins. Trends Biochem Sci 1995;20(5):187–90.
47. Helin K. Regulation of cell proliferation by the E2F transcription factors. Curr Opin Genet Dev 1998;8:28–35.

48. Bernards R. CDK-independent activities of D type cyclins. Biochim Biophys Acta 1999;1424(2–3):M17–22.
49. Neuman E, Ladha MH, Lin N, et al. Cyclin D1 stimulation of estrogen receptor transcriptional activity independent of cdk4. Mol Cell Biol 1997;17:5338–47.
50. Zwijsen RM, Buckle RS, Hijmans EM, et al. Ligand-independent recruitment of steroid receptor coactivators to estrogen receptor by cyclin D1. Genes Dev 1998;12:3488–98.
51. Zwijsen RM, Wientjens E, Klompmaker R, et al. Cdk-independent activation of estrogen receptor by cyclin D1. Cell 1997;88:405–15.
52. McMahon C, Suthiphongchai T, DiRenzo J, et al. P/CAF associates with cyclin D1 and potentiates its activation of the estrogen receptor. Proc Natl Acad Sci U S A 1999;96(10):5382–7.
53. Sicinski P, Donaher JL, Parker SB, et al. Cyclin D1 provides a link between development and oncogenesis in the retina and breast. Cell 1995;82:621–30.
54. Fantl V, Stamp G, Andrews A, et al. Mice lacking cyclin D1 are small and show defects in eye and mammary gland development. Genes Dev 1995;9(19):2364–72.
55. Brisken C, Ayyannan A, Nguyen C, et al. IGF-2 is a mediator of prolactin-induced morphogenesis in the breast. Dev Cell 2002;3(6):877–87.
56. Yu Q, Geng Y, Sicinski P. Specific protection against breast cancers by cyclin D1 ablation. Nature 2001;411(6841):1017–21.
57. Wang T, Cardiff RD, Zukerberg L, et al. Mammary hyperplasia and carcinoma in MMTV-cyclin D1 transgenic mice. Nature 1994;369:669–71.
58. Stendahl M, Kronblad A, Ryden L, et al. Cyclin D1 overexpression is a negative predictive factor for tamoxifen response in postmenopausal breast cancer patients. Br J Cancer 2004;90(10):1942–8.
59. Jirstrom K, Stendahl M, Ryden L, et al. Adverse effect of adjuvant tamoxifen in premenopausal breast cancer with cyclin d1 gene amplification. Cancer Res 2005;65(17):8009–16.
60. Ishii Y, Waxman S, Germain D. Tamoxifen stimulates the growth of cyclin D1-overexpressing breast cancer cells by promoting the activation of signal transducer and activator of transcription 3. Cancer Res 2008;68(3):852–60.
61. Fuqua SA, Wiltschke C, Zhang QX, et al. A hypersensitive estrogen receptor-alpha mutation in premalignant breast lesions. Cancer Res 2000;60(15):4026–9.
62. Herynk MH, Fuqua SA. Estrogen receptor mutations in human disease. Endocr Rev 2004;25(6):869–98.
63. Kohler MF, Berkholz A, Risinger JI, et al. Mutational analysis of the estrogen-receptor gene in endometrial carcinoma. Obstet Gynecol 1995;86(1):33–7.
64. Levin ER, Pietras RJ. Estrogen receptors outside the nucleus in breast cancer. Breast Cancer Res Treat 2008;108(3):351–61.
65. Witters LM, Kumar R, Chinchilli VM, et al. Enhanced anti-proliferative activity of the combination of tamoxifen plus HER-2-neu antibody. Breast Cancer Res Treat 1997;42(1):1–5.
66. Kunisue H, Kurebayashi J, Otsuki T, et al. Anti-HER2 antibody enhances the growth inhibitory effect of anti-oestrogen on breast cancer cells expressing both oestrogen receptors and HER2. Br J Cancer 2000;82(1):46–51.
67. Nicholson RI, Hutcheson IR, Harper ME, et al. Modulation of epidermal growth factor receptor in endocrine-resistant, oestrogen receptor-positive breast cancer. Endocr Relat Cancer 2001;8(3):175–82.
68. Liddle FJ, Alvarez JV, Poli V, et al. Tyrosine phosphorylation is required for functional activation of disulfide-containing constitutively active STAT mutants. Biochemistry 2006;45(17):5599–605.

Hormonal Mechanisms Underlying the Relationship Between Obesity and Breast Cancer

Claire M. Perks, PhD*, Jeff M.P. Holly, PhD

KEYWORDS

- Breast cancer • Obesity • Adipokines • IGFs
- Estrogen receptor

OBESITY TRENDS

Obesity affects more than one-third of the adult American population (approximately 72 million Americans).[1] The number of overweight and obese Americans has increased dramatically since 1960, and this is a continuing trend. Currently 66.3% of adult Americans (approximately 200 million) are categorized as overweight or obese. Obesity is defined as excess adipose (fat) tissue and there are several different methods for assessing excess adipose tissue; the most common is estimating body mass index (BMI). Overweight and obesity are defined by the World Health Organization as a BMI of less than or equal to 25 kg/m^2 and less than or equal to 30 kg/m^2, respectively. Normal body fat percentages for an average population are 9% to19% for men and 14% to 25% in women, but it may be as much as 60% to 70% in morbidly obese individuals (NIDDK.nih.gov). Obesity is increasing around the world and high BMI now ranks with other major global health problems, such as high blood pressure, high cholesterol, and smoking. Each year, obesity causes at least 112,000 excess deaths in the United States[2] and health care costs of American adults with obesity amount to approximately $147 billion.[3]

The authors have nothing to disclose.

Funding: We acknowledge the Breast Cancer Campaign and The European Foundation for the study of Diabetes for supporting our work.

School of Clinical Sciences, University of Bristol, Research & Learning Building, Southmead Hospital, Bristol BS10 5NB, UK

* Corresponding author.

E-mail address: Claire.m.perks@bristol.ac.uk

Endocrinol Metab Clin N Am 40 (2011) 485–507

doi:10.1016/j.ecl.2011.05.010

0889-8529/11/$ – see front matter © 2011 Elsevier Inc. All rights reserved.

endo.theclinics.com

OBESITY AND BREAST CANCER

Studies of life course epidemiology have provided evidence that obesity has different impacts on the risk and progression of breast cancer depending on when a woman is exposed to increased levels of adiposity. Studies examining associations between birthweight and breast cancer have generally found positive associations, with higher risk associated with heavier babies. In the Nurses' Health Study,[4] a UK 1946 birth cohort[5] and a Swedish cohort,[6] approximately twofold higher risks were observed in women born weighing over 4 kg compared with those born weighing under 3 kg. A study in twins also found a higher risk of breast cancer among higher birthweight twins.[7] A higher birthweight is also associated with increased levels of insulin-like growth factor (IGF)-1 and decreased IGF binding protein (IGFBP)-3 in premenopausal women,[8–10] which could therefore mediate the observed associations between birthweight and breast cancer. Other studies suggest that greater body fatness at young ages, before adulthood, confers a long-term protective effect against developing breast cancer.[11,12] A recent prospective epidemiology study analyzing data from the Nurses' Health Study I and II confirmed these data and indicated that early life adiposity conferred a permanent protective effect against the risk of developing both premenopausal and postmenopausal breast cancer, which was independent of current BMI. The association was stronger for female infants with a birthweight of less than 8.5 pounds and for estrogen receptor (ER)-negative tumors compared with ER-positive tumors, and it was concluded that the association was not mediated by adult BMI or endogenous sex hormones and was therefore probably mediated by an alternative biologic pathway.[13]

It is generally accepted that adult obese women have an increased risk for postmenopausal but not premenopausal breast cancer.[14,15] Once a woman has developed breast cancer, however, either premenopausally or postmenopausally, being overweight or obese has significant adverse consequences.[15–17] One study examined associations between overweight or obesity and mortality from cancer in 495,477 US women over a 16-year period and found that obese women in the highest quintile of BMI had double the death rate (relative risk 2.12) from breast cancer compared with women in the lowest quintile of BMI.[18] When investigating the epidemiology of breast cancer subtypes in two prospective cohort studies of breast cancer survivors, it was observed that among premenopausal women, the women with triple-negative breast cancers compared with those with luminal A breast cancer were more likely to be overweight or obese.[19] In addition, it has been shown that obese breast cancer patients seem to have a higher risk for lymph node metastasis, large tumors, and death when compared with nonobese breast cancer patients.[18,20,21]

Obesity in women with a family history of breast cancer has been shown to significantly increase the risk of developing postmenopausal breast cancer compared with slimmer women.[22] Furthermore, women with a familial genetic predisposition to developing breast cancer (BRCA mutation carriers) are additionally affected by weight gain: in a study of French Canadian families with inherited BRCA1/2 mutations, the risk of developing breast cancer was not related to BMI but was related to weight gain since the age of 18 years.[23]

The following sections document the many potential direct effects of adipose-derived hormones and indirect effects of disturbances to systemic hormone levels caused by obesity, which may mediate the poor prognosis observed for obese women with breast cancer. That adiposity in early life may have different, more complex, and sometimes counterintuitive effects on breast cancer much later in life is probably less related to immediate hormonal effects and more to long-term programming effects that metabolic disturbance in infancy and childhood have on hormonal status much later in life. Both nutrition[24] and adiposity[25] in childhood have long-term effects on the systemic IGF-system that can be detected up to 65 years later in adult life and which can differ from the immediate effects that the same exposures have in adult life. The effects of adiposity in infancy and childhood, when there is still plasticity in hormonal settings, may affect later breast cancer by affecting mammary gland development throughout puberty or through these very long-term effects on programming hormonal levels throughout later adult life.

HORMONAL MECHANISMS THAT UNDERLIE THE RELATIONSHIP BETWEEN OBESITY AND BREAST CANCER
Role of Estrogen Receptor

ERs are members of the nuclear receptor superfamily and mediate the effects of the steroid hormone estrogen in a wide range of developmental and physiologic processes.[26] The ER has two isoforms, α and β, each encoded by separate genes.[27,28] Most premalignant breast lesions express high levels of ER-α and these lesions proliferate in response to estrogen and conversely regress when estrogen is removed.[29] ER-β has an overall antiproliferative effect, thereby antagonizing ER-α function in the breast and as such is downregulated in malignant breast tissue compared with normal nonmalignant mammary tissue.[30] Approximately 80% of breast carcinomas are positive for ER and therefore could be influenced by plasma estrogens.

Testosterone and androstenedione are the principal androgens, the circulating levels of which are much higher than circulating levels of estrogens in postmenopausal women[31]; these androgens are converted to estradiol and estrone, respectively, via enzymes called aromatases. Premenopausal women mainly synthesize estrogens in the ovary and this is the principal source of circulating sex steroids. In postmenopausal women, ovarian biosynthesis is replaced by synthesis in peripheral tissues, and in obese postmenopausal women, adipose tissue is the main source of estrogen biosynthesis via aromatisation of androgens. Aromatase is also found in adipose tissue in the breast as well as in tumor tissue itself[32] and these convert androgens produced by the adrenal cortex into estrogens. This mechanism of estrogen production can lead to local estrogen levels in breast tumors that are as much as 10-fold higher compared with those in the circulation.[33] The lack of functional BRCA1 protein has been found to correlate with higher aromatase levels in 85% of BRCA1 mutation carriers, which is mediated by aberrant transcriptional regulation of aromatase.[34]

Lower concentrations of sex hormone–binding globulin (SHBG), which binds to estradiol and decreases its bioavailability, have also been associated with a higher risk for breast cancer.[35] Circulating SHBG is derived from the liver where its production is suppressed by insulin[36]; increased adiposity results in insulin resistance and consequently raised insulin levels; hepatic SHBG production, however, remains sensitive to insulin and hence SHBG levels are reduced in obese subjects.[37] Obese postmenopausal women have significantly lower levels of SHBG, which are associated with increased risk of breast cancer.[38] Concentrations of estradiol are higher in malignant breast tissue compared with nonmalignant breast tissue.[39] The dense layer of fibroblasts that make up the capsule surrounding the premalignant or cancerous breast lesion have increased aromatase activity, adding to enhanced estrogen biosynthesis.[40]

With postmenopausal women, the Endogenous Hormones and Breast Cancer Collaborative Group analyzed prospective data from nine trials and found that the relative risk for women whose estradiol levels were in the top quintile compared with the bottom was 2.0 and the overall estimate of relative risk of breast cancer associated with the doubling of estradiol was 1.29. This implicates raised estradiol levels as linked to breast cancer development, not as a consequence of the preclinical cancer.[41] These were also the findings of the Nurses' Health Study.[42] In the European Prospective Investigation into Cancer and Nutrition study, blood samples collected 3 years before diagnosis were found to contain significantly higher levels of total estradiol and free estradiol than controls.[43] Higher endogenous estrogen levels have also been shown associated with a decrease in the disease-free interval before recurrence in postmenopausal women with breast cancer.[44] For postmenopausal women, increased BMI is associated with increased levels of estrone and estradiol.[38,45,46] With premenopausal women, one study found that estrogen levels were similar between obese and lean women.[47] In a recent large nested case-control study, involving 18,521 premenopausal women with 197 cases of breast cancer, women with the highest quartiles of menstrual cycle follicular phase total estradiol and free estradiol levels had a significantly increased risk for breast cancer, which was stronger for invasive and estrogen-positive and progesterone receptor–positive breast cancer.[48]

Role of Insulin/IGF Axis

Insulin and IGF-1 and IGF-2 belong to a phylogenetically ancient family of peptide hormones and growth factors that play a fundamental role in the control of essential cellular processes, such as the cell cycle, survival or apoptosis, cell migration, proliferation, and differentiation as well as physiologic processes, such as body growth, metabolism, reproduction, and longevity.

The IGF system consists of 2 ligands (IGF-1 and IGF-2), 2 receptors (type 1 IGF-1R and IGF-2/mannose 6-phosphate receptor), and at least 6 high-affinity IGFBPs (IGFBP-1 to IGFBP-6).[49] Insulin interacts with its own receptor (InsR), which is structurally homologous to the type 1 IGF receptor but can also interact with the IGF-1R with low affinity, whereas IGFs may also interact with the InsR. There is further complexity as the insulin receptor has two isoforms, IR-A and IR-B, of which IR-A has an affinity for IGF-2 (which is overexpressed in most cancers) comparable with that of insulin. In addition to the marked structural similarities at both ligand and receptor levels, the vast majority of the signaling modules downstream of IGF-1R, InsR (A and B isoforms), and IGF-1R-InsR hybrid receptors (composed of an IGF-1R hemireceptor linked to an InsR hemireceptor) are shared by all of these receptors.[50]

As described previously, obesity is a risk factor for postmenopausal breast cancer and predicts a bad prognosis for women with either premenopausal or postmenopausal breast cancer. Obesity is also a strong risk factor for adult-onset diabetes. Obesity is known to induce insulin resistance, a condition whereby some organs become resistant to the effect of insulin to shuttle glucose into cells, especially after a meal high in carbohydrates. To compensate for this resistance to insulin, the pancreas produces more insulin, which leads to an increase in circulating insulin levels.[51] Postmenopausal women with raised BMI, therefore, have not only increased estrogen production but also increased insulin concentrations. The pancreatic compensation may continue for many years, but the pancreas cannot maintain this high insulin output indefinitely, especially in some susceptible individuals. Blood sugar levels, which are increased due to insulin resistance, then increase further as the pancreas fails and insulin levels decrease. The link between insulin resistance and cancer may be related to the compensatory high levels of insulin. Insulin is an important growth factor for body tissues and has been shown to increase proliferation of ER-positive MCF-7 and ZR-751 but not ER-negative MDA-MB-231 cells.[52,53] Insulin may signal cells to proliferate through a variety of mechanisms either directly[52] or indirectly by increasing the levels and bioactivity of other more potent growth factors, such as IGFs. Insulin is able to decrease IGFBPs, such as IGFBP-1 (which is coordinately regulated with SHBG[36]) with a consequent increase in IGF bioactivity,[54] or it can make cells more sensitive to other growth factors, such as estradiol.[55] Insulin also regulates the levels of growth hormone receptors on hepatocytes,[56] which are the main source of circulating IGF-1 and hence may also act indirectly via increasing IGF-1 production. Although insulin resistance is characterized by cells becoming less sensitive to the effects of insulin to transport glucose into cells, insulin insensitivity does not seem to lower the growth promoting properties of insulin. Thus, in an insulin-resistant state, such as induced by obesity, the higher circulating levels of insulin may have a cancer-promoting influence for at least some tissues. In terms of circulating concentrations of IGF-1, in contrast to insulin, there is not such a direct relationship between IGF-1 and the level of adiposity. A nonlinear association between circulating IGF-1 and BMI has been found in studies with sufficient power to detect such an association, with the highest IGF-1 levels in women with BMI between 24 and 25 kg/m^2 and lower levels in those at either extreme of the BMI range.[57,58] The relationship between the IGF axis and the risk of development of breast cancer however is compelling. A recent study that pooled 17 prospective studies indicated that IGF-1 was associated with an increased risk of both premenopausal and postmenopausal breast cancer, although these associations seemed predominantly confined to ER-positive tumors.[59] The IGF-1R seems to play a critical role in malignant transformation and in the maintenance of a transformed cell phenotype.[60] This is due, in part to the efficacy with which the IGF-1R can maintain cell survival and protect cells from apoptosis via multiple signaling pathways.[61] It is also suggested that IGFs can modulate integrin-mediated processes because they regulate cell-cell adhesion[62] and cell migration and motility of both normal and cancer cells, including those in the breast.[63,64]

Role of Other Hormones

Glucocorticoids

Glucocorticoids play an important role in the development and function of the mammary gland: they can induce differentiation of mammary epithelial cells in primary culture[65] and are thought to be vital for the initiation and maintenance of lactation.[66] Their role in breast cancer, however, is still unclear: some studies report that glucocorticoids have inhibitory effects on breast cancer cells,[67,68] whereas others observed that glucocorticoids decreased the efficacy of chemotherapy.[69] Inactive cortisone is converted to active cortisol by the enzyme 11β–hydroxysteroid dehydrogenase type 1, and a recent study observed that this enzyme was significantly lower in breast cancer specimens relative to normal adjacent tissues, implying a lower production of cortisol may be advantageous for the tumor cells.[70] This enzyme has also been identified from a genome-wide linkage analysis as a possible candidate gene for breast cancer development in postmenopausal women.[71] Glucocorticoids exert their effects by binding to the glucocorticoid receptor.[72] Glucocorticoid receptor expression was found lower in breast cancer relative to normal cells[70] but an earlier study showed a lack of glucocorticoid receptor expression in cancer cells in the majority of nonmetaplastic carcinomas but strong expression in metaplastic carcinomas.[73] Although the impact of obesity on the levels of glucocorticoids and the glucocorticoid receptors in breast tissue is unclear, reports show that in obese women, serum levels of glucocorticoids are unaltered but the activity of 11β–hydroxysteroid dehydrogenase in adipose tissue is increased.[74,75] This may suggest that obesity-induced changes in the production of cortisol from adipose tissue may be able to have an impact on breast tumorigenesis.

Ghrelin and obestatin

Ghrelin and obestatin are two gastrointestinal hormones obtained by post-translational processing of the transcript from the same gene, preproghrelin.[76] The acylation of ghrelin is required before it can activate its receptor, the growth hormone secretagogue receptor (GHS-R). Ghrelin has emerged as the first identified circulating hunger hormone increasing food intake and fat mass[77,78] by an action exerted at the level of the hypothalamus. Obestatin was originally identified as ananorectic peptide, antagonizing growth hormone secretion and food intake induced by ghrelin.[79] It was originally proposed that GPR39 functioned as an obestatin receptor; however, more recent findings suggest that this is unlikely.[80] Little is known with respect to obestatin and breast cancer, whereas ghrelin production has been reported in both nonmalignant breast tissues[81,82] and breast carcinomas.[83] The truncated isoform of the receptor, GHS-R1b, was reported as highly expressed in breast cancer tissues compared with normal breast, and ghrelin, at physiologic levels, has been shown to increase breast cancer cell proliferation (in vitro).[84] A case control study of 1359 breast cancer cases nested within the European Prospective Investigation into Cancer and Nutrition found evidence for associations of ghrelin polymorphisms with circulating IGF-1 levels and with breast cancer risk.[85] There are conflicting studies regarding the effects of obesity on ghrelin and obestatin levels. Studies generally agree that ghrelin levels in the plasma of obese individuals are lower than those in leaner individuals.[86,87] Levels of obestatin have been observed to either increase or decrease. A recent meta-analysis reported that obestatin and total and active ghrelin levels were all significantly higher in normal weight compared with obese individuals and that the ghrelin/obestatin ratio was also higher but this was not significant.[88] Another study, however, reported that obestatin levels were lower in normal weight compared with obese women.[89] With regard to breast cancer progression, the impact of obesity in women on local levels of ghrelin and its receptors and the impact of obesity on altering the normal balance that exists between ghrelin and obsestatin remain to be elucidated.

Role of Adipocytes

Adipocytes were originally considered simple energy depots but recently it has been recognized that these cells also act as endocrine cells, secreting molecules that can influence the cells around them. Mature adipocytes are a major component of the breast tissue and crosstalk exists between tumor cells, surrounding normal cells and adipocytes that may promote tumor progression. In obese women it is likely that this is amplified and could contribute to the poor prognosis for obese women with breast cancer. In support of this, several studies have shown that adipocyte cell culture media increases invasiveness of breast cancer cells.[90–92] There is, however, a conundrum because one of the strongest risk factors for breast cancer is mammographic breast density[93] and a high breast density is due to a greater ratio of glandular tissue compared with adipose tissue, which may argue against breast adipose tissue being a strong influence. Loss of BRCA1 has also been shown to promote aromatase activity in preadipocytes,[94] and the positive relationship between breast density and breast cancer risk is absent in women with BRCA mutations,[95] which could indicate an altered relationship with adipose tissue. The influence that preadipocytes might exert is not clear since Johnston and colleagues[96] found that 3T3 L1 preadipocytes conditioned media inhibited the growth of MCF-7 breast cancer cells, whereas Chamras and colleagues[97] found that it promoted the growth of MCF-7, MDA-MB-231, and MDA-MB-436 cells, and Manabe and colleagues[90] found that it had no effect on breast cancer cells.

Role of Adipokines

Adipokines are secreted from adipose tissue and are thought to contribute to the mechanisms by which obesity and related metabolic disorders influence breast cancer development. Obesity is associated with increased levels of leptin, hepatocyte growth factor (HGF), tumor necrosis factor α (TNF-α), and interleukin 6 (IL-6). In contrast, levels of adiponectin are decreased. The impact of obesity-induced changes in relation to breast cancer is discussed in the following sections.

Leptin

Leptin is a 16-kDa cytokine that circulates predominantly bound to a soluble form of its receptor and exerts its effects on the transmembrane leptin receptor (Ob-R) of which there are many isoforms, the two main ones being the long isoform (Ob-R1/Rb) that activates JAK2, Ras, and PI3-K pathways and the short isoform (Ob-Rs/Ra) that mainly activates MAPK.[98] Leptin is primarily synthesized in preadipocytes and adipocytes[99,100] but can also be made by mammary epithelial cells.[101] Leptin acts on the hypothalamus to regulate food intake.[102] In obese ob/ob mice, where leptin is deficient, leptin treatment decreases food intake and body weight.[103] Mutations in functional leptin or in Ob-R results in extreme obesity in humans.[104] A rise in circulating leptin was, therefore, anticipated to prevent obesity by decreasing appetite but in most cases of human obesity circulating leptin levels are increased,[105,106] indicating that obesity is associated with a resistance to the normal effects of leptin.

Leptin receptors are found on breast cancer cells[107] and leptin exerts a stimulatory effect promoting their survival, proliferation, migration, and invasion.[108–110] Consistent with these studies, leptin has been shown to upregulate vascular endothelial growth factor (via hypoxia-inducible factor-1a [HIF-1a] and nuclear factor κb [NFκB]),[111] telomerase activity, and transcription of human telomerase reverse transcriptase in MCF-7 breast cancer cells.[112] Leptin has also been shown to transactivate HER2 in breast cancer cells.[113] Leptin levels are higher in breast cancer tissue than normal breast tissue.[114] When found in breast tumors, both leptin and leptin receptor are strongly associated with poorer prognosis, having greater occurrence in distant metastases and linked with lower survival[115] and positively correlating with breast cancer stage and lymph node metastasis.[116] Ob-R expression also correlates positively with tumor size.[117] Leptin receptors were not detectable in normal mammary epithelial cells by immunohistochemistry, whereas cancer cells showed positive staining in 83% of cases. Leptin was also expressed in 92% of breast carcinomas but none of the normal tissue examined.[115] Serum leptin levels show strong correlation with BMI and are significantly greater in breast cancer patients than in controls.[118] Results from epidemiologic studies, however, have provided little evidence for an association of breast cancer risk with circulating leptin levels.[119–121]

An area of increasing interest is the impact of polymorphisms in leptin and its receptor and their associations with tumor progression. The American Cancer Society Cancer Prevention Study II, a nested case control study, reported that single nucleotide polymorphisms in leptin did not seem to affect postmenopausal breast cancer risk.[122] In contrast the Long Island Breast Cancer Study Group, a population-based study of European American women, observed that a common variant in leptin may be associated with the risk of developing breast cancer: the LEP-2548AA genotype was associated with a 30% increased risk of developing breast cancer but was not associated with survival among those diagnosed with breast cancer. Another variant, LEP-0223R polymorphism, showed no correlation.[123] A study by Terrasi and colleagues[124] looking in vitro and in vivo found that the LEP-2548G/A genotype was identified in a homozygous conformation in BT-474 and SK-BR-3 breast cancer cells, in a heterozygous conformation in MDA-MB-231 cells, and a wild-type LEP-2548G/G sequence was found in MCF-7 and ZR-75-1 cells. They also reported that 14 tumors expressing LEP-2548A/A were associated with high leptin levels. Polymorphisms of the leptin receptor, specifically LEP-R-109 in premenopausal women, have also been associated with obesity and with tumor progression.[125]

Adiponectin

Adiponectin is an adipocyte-secreted, insulin-sensitizing hormone involved in glucose regulation and fatty acid catabolism.[126] It can act via two receptors, ADIPOR1 and ADIPOR2,[127] both of which are present on breast cancer cells.[128] Adiponectin biosynthesis is downregulated in obesity, = so circulating concentrations are decreased.[129] The majority of studies report that low serum adiponectin levels are significantly associated with increased risk of breast cancer[130–132] particularly postmenopausal.[133] A case-control study showed that women with the highest circulating levels of adiponectin had a significantly reduced risk of breast cancer.[134] One recent study, however, showed low levels of adiponectin measured in prospectively collected serum from postmenopausal women were associated with increasing BMI but not breast cancer risk.[135] Because the levels of adiponectin are inversely correlated with adiposity,[129] it has been suggested that decreased levels of adiponectin may explain the increased risk of postmenopausal breast cancer in obese women. To support this, breast cancer cell lines were found to express both adiponectin receptors ADIPOR1 and ADIPOR2,[134,136] and a large body of evidence indicates that exposure of breast cancer cells to adiponectin significantly inhibited their proliferation and migration.[40,137–139] LKB1 has been suggested as required for adiponectin-mediated modulation of adenosine monophosphate–activated protein kinase (AMPK)-S6K and its consequent growth inhibitory effects on breast cancer cells.[137,140]

Hepatocyte growth factor

The adipocytes also synthesize HGF,[141] and serum HGF levels positively correlate with BMI.[142] In vitro studies in the rat showed that HGF in adipocyte culture medium was the major growth promoter of mammary epithelial cells.[143] Patients with more advanced TNM staging were shown to have higher serum soluble HGF.[144]

Tumor necrosis factor α

Several studies have shown that obesity is characterized by an abnormal inflammatory response, particularly in the liver, muscle, and adipose tissue, which culminates in higher than normal levels of TNF-α.[145,146] Both in experimental models and in humans, adipose tissue expression of TNF-α increases with obesity and is positively correlated with the amount of adipose tissue and degree of insulin-resistance.[145] Adipocyte culture medium with increased abundance of TNF-α promoted the migration and invasiveness of MDA-MB-231 breast cancer cells.[92] Conversely, breast cancer cells are also able to secrete TNF-α, which seems to be involved in desmoplasia, which brings about a fibrotic response with reversion of adipocyte cells to fibroblasts.[147] Invasion of malignant neoplasms into adjacent normal tissues is fundamental to the neoplastic process and includes the ability to induce a desmoplastic response of the host tissues at the site of primary invasion. The impact of adipocyte-derived TNF-α compared with tumor-derived TNF-α may have different impacts depending on tumor grade and the overall balance of TNF-α in the microenvironment may affect the development of the cancer.

Interleukin 6

Obesity is also associated with higher circulating levels of IL-6,[148] which is mainly produced by visceral fat.[149] High levels of serum IL-6 were significantly correlated to poor survival in patients with hormone-refractory breast cancer.[150] Conditioned media from MDA-MB-231 breast cancer cells caused bone cells to secrete IL-6, which is thought to promote the ability of breast cancer cells to metastasize to bone.[151] Studies suggest that IL-6 polymorphisms play a limited role in breast cancer. A recent study conducted within The European Prospective Investigation into Cancer and Nutrition genotyped 27 polymorphisms in 6292 breast cancer cases and 8135 matched controls. One IL-6 polymorphism (re6949149) was marginally associated with breast cancer risk, and an increased risk of breast cancer was observed for the PTGS2 polymorphism rs7550380.[85] An earlier study looked at 5 polymorphisms in the IL-6 gene and did not detect significant associations between IL-6 genotypes and BMI. They detected significant interactions, however, between waist-to-hip ratio and IL-6 rs1800795 but only in postmenopausal women. These data suggested that IL6 genotypes may influence breast cancer risk in conjunction with central adiposity.[152]

CROSSTALK BETWEEN INSULIN/IGF AND ESTROGEN SIGNALING PATHWAYS AND IMPACT OF ADIPOKINES

Crosstalk exists between estrogen and insulin/IGF signaling.[153] Estrogen and insulin/IGF-1 synergize to increase cell proliferation.[55] Estrogen can increase levels of the IGF-1R[154] whereas in ER-negative tumors IGF-I has been reported to lack mitogenic activity.[155] Insulin/IGF-1 can activate the ER independently of estrogen and increase the expression of target genes,[156] and re-expression of ER-α in ER-negative MCF-7 cells restores both ER and IGF-1–mediated signaling and growth.[157] It seems that these pathways are further enhanced through the influence of adipokines. Leptin has also been shown to affect ER signaling in xenografts of MCF7 breast cancer cells in nude mice; leptin was found to increase ER-α and decrease ER-β abundance[158]; and in MCF-7 and MDA-MB-231 breast cancer cells, correlations in expression between ER-α and leptin receptors have been identified.[159] In addition, some of the effects of ER-α on breast cancer development have been found dependent on leptin-induction of STAT3.[160] Leptin has also been shown to increase aromatase activity in MCF-7 breast cancer cells.[161] There does not, however, seem to be an association of leptin with breast density (a strong risk factor for breast cancer).[162] In a prospective observational study, serum levels of leptin reflected total amount of fat mass, which correlated to aromatase activity and subsequent levels of estrogens.[163] Bidirectional crosstalk also exists between leptin and IGF-1 signaling promoting invasion and migration of breast cancer cells via transactivation of epidermal growth factor receptors.[164] Studies have demonstrated that TNF-α regulates IL-6 synthesis and both may increase aromatase expression in the adipose tissue, thus stimulating estrogen production.[165,166]

EFFECTS OF PHYSICAL ACTIVITY AND DIET ON RISK AND DEVELOPMENT OF BREAST CANCER AND POTENTIAL MECHANISMS OF ACTIONS

As discussed previously, evidence indicates that obesity is associated with increased risk of postmenopausal breast cancer and is detrimental for breast cancer patients both premenopausally and postmenopausally. Obesity is a modifiable risk factor, so it would be anticipated that decreasing levels of adiposity would have a beneficial effect on breast cancer risk and development. Two potential ways of achieving this are through modifications in levels of exercise and in diet, thus either increasing energy expenditure or reducing energy intake. The World Cancer Research Fund with the American Association for Cancer Research recently reviewed the literature and concluded that there was a large body of evidence from prospective epidemiology studies suggesting that physical activity (total physical activity, occupational, and recreational) is protective for breast cancer in premenopausal and postmenopausal women, although the evidence is stronger for this relationship in postmenopausal women (WCRF/AICR report 2007).[167] Physical activity also promotes a lower risk for breast cancer in women of diverse races and ethnicities.[168–171] Physical activity in adolescence has also been observed to be associated with a delayed age of breast cancer onset among women with substantially increased risk for breast cancer due to mutations in tumor suppressor genes, BRCA1 and BRCA2.[172] Physical activity has also been shown to increase survival in women with pre-existing breast cancer.[173–176]

Evidence suggests that diet modifications (increasing fruit, vegetables, and fiber and reducing fat intake) may only significantly reduce breast cancer risk or increase relapse-free survival if they are associated with weight loss. A prospective cohort study within the Nurses' Health Study found that weight loss after menopause is associated with a decreased risk of breast cancer.[48] Results from the Women's Intervention Nutrition Study achieved a modest but significant weight loss in the dietary intervention arm and this was associated with increased relapse-free survival.[177,178] This is in contrast to the Women's Healthy Eating and Living Study, a randomized trial, that found no difference in the dietary intervention arm in relation to relapse-free surviva, l but unlike in Women's Intervention Nutrition Study, this study reported no weight loss in the dietary intervention group.[179]

In the Women's Health Initiative Dietary Modification Trial, mean levels of estrone were reduced in obese women who increased their physical activity,[38] which may have contributed to the observed reduction in risk of breast cancer with increased physical activity. Abdominal obesity and physical inactivity throughout life were associated with low serum adiponectin and increased breast cancer risk.[131] Serum HGF levels positively correlate with BMI and decrease after weight loss.[142] A clinical trial, the Yale Exercise and Survivorship Study, in breast cancer survivors assessed the effects of 4 to 6 months of aerobic exercise interventions and found that it significantly reduced insulin and IGF-1 levels but did not affect levels of leptin or adiponectin,[180–182] which they suggested could have a big impact on breast cancer prognosis.

IMPLICATIONS FOR THERAPY, TREATMENT, AND PREVENTION

As discussed in this review, evidence shows that circulating and tissue levels of estrogens differ according to BMI and metabolic status. Obese postmenopausal women have an increase in circulating and local levels of estrogen and aromatase activity compared with slimmer women. As a result, antiestrogen therapy and aromatase inhibitors may show increased efficacy in obese breast cancer patients and perhaps should be considered as chemopreventive in obese postmenopausal women.

Currently, antiestrogens, such as tamoxifen, are the mainstay of treatment for managing hormonally responsive breast cancers. They classically inhibit estrogen-stimulated cancer cell growth by blocking estrogen acting at its receptor. Aromatase inhibitors bind reversibly or irreversibly to the aromatase enzyme, leading to undetectable levels of estrogen in postmenopausal women. Several different aromatase inhibitors are currently used to control the peripheral production of estrogens in women who have had breast cancer, and additional applications for the aromatase inhibitors are being evaluated.[183] A collection of studies determined that the effectiveness of aromatase inhibitors is dependent on the suppression of intratumoral estrogen levels but that this suppression is mainly due to lowering plasma estradiol concentrations as opposed to inhibiting intratumoral estrogen synthesis. Haynes and colleagues[184] found that intratumoral concentrations of aromatase mRNA correlated with ER-α levels but not with intratumoral estrogen concentrations. In addition, plasma estradiol levels correlated strongly with the expression of estrogen-responsive genes in ER-α–positive tumors.[185] Furthermore, after presurgical treatment with aromatase inhibitors (letrozole and anastrozole), baseline estradiol measurements correlated with the degree of Ki67 reduction (a marker of proliferation and intermediate marker of benefit from endocrine therapy).[185,186] Targeting the IGF-1R may also be of greater benefit in obese postmenopausal women who exhibit increased circulating levels of insulin and IGF-1. The IGFs acting via the type 1 IGF receptor (IGF-1R) regulate cancer cell proliferation, survival, metabolism, and metastasis. Drugs targeting the IGF-1R are being tested in clinical trials for cancer therapy and it seems likely that this class of drugs could be approved soon. Data also suggest that the insulin receptor, closely related to IGF-1R, may also be a target and may need to be inhibited to maximally suppress the intracellular pathways that are activated by both IGF-1R and insulin receptors (see review by Sachdev and colleageus[187]). The importance of the IGF axis is highlighted further by data showing that tamoxifen is additionally effective through it ability to reduce levels of IGF-1.[188] Breast cancer risk can be reduced by prophylactic use of tamoxifen that lowers circulating IGF-1 concentrations.[189] In addition, in vitro data shows that combined use of IGF-1 receptor inhibitors and an aromatase inhibitor, letrozole, synergistically increase the induction of apoptosis in breast cancer cell lines.[190]

There has recently been a surge of interest in the potential of insulin-sensitizing drugs, in particular, metformin, as effective anticancer agents. Metformin activates the key cellular metabolism enzyme, AMPK; once activated, this enzyme signals for reduced protein synthesis and gluconeogenesis, which in cancer cells may culminate in cell growth inhibition and the induction of apoptosis. Several studies have indicated that diabetes is associated with poor prognosis and an increase in cancer mortality and can also affect cancer therapy[191,192] and that these affects are ameliorated when breast cancer patients concomitantly take metformin.[193] There are several purported mechanisms by which metformin could affect tumor growth, such as reducing signaling through the IGF-1R and ER-α or through lowering insulin resistance (reviewed by Jalving and colleagues[194]). These investigations have led to the initiation of many ongoing prospective clinical studies with a view to developing metformin as an anticancer agent, particularly in breast cancer patients.

Leptin is potentially a therapeutic target for breast cancer prevention and treatment. Peptide-based leptin receptor antagonists have been proposed, which in immunocompromised mice decreased the growth of proliferating orthotic human breast cancer xenografts by 50%.[195] In addition, use of a pegylated leptin peptide receptor antagonist 2 (PEG LPrA2) in severe immunodeficient mice hosting established ER-positive and ER-negative breast cancer xenografts showed that leptin was involved in the growth of both.[196] With a role for inflammation-associated signaling pathways (regulated by IL-6 and TNF-α) in breast tumor growth and disease outcome having been identified, several studies have investigated the use of aspirin and nonsteroidal anti-inflammatory drugs in reducing breast cancer risk and prevention.[197–199] It has been suggested that aspirin and other cyclooxygenase-2 inhibitors may reduce the risk of breast cancer by inhibiting aromatase activity.[200]

Human and animal studies have clearly demonstrated that dietary energy restriction brings about favorable changes in all the factors that have been described in this article. Adverse changes in these same factors may be involved in the increased risk and poor progression of breast cancer in obese women. Realistically achieving and maintaining dietary energy restriction would be a challenge. Others have investigated the potential benefits of intermittent energy restriction on a long-term basis and initial animal and human studies suggest it may have cancer preventive effects but requires further study (see review by Harvie and Howell[201]). Intermittent energy restriction may, therefore, prove a strategy for breast cancer prevention.

SUMMARY

Breast cancer continues to be a major health problem worldwide with obesity inevitably an increasingly common comorbidity for many women. This article discusses several molecular pathways that underlie the link between obesity and breast cancer and describes the impact of obesity on breast cancer risk and progression. A better understanding of these pathways may enable the optimization of current treatments for obese women. Evidence would also suggest that women could reduce their risk of developing breast cancer through the maintenance of a lean body mass.

REFERENCES

1. Ogden CL, Carroll MD, McDowell MA, et al. Obesity among adults in the United States—no statistically significant chance since 2003–2004. NCHS Data Brief 2007;(1):1–8.
2. Flegal KM. Epidemiologic aspects of overweight and obesity in the United States. Physiol Behav 2005;86(5):599–602.
3. Finkelstein EA, Trogdon JG, Cohen JW, et al. Annual medical spending attributable to obesity: payer-and service-specific estimates. Health Aff (Millwood) 2009;28(5):w822–31.
4. Michels KB, Trichopoulos D, Robins JM, et al. Birthweight as a risk factor for breast cancer. Lancet 1996;348(9041):1542–6.
5. dos Santos Silva I, De Stavola BL, Hardy RJ, et al. Is the association of birth weight with premenopausal breast cancer risk mediated through childhood growth? Br J Cancer 2004;91(3):519–24.
6. Andersson SW, Bengtsson C, Hallberg L, et al. Cancer risk in Swedish women: the relation to size at birth. Br J Cancer 2001;84(9):1193–8.
7. Hubinette A, Lichtenstein P, Ekbom A, et al. Birth characteristics and breast cancer risk: a study among like-sexed twins. Int J Cancer 2001;91(2):248–51.
8. Schernhammer ES, Tworoger SS, Eliassen AH, et al. Body shape throughout life and correlations with IGFs and GH. Endocr Relat Cancer 2007;14(3):721–32.
9. Boyne MS, Thame M, Bennett FI, et al. The relationship among circulating insulin-like growth factor (IGF)-I, IGF-binding proteins-1 and -2, and birth anthropometry: a prospective study. J Clin Endocrinol Metab 2003;88(4):1687–91.
10. Vatten LJ, Maehle BO, Lund Nilsen TI, et al. Birth weight as a predictor of breast cancer: a case-control study in Norway. Br J Cancer 2002;86(1):89–91.
11. Bardia A, Vachon CM, Olson JE, et al. Relative weight at age 12 and risk of postmenopausal breast cancer. Cancer Epidemiol Biomarkers Prev 2008;17(2):374–8.
12. Michels KB, Terry KL, Willett WC. Longitudinal study on the role of body size in premenopausal breast cancer. Arch Intern Med 2006;166(21):2395–402.
13. Baer HJ, Tworoger SS, Hankinson SE, et al. Body fatness at young ages and risk of breast cancer throughout life. Am J Epidemiol 2010;171(11):1183–94.

14. van den Brandt PA, Spiegelman D, Yaun SS, et al. Pooled analysis of prospective cohort studies on height, weight, and breast cancer risk. Am J Epidemiol 2000;152(6):514–27.
15. Reeves GK, Pirie K, Beral V, et al. Cancer incidence and mortality in relation to body mass index in the Million Women Study: cohort study. BMJ 2007; 335(7630):1134.
16. Barnett GC, Shah M, Redman K, et al. Risk factors for the incidence of breast cancer: do they affect survival from the disease? J Clin Oncol 2008;26(20): 3310–6.
17. Dal Maso L, Zucchetto A, Talamini R, et al. Effect of obesity and other lifestyle factors on mortality in women with breast cancer. Int J Cancer 2008;123(9): 2188–94.
18. Calle EE, Rodriguez C, Walker-Thurmond K, et al. Overweight, obesity, and mortality from cancer in a prospectively studied cohort of U.S. adults. N Engl J Med 2003;348(17):1625–38.
19. Kwan ML, Kushi LH, Weltzien E, et al. Epidemiology of breast cancer subtypes in two prospective cohort studies of breast cancer survivors. Breast Cancer Res 2009;11(3):R31.
20. Berclaz G, Li S, Price KN, et al. Body mass index as a prognostic feature in operable breast cancer: the International Breast Cancer Study Group experience. Ann Oncol 2004;15(6):875–84.
21. Feigelson HS, Patel AV, Teras LR, et al. Adult weight gain and histopathologic characteristics of breast cancer among postmenopausal women. Cancer 2006;107(1):12–21.
22. Carpenter CL, Ross RK, Paganini-Hill A, et al. Effect of family history, obesity and exercise on breast cancer risk among postmenopausal women. Int J Cancer 2003;106(1):96–102.
23. Nkondjock A, Robidoux A, Paredes Y, et al. Diet, lifestyle and BRCA-related breast cancer risk among French-Canadians. Breast Cancer Res Treat 2006; 98(3):285–94.
24. Martin RM, Holly JM, Middleton N, et al. Childhood diet and insulin-like growth factors in adulthood: 65-year follow-up of the Boyd Orr Cohort. Eur J Clin Nutr 2007;61(11):1281–92.
25. Martin RM, Holly JM, Davey Smith G, et al. Associations of adiposity from childhood into adulthood with insulin resistance and the insulin-like growth factor system: 65-year follow-up of the Boyd Orr Cohort. J Clin Endocrinol Metab 2006;91(9):3287–95.
26. Mangelsdorf DJ, Thummel C, Beato M, et al. The nuclear receptor superfamily: the second decade. Cell 1995;83(6):835–9.
27. Nilsson S, Makela S, Treuter E, et al. Mechanisms of estrogen action. Physiol Rev 2001;81(4):1535–65.
28. Fox EM, Davis RJ, Shupnik MA. ERbeta in breast cancer—onlooker, passive player, or active protector? Steroids 2008;73(11):1039–51.
29. Fuqua SA. The role of estrogen receptors in breast cancer metastasis. J Mammary Gland Biol Neoplasia 2001;6(4):407–17.
30. Hartman J, Strom A, Gustafsson JA. Estrogen receptor beta in breast cancer—diagnostic and therapeutic implications. Steroids 2009;74(8):635–41.
31. Siiteri PK. Adipose tissue as a source of hormones. Am J Clin Nutr 1987; 45(Suppl 1):277–82.
32. Miller WR. Aromatase and the breast: regulation and clinical aspects. Maturitas 2006;54(4):335–41.

33. Lonning PE, Helle H, Duong NK, et al. Tissue estradiol is selectively elevated in receptor positive breast cancers while tumour estrone is reduced independent of receptor status. J Steroid Biochem Mol Biol 2009;117(1–3):31–41.

34. Chand AL, Simpson ER, Clyne CD. Aromatase expression is increased in BRCA1 mutation carriers. BMC Cancer 2009;9:148.

35. Zhu BT, Conney AH. Functional role of estrogen metabolism in target cells: review and perspectives. Carcinogenesis 1998;19(1):1–27.

36. Holly JM, Smith CP, Dunger DB, et al. Relationship between the pubertal fall in sex hormone binding globulin and insulin-like growth factor binding protein-I. A synchronized approach to pubertal development? Clin Endocrinol (Oxf) 1989; 31(3):277–84.

37. Weaver JU, Holly JM, Kopelman PG, et al. Decreased sex hormone binding globulin (SHBG) and insulin-like growth factor binding protein (IGFBP-1) in extreme obesity. Clin Endocrinol (Oxf) 1990;33(3):415–22.

38. McTiernan A, Wu L, Chen C, et al. Relation of BMI and physical activity to sex hormones in postmenopausal women. Obesity (Silver Spring) 2006;14(9):1662–77.

39. Yager JD, Davidson NE. Estrogen carcinogenesis in breast cancer. N Engl J Med 2006;354(3):270–82.

40. Vona-Davis L, Rose DP. Adipokines as endocrine, paracrine, and autocrine factors in breast cancer risk and progression. Endocr Relat Cancer 2007; 14(2):189–206.

41. Key T, Appleby P, Barnes I, et al. Endogenous sex hormones and breast cancer in postmenopausal women: reanalysis of nine prospective studies. J Natl Cancer Inst 2002;94(8):606–16.

42. Hankinson SE, Willett WC, Manson JE, et al. Plasma sex steroid hormone levels and risk of breast cancer in postmenopausal women. J Natl Cancer Inst 1998; 90(17):1292–9.

43. Kaaks R, Rinaldi S, Key TJ, et al. Postmenopausal serum androgens, oestrogens and breast cancer risk: the European prospective investigation into cancer and nutrition. Endocr Relat Cancer 2005;12(4):1071–82.

44. Lonning PE. Aromatase inhibition for breast cancer treatment. Acta Oncol 1996; 35(Suppl 5):38–43.

45. Hankinson SE, Willett WC, Manson JE, et al. Alcohol, height, and adiposity in relation to estrogen and prolactin levels in postmenopausal women. J Natl Cancer Inst 1995;87(17):1297–302.

46. Bezemer ID, Rinaldi S, Dossus L, et al. C-peptide, IGF-I, sex-steroid hormones and adiposity: a cross-sectional study in healthy women within the European Prospective Investigation into Cancer and Nutrition (EPIC). Cancer Causes Control 2005;16(5):561–72.

47. Cento RM, Proto C, Spada RS, et al. Leptin levels in menopause: effect of estrogen replacement therapy. Horm Res 1999;52(6):269–73.

48. Eliassen AH, Missmer SA, Tworoger SS, et al. Endogenous steroid hormone concentrations and risk of breast cancer among premenopausal women. J Natl Cancer Inst 2006;98(19):1406–15.

49. Perks CM, Holly JM. IGF binding proteins (IGFBPs) and regulation of breast cancer biology. J Mammary Gland Biol Neoplasia 2008;13(4):455–69.

50. Belfiore A, Frasca F, Pandini G, et al. Insulin receptor isoforms and insulin receptor/insulin-like growth factor receptor hybrids in physiology and disease. Endocr Rev 2009;30(6):586–623.

51. Grundy SM. What is the contribution of obesity to the metabolic syndrome? Endocrinol Metab Clin North Am 2004;33(2):267–82.

52. Godden J, Leake R, Kerr DJ. The response of breast cancer cells to steroid and peptide growth factors. Anticancer Res 1992;12(5):1683–8.
53. De Leon DD, Wilson DM, Powers M, et al. Effects of insulin-like growth factors (IGFs) and IGF receptor antibodies on the proliferation of human breast cancer cells. Growth Factors 1992;6(4):327–36.
54. Taylor AM, Dunger DB, Preece MA, et al. The growth hormone independent insulin-like growth factor-I binding protein BP-28 is associated with serum insulin-like growth factor-I inhibitory bioactivity in adolescent insulin-dependent diabetics. Clin Endocrinol (Oxf) 1990;32(2):229–39.
55. Mawson A, Lai A, Carroll JS, et al. Estrogen and insulin/IGF-1 cooperatively stimulate cell cycle progression in MCF-7 breast cancer cells through differential regulation of c-Myc and cyclin D1. Mol Cell Endocrinol 2005;229(1–2):161–73.
56. Baxter RC, Brown AS, Turtle JR. Association between serum insulin, serum somatomedin and liver receptors for human growth hormone in streptozotocin diabetes. Horm Metab Res 1980;12(8):377–81.
57. Lukanova A, Lundin E, Zeleniuch-Jacquotte A, et al. Body mass index, circulating levels of sex-steroid hormones, IGF-I and IGF-binding protein-3: a cross-sectional study in healthy women. Eur J Endocrinol 2004;150(2):161–71.
58. Allen NE, Appleby PN, Kaaks R, et al. Lifestyle determinants of serum insulin-like growth-factor-I (IGF-I), C-peptide and hormone binding protein levels in British women. Cancer Causes Control 2003;14(1):65–74.
59. Key TJ, Appleby PN, Reeves GK, et al. Insulin-like growth factor 1 (IGF1), IGF binding protein 3 (IGFBP3), and breast cancer risk: pooled individual data analysis of 17 prospective studies. Lancet Oncol 2010;11(6):530–42.
60. Valentinis B, Baserga R. IGF-I receptor signalling in transformation and differentiation. Mol Pathol 2001;54(3):133–7.
61. Peruzzi F, Prisco M, Dews M, et al. Multiple signaling pathways of the insulin-like growth factor 1 receptor in protection from apoptosis. Mol Cell Biol 1999;19(10): 7203–15.
62. Mauro L, Salerno M, Morelli C, et al. Role of the IGF-I receptor in the regulation of cell-cell adhesion: implications in cancer development and progression. J Cell Physiol 2003;194(2):108–16.
63. Doerr ME, Jones JI. The roles of integrins and extracellular matrix proteins in the insulin-like growth factor I-stimulated chemotaxis of human breast cancer cells. J Biol Chem 1996;271(5):2443–7.
64. Guvakova MA, Adams JC, Boettiger D. Functional role of alpha-actinin, PI 3-kinase and MEK1/2 in insulin-like growth factor I receptor kinase regulated motility of human breast carcinoma cells. J Cell Sci 2002;115(Pt 21):4149–65.
65. Darcy KM, Shoemaker SF, Lee PP, et al. Hydrocortisone and progesterone regulation of the proliferation, morphogenesis, and functional differentiation of normal rat mammary epithelial cells in three dimensional primary culture. J Cell Physiol 1995;163(2):365–79.
66. Lyons WR. Hormonal synergism in mammary growth. Proc R Soc Lond B Biol Sci 1958;149(936):303–25.
67. Goya L, Maiyar AC, Ge Y, et al. Glucocorticoids induce a G1/G0 cell cycle arrest of Con8 rat mammary tumor cells that is synchronously reversed by steroid withdrawal or addition of transforming growth factor-alpha. Mol Endocrinol 1993; 7(9):1121–32.
68. Gong H, Jarzynka MJ, Cole TJ, et al. Glucocorticoids antagonize estrogens by glucocorticoid receptor-mediated activation of estrogen sulfotransferase. Cancer Res 2008;68(18):7386–93.

69. Pang D, Kocherginsky M, Krausz T, et al. Dexamethasone decreases xenograft response to Paclitaxel through inhibition of tumor cell apoptosis. Cancer Biol Ther 2006;5(8):933–40.
70. Lu L, Zhao G, Luu-The V, et al. Expression of 11beta-hydroxysteroid Dehydrogenase Type 1 in Breast cancer and adjacent non-malignant tissue. An Immunocytochemical Study. Pathol Oncol Res 2011. [Epub ahead of print].
71. Feigelson HS, Teras LR, Diver WR, et al. Genetic variation in candidate obesity genes ADRB2, ADRB3, GHRL, HSD11B1, IRS1, IRS2, and SHC1 and risk for breast cancer in the Cancer Prevention Study II. Breast Cancer Res 2008; 10(4):R57.
72. Beato M, Herrlich P, Schutz G. Steroid hormone receptors: many actors in search of a plot. Cell 1995;83(6):851–7.
73. Lien HC, Lu YS, Cheng AL, et al. Differential expression of glucocorticoid receptor in human breast tissues and related neoplasms. J Pathol 2006; 209(3):317–27.
74. Rask E, Walker BR, Soderberg S, et al. Tissue-specific changes in peripheral cortisol metabolism in obese women: increased adipose 11beta-hydroxysteroid dehydrogenase type 1 activity. J Clin Endocrinol Metab 2002;87(7):3330–6.
75. Stimson RH, Walker BR. Glucocorticoids and 11beta-hydroxysteroid dehydrogenase type 1 in obesity and the metabolic syndrome. Minerva Endocrinol 2007;32(3):141–59.
76. Gualillo O, Lago F, Casanueva FF, et al. One ancestor, several peptides post-translational modifications of preproghrelin generate several peptides with antithetical effects. Mol Cell Endocrinol 2006;256(1–2):1–8.
77. Lall S, Tung LY, Ohlsson C, et al. Growth hormone (GH)-independent stimulation of adiposity by GH secretagogues. Biochem Biophys Res Commun 2001; 280(1):132–8.
78. Tschop M, Smiley DL, Heiman ML. Ghrelin induces adiposity in rodents. Nature 2000;407(6806):908–13.
79. Hassouna R, Zizzari P, Tolle V. The ghrelin/obestatin balance in the physiological and pathological control of growth hormone secretion, body composition and food intake. J Neuroendocrinol 2010;22(7):793–804.
80. Dong XY, He JM, Tang SQ, et al. Is GPR39 the natural receptor of obestatin? Peptides 2009;30(2):431–8.
81. Gnanapavan S, Kola B, Bustin SA, et al. The tissue distribution of the mRNA of ghrelin and subtypes of its receptor, GHS-R, in humans. J Clin Endocrinol Metab 2002;87(6):2988.
82. Kierson JA, Dimatteo DM, Locke RG, et al. Ghrelin and cholecystokinin in term and preterm human breast milk. Acta Paediatr 2006;95(8):991–5.
83. Cassoni P, Papotti M, Ghe C, et al. Identification, characterization, and biological activity of specific receptors for natural (ghrelin) and synthetic growth hormone secretagogues and analogs in human breast carcinomas and cell lines. J Clin Endocrinol Metab 2001;86(4):1738–45.
84. Jeffery PL, Murray RE, Yeh AH, et al. Expression and function of the ghrelin axis, including a novel preproghrelin isoform, in human breast cancer tissues and cell lines. Endocr Relat Cancer 2005;12(4):839–50.
85. Dossus L, McKay JD, Canzian F, et al. Polymorphisms of genes coding for ghrelin and its receptor in relation to anthropometry, circulating levels of IGF-I and IGFBP-3, and breast cancer risk: a case-control study nested within the European Prospective Investigation into Cancer and Nutrition (EPIC). Carcinogenesis 2008;29(7):1360–6.

86. Tschop M, Weyer C, Tataranni PA, et al. Circulating ghrelin levels are decreased in human obesity. Diabetes 2001;50(4):707–9.

87. Cummings DE, Weigle DS, Frayo RS, et al. Plasma ghrelin levels after diet-induced weight loss or gastric bypass surgery. N Engl J Med 2002;346(21): 1623–30.

88. Zhang N, Yuan C, Li Z, et al. Meta-analysis of the relationship between obestatin and ghrelin levels and the ghrelin/obestatin ratio with respect to obesity. Am J Med Sci 2011;341(1):48–55.

89. Vicennati V, Genghini S, De Iasio R, et al. Circulating obestatin levels and the ghrelin/obestatin ratio in obese women. Eur J Endocrinol 2007;157(3):295–301.

90. Manabe Y, Toda S, Miyazaki K, et al. Mature adipocytes, but not preadipocytes, promote the growth of breast carcinoma cells in collagen gel matrix culture through cancer-stromal cell interactions. J Pathol 2003;201(2):221–8.

91. Iyengar P, Espina V, Williams TW, et al. Adipocyte-derived collagen VI affects early mammary tumor progression in vivo, demonstrating a critical interaction in the tumor/stroma microenvironment. J Clin Invest 2005;115(5):1163–76.

92. Kim KY, Baek A, Park YS, et al. Adipocyte culture medium stimulates invasiveness of MDA-MB-231 cell via CCL20 production. Oncol Rep 2009;22(6): 1497–504.

93. Martin LJ, Boyd NF. Mammographic density. Potential mechanisms of breast cancer risk associated with mammographic density: hypotheses based on epidemiological evidence. Breast Cancer Res 2008;10(1):201.

94. Hu Y, Ghosh S, Amleh A, et al. Modulation of aromatase expression by BRCA1: a possible link to tissue-specific tumor suppression. Oncogene 2005;24(56): 8343–8.

95. Passaperuma K, Warner E, Hill KA, et al. Is mammographic breast density a breast cancer risk factor in women with BRCA mutations? J Clin Oncol 2010;28(23):3779–83.

96. Johnston PG, Rondinone CM, Voeller D, et al. Identification of a protein factor secreted by 3T3-L1 preadipocytes inhibitory for the human MCF-7 breast cancer cell line. Cancer Res 1992;52(24):6860–5.

97. Chamras H, Bagga D, Elstner E, et al. Preadipocytes stimulate breast cancer cell growth. Nutr Cancer 1998;32(2):59–63.

98. Bjorbaek C, Uotani S, da Silva B, et al. Divergent signaling capacities of the long and short isoforms of the leptin receptor. J Biol Chem 1997;272(51):32686–95.

99. Phrakonkham P, Viengchareun S, Belloir C, et al. Dietary xenoestrogens differentially impair 3T3-L1 preadipocyte differentiation and persistently affect leptin synthesis. J Steroid Biochem Mol Biol 2008;110(1–2):95–103.

100. Simon PA, Frye DM. Obesity and longevity. N Engl J Med 2005;352(24):2555 [author reply: 2556–7].

101. Smith-Kirwin SM, O'Connor DM, De Johnston J, et al. Leptin expression in human mammary epithelial cells and breast milk. J Clin Endocrinol Metab 1998;83(5):1810–3.

102. Ahima RS, Prabakaran D, Mantzoros C, et al. Role of leptin in the neuroendocrine response to fasting. Nature 1996;382(6588):250–2.

103. Weigle DS, Bukowski TR, Foster DC, et al. Recombinant ob protein reduces feeding and body weight in the ob/ob mouse. J Clin Invest 1995;96(4):2065–70.

104. Montague CT, Farooqi IS, Whitehead JP, et al. Congenital leptin deficiency is associated with severe early-onset obesity in humans. Nature 1997;387(6636):903–8.

105. Considine RV, Caro JF. Leptin in humans: current progress and future directions. Clin Chem 1996;42(6 Pt 1):843–4.

106. Maffei M, Halaas J, Ravussin E, et al. Leptin levels in human and rodent: measurement of plasma leptin and ob RNA in obese and weight-reduced subjects. Nat Med 1995;1(11):1155–61.
107. Dieudonne MN, Machinal-Quelin F, Serazin-Leroy V, et al. Leptin mediates a proliferative response in human MCF7 breast cancer cells. Biochem Biophys Res Commun 2002;293(1):622–8.
108. Lautenbach A, Budde A, Wrann CD, et al. Obesity and the associated mediators leptin, estrogen and IGF-I enhance the cell proliferation and early tumorigenesis of breast cancer cells. Nutr Cancer 2009;61(4):484–91.
109. Naviglio S, Di Gesto D, Illiano F, et al. Leptin potentiates antiproliferative action of cAMP elevation via protein kinase A down-regulation in breast cancer cells. J Cell Physiol 2010;225(3):801–9.
110. Jiang H, Yu J, Guo H, et al. Upregulation of survivin by leptin/STAT3 signaling in MCF-7 cells. Biochem Biophys Res Commun 2008;368(1):1–5.
111. Gonzalez-Perez RR, Xu Y, Guo S, et al. Leptin upregulates VEGF in breast cancer via canonic and non-canonical signalling pathways and NFkappaB/HIF-1alpha activation. Cell Signal 2010;22(9):1350–62.
112. Ren H, Zhao T, Wang X, et al. Leptin upregulates telomerase activity and transcription of human telomerase reverse transcriptase in MCF-7 breast cancer cells. Biochem Biophys Res Commun 2010;394(1):59–63.
113. Soma D, Kitayama J, Yamashita H, et al. Leptin augments proliferation of breast cancer cells via transactivation of HER2. J Surg Res 2008;149(1):9–14.
114. Karaduman M, Bilici A, Ozet A, et al. Tissue leptin levels in patients with breast cancer. J BUON 2010;15(2):369–72.
115. Ishikawa M, Kitayama J, Nagawa H. Enhanced expression of leptin and leptin receptor (OB-R) in human breast cancer. Clin Cancer Res 2004;10(13):4325–31.
116. Xia XH, Gu JC, Bai QY, et al. Overexpression of leptin and leptin receptors in breast cancer positively correlates with clinicopathological features. Chin Med J (Engl) 2009;122(24):3078–81.
117. Jarde T, Caldefie-Chezet F, Damez M, et al. Leptin and leptin receptor involvement in cancer development: a study on human primary breast carcinoma. Oncol Rep 2008;19(4):905–11.
118. Hancke K, Grubeck D, Hauser N, et al. Adipocyte fatty acid-binding protein as a novel prognostic factor in obese breast cancer patients. Breast Cancer Res Treat 2010;119(2):367–77.
119. Falk RT, Brinton LA, Madigan MP, et al. Interrelationships between serum leptin, IGF-1, IGFBP3, C-peptide and prolactin and breast cancer risk in young women. Breast Cancer Res Treat 2006;98(2):157–65.
120. Petridou E, Papadiamantis Y, Markopoulos C, et al. Leptin and insulin growth factor I in relation to breast cancer (Greece). Cancer Causes Control 2000;11(5):383–8.
121. Stattin P, Soderberg S, Biessy C, et al. Plasma leptin and breast cancer risk: a prospective study in northern Sweden. Breast Cancer Res Treat 2004;86(3):191–6.
122. Teras LR, Goodman M, Patel AV, et al. No association between polymorphisms in LEP, LEPR, ADIPOQ, ADIPOR1, or ADIPOR2 and postmenopausal breast cancer risk. Cancer Epidemiol Biomarkers Prev 2009;18(9):2553–7.
123. Cleveland RJ, Gammon MD, Long CM, et al. Common genetic variations in the LEP and LEPR genes, obesity and breast cancer incidence and survival. Breast Cancer Res Treat 2010;120(3):745–52.
124. Terrasi M, Fiorio E, Mercanti A, et al. Functional analysis of the -2548G/A leptin gene polymorphism in breast cancer cells. Int J Cancer 2009;125(5):1038–44.

125. Liu CL, Chang YC, Cheng SP, et al. The roles of serum leptin concentration and polymorphism in leptin receptor gene at codon 109 in breast cancer. Oncology 2007;72(1–2):75–81.

126. Diez JJ, Iglesias P. The role of the novel adipocyte-derived hormone adiponectin in human disease. Eur J Endocrinol 2003;148(3):293–300.

127. Yamauchi T, Kamon J, Ito Y, et al. Cloning of adiponectin receptors that mediate antidiabetic metabolic effects. Nature 2003;423(6941):762–9.

128. Pfeiler GH, Buechler C, Neumeier M, et al. Adiponectin effects on human breast cancer cells are dependent on 17-beta estradiol. Oncol Rep 2008; 19(3):787–93.

129. Kern PA, Di Gregorio GB, Lu T, et al. Adiponectin expression from human adipose tissue: relation to obesity, insulin resistance, and tumor necrosis factor-alpha expression. Diabetes 2003;52(7):1779–85.

130. Miyoshi Y, Funahashi T, Kihara S, et al. Association of serum adiponectin levels with breast cancer risk. Clin Cancer Res 2003;9(15):5699–704.

131. Shahar S, Salleh RM, Ghazali AR, et al. Roles of adiposity, lifetime physical activity and serum adiponectin in occurrence of breast cancer among Malaysian women in Klang Valley. Asian Pac J Cancer Prev 2010;11(1):61–6.

132. Chen DC, Chung YF, Yeh YT, et al. Serum adiponectin and leptin levels in Taiwanese breast cancer patients. Cancer Lett 2006;237(1):109–14.

133. Mantzoros C, Petridou E, Dessypris N, et al. Adiponectin and breast cancer risk. J Clin Endocrinol Metab 2004;89(3):1102–7.

134. Korner A, Pazaitou-Panayiotou K, Kelesidis T, et al. Total and high-molecular-weight adiponectin in breast cancer: in vitro and in vivo studies. J Clin Endocrinol Metab 2007;92(3):1041–8.

135. Gaudet MM, Falk RT, Gierach GL, et al. Do adipokines underlie the association between known risk factors and breast cancer among a cohort of United States women? Cancer Epidemiol 2010;34(5):580–6.

136. Dos Santos E, Benaitreau D, Dieudonne MN, et al. Adiponectin mediates an antiproliferative response in human MDA-MB 231 breast cancer cells. Oncol Rep 2008;20(4):971–7.

137. Saxena NK, Sharma D. Metastasis suppression by adiponectin: LKB1 rises up to the challenge. Cell Adh Migr 2010;4(3):358–62.

138. Jarde T, Caldefie-Chezet F, Goncalves-Mendes N, et al. Involvement of adiponectin and leptin in breast cancer: clinical and in vitro studies. Endocr Relat Cancer 2009;16(4):1197–210.

139. Arditi JD, Venihaki M, Karalis KP, et al. Antiproliferative effect of adiponectin on MCF7 breast cancer cells: a potential hormonal link between obesity and cancer. Horm Metab Res 2007;39(1):9–13.

140. Taliaferro-Smith L, Nagalingam A, Zhong D, et al. LKB1 is required for adiponectin-mediated modulation of AMPK-S6K axis and inhibition of migration and invasion of breast cancer cells. Oncogene 2009;28(29):2621–33.

141. Bell LN, Ward JL, Degawa-Yamauchi M, et al. Adipose tissue production of hepatocyte growth factor contributes to elevated serum HGF in obesity. Am J Physiol Endocrinol Metab 2006;291(4):E843–8.

142. Rehman J, Considine RV, Bovenkerk JE, et al. Obesity is associated with increased levels of circulating hepatocyte growth factor. J Am Coll Cardiol 2003;41(8):1408–13.

143. Rahimi N, Saulnier R, Nakamura T, et al. Role of hepatocyte growth factor in breast cancer: a novel mitogenic factor secreted by adipocytes. DNA Cell Biol 1994;13(12):1189–97.

144. Sheen-Chen SM, Liu YW, Eng HL, et al. Serum levels of hepatocyte growth factor in patients with breast cancer. Cancer Epidemiol Biomarkers Prev 2005; 14(3):715–7.

145. Ruan H, Lodish HF. Insulin resistance in adipose tissue: direct and indirect effects of tumor necrosis factor-alpha. Cytokine Growth Factor Rev 2003; 14(5):447–55.

146. Bastard JP, Maachi M, Lagathu C, et al. Recent advances in the relationship between obesity, inflammation, and insulin resistance. Eur Cytokine Netw 2006;17(1):4–12.

147. Guerrero J, Tobar N, Caceres M, et al. Soluble factors derived from tumor mammary cell lines induce a stromal mammary adipose reversion in human and mice adipose cells. Possible role of TGF-beta1 and TNF-alpha. Breast Cancer Res Treat 2010;119(2):497–508.

148. Mohamed-Ali V, Pinkney JH, Coppack SW. Adipose tissue as an endocrine and paracrine organ. Int J Obes Relat Metab Disord 1998;22(12):1145–58.

149. Fried SK, Bunkin DA, Greenberg AS. Omental and subcutaneous adipose tissues of obese subjects release interleukin-6: depot difference and regulation by glucocorticoid. J Clin Endocrinol Metab 1998;83(3):847–50.

150. Bachelot T, Ray-Coquard I, Menetrier-Caux C, et al. Prognostic value of serum levels of interleukin 6 and of serum and plasma levels of vascular endothelial growth factor in hormone-refractory metastatic breast cancer patients. Br J Cancer 2003;88(11):1721–6.

151. Grano M, Mori G, Minielli V, et al. Breast cancer cell line MDA-231 stimulates osteoclastogenesis and bone resorption in human osteoclasts. Biochem Biophys Res Commun 2000;270(3):1097–100.

152. Slattery ML, Curtin K, Sweeney C, et al. Modifying effects of IL-6 polymorphisms on body size-associated breast cancer risk. Obesity (Silver Spring) 2008;16(2): 339–47.

153. Pollak M. Insulin and insulin-like growth factor signalling in neoplasia. Nat Rev Cancer 2008;8(12):915–28.

154. Maor S, Mayer D, Yarden RI, et al. Estrogen receptor regulates insulin-like growth factor-I receptor gene expression in breast tumor cells: involvement of transcription factor Sp1. J Endocrinol 2006;191(3):605–12.

155. Surmacz E, Bartucci M. Role of estrogen receptor alpha in modulating IGF-I receptor signaling and function in breast cancer. J Exp Clin Cancer Res 2004;23(3):385–94.

156. Yee D, Lee AV. Crosstalk between the insulin-like growth factors and estrogens in breast cancer. J Mammary Gland Biol Neoplasia 2000;5(1):107–15.

157. Oesterreich S, Zhang P, Guler RL, et al. Re-expression of estrogen receptor alpha in estrogen receptor alpha-negative MCF-7 cells restores both estrogen and insulin-like growth factor-mediated signaling and growth. Cancer Res 2001;61(15):5771–7.

158. Yu W, Gu JC, Liu JZ, et al. Regulation of estrogen receptors alpha and beta in human breast carcinoma by exogenous leptin in nude mouse xenograft model. Chin Med J (Engl) 2010;123(3):337–43.

159. Fusco R, Galgani M, Procaccini C, et al. Cellular and molecular crosstalk between leptin receptor and estrogen receptor-{alpha} in breast cancer: molecular basis for a novel therapeutic setting. Endocr Relat Cancer 2010;17(2):373–82.

160. Binai NA, Damert A, Carra G, et al. Expression of estrogen receptor alpha increases leptin-induced STAT3 activity in breast cancer cells. Int J Cancer 2010;127(1):55–66.

161. Catalano S, Marsico S, Giordano C, et al. Leptin enhances, via AP-1, expression of aromatase in the MCF-7 cell line. J Biol Chem 2003;278(31):28668–76.
162. Maskarinec G, Woolcott C, Steude JS, et al. The relation of leptin and adiponectin with breast density among premenopausal women. Eur J Cancer Prev 2010; 19(1):55–60.
163. Maccio A, Madeddu C, Gramignano G, et al. Correlation of body mass index and leptin with tumor size and stage of disease in hormone-dependent postmenopausal breast cancer: preliminary results and therapeutic implications. J Mol Med 2010;88(7):677–86.
164. Saxena NK, Taliaferro-Smith L, Knight BB, et al. Bidirectional crosstalk between leptin and insulin-like growth factor-I signaling promotes invasion and migration of breast cancer cells via transactivation of epidermal growth factor receptor. Cancer Res 2008;68(23):9712–22.
165. Purohit A, Newman SP, Reed MJ. The role of cytokines in regulating estrogen synthesis: implications for the etiology of breast cancer. Breast Cancer Res 2002;4(2):65–9.
166. Suarez-Cuervo C, Harris KW, Kallman L, et al. Tumor necrosis factor-alpha induces interleukin-6 production via extracellular-regulated kinase 1 activation in breast cancer cells. Breast Cancer Res Treat 2003;80(1):71–8.
167. World Cancer Research Fund/American Institute for Cancer Research. Food, nutrition, physical activity, and the prevention of cancer: a global perspective. Washington, DC: AICR; 2007.
168. John EM, Horn-Ross PL, Koo J. Lifetime physical activity and breast cancer risk in a multiethnic population: the San Francisco Bay area breast cancer study. Cancer Epidemiol Biomarkers Prev 2003;12(11 Pt 1):1143–52.
169. Matthews CE, Shu XO, Jin F, et al. Lifetime physical activity and breast cancer risk in the Shanghai Breast Cancer Study. Br J Cancer 2001;84(7):994–1001.
170. Ueji M, Ueno E, Osei-Hyiaman D, et al. Physical activity and the risk of breast cancer: a case-control study of Japanese women. J Epidemiol 1998;8(2):116–22.
171. Yang D, Bernstein L, Wu AH. Physical activity and breast cancer risk among Asian-American women in Los Angeles: a case-control study. Cancer 2003; 97(10):2565–75.
172. King MC, Marks JH, Mandell JB. Breast and ovarian cancer risks due to inherited mutations in BRCA1 and BRCA2. Science 2003;302(5645):643–6.
173. Abrahamson PE, Gammon MD, Lund MJ, et al. Recreational physical activity and survival among young women with breast cancer. Cancer 2006;107(8):1777–85.
174. Holick CN, Newcomb PA, Trentham-Dietz A, et al. Physical activity and survival after diagnosis of invasive breast cancer. Cancer Epidemiol Biomarkers Prev 2008;17(2):379–86.
175. Irwin ML, Mayne ST. Impact of nutrition and exercise on cancer survival. Cancer J 2008;14(6):435–41.
176. Sternfeld B, Weltzien E, Quesenberry CP Jr, et al. Physical activity and risk of recurrence and mortality in breast cancer survivors: findings from the LACE study. Cancer Epidemiol Biomarkers Prev 2009;18(1):87–95.
177. Chlebowski RT, Blackburn GL, Thomson CA, et al. Dietary fat reduction and breast cancer outcome: interim efficacy results from the Women's Intervention Nutrition Study. J Natl Cancer Inst 2006;98(24):1767–76.
178. Hoy MK, Winters BL, Chlebowski RT, et al. Implementing a low-fat eating plan in the Women's Intervention Nutrition Study. J Am Diet Assoc 2009;109(4):688–96.

179. Pierce JP, Natarajan L, Caan BJ, et al. Influence of a diet very high in vegetables, fruit, and fiber and low in fat on prognosis following treatment for breast cancer: the Women's Healthy Eating and Living (WHEL) randomized trial. JAMA 2007;298(3):289–98.

180. Ligibel JA, Giobbie-Hurder A, Olenczuk D, et al. Impact of a mixed strength and endurance exercise intervention on levels of adiponectin, high molecular weight adiponectin and leptin in breast cancer survivors. Cancer Causes Control 2009; 20(8):1523–8.

181. Irwin ML. Physical activity interventions for cancer survivors. Br J Sports Med 2009;43(1):32–8.

182. Ligibel JA, Campbell N, Partridge A, et al. Impact of a mixed strength and endurance exercise intervention on insulin levels in breast cancer survivors. J Clin Oncol 2008;26(6):907–12.

183. Miller WR. Aromatase inhibitors and breast cancer. Minerva Endocrinol 2006; 31(1):27–46.

184. Haynes BP, Straume AH, Geisler J, et al. Intratumoral estrogen disposition in breast cancer. Clin Cancer Res 2010;16(6):1790–801.

185. Dunbier AK, Anderson H, Ghazoui Z, et al. Relationship between plasma estradiol levels and estrogen-responsive gene expression in estrogen receptor-positive breast cancer in postmenopausal women. J Clin Oncol 2010;28(7): 1161–7.

186. Ellis MJ, Miller WR, Tao Y, et al. Aromatase expression and outcomes in the P024 neoadjuvant endocrine therapy trial. Breast Cancer Res Treat 2009;116(2): 371–8.

187. Sachdev D, Zhang X, Matise I, et al. The type I insulin-like growth factor receptor regulates cancer metastasis independently of primary tumor growth by promoting invasion and survival. Oncogene 2010;29(2):251–62.

188. Helle SI, Holly JM, Tally M, et al. Influence of treatment with tamoxifen and change in tumor burden on the IGF-system in breast cancer patients. Int J Cancer 1996;69(4):335–9.

189. Pollak MN, Huynh HT, Lefebvre SP. Tamoxifen reduces serum insulin-like growth factor I (IGF-I). Breast Cancer Res Treat 1992;22(1):91–100.

190. Lisztwan J, Pornon A, Chen B, et al. The aromatase inhibitor letrozole and inhibitors of insulin-like growth factor I receptor synergistically induce apoptosis in in vitro models of estrogen-dependent breast cancer. Breast Cancer Res 2008;10(4):R56.

191. Wolf I, Sadetzki S, Catane R, et al. Diabetes mellitus and breast cancer. Lancet Oncol 2005;6(2):103–11.

192. Richardson LC, Pollack LA. Therapy insight: influence of type 2 diabetes on the development, treatment and outcomes of cancer. Nat Clin Pract Oncol 2005; 2(1):48–53.

193. Goodwin PJ, Stambolic V, Lemieux J, et al. Evaluation of metformin in early breast cancer: a modification of the traditional paradigm for clinical testing of anti-cancer agents. Breast Cancer Res Treat 2011;126(1):215–20.

194. Jalving M, Gietema JA, Lefrandt JD, et al. Metformin: taking away the candy for cancer? Eur J Cancer 2010;46(13):2369–80.

195. Otvos L Jr, Kovalszky I, Scolaro L, et al. Peptide-based leptin receptor antagonists for cancer treatment and appetite regulation. Peptide Science 2011;96:117–25.

196. Rene Gonzalez R, Watters A, Xu Y, et al. Leptin-signaling inhibition results in efficient anti-tumor activity in estrogen receptor positive or negative breast cancer. Breast Cancer Res 2009;11(3):R36.

197. Terry MB, Gammon MD, Zhang FF, et al. Association of frequency and duration of aspirin use and hormone receptor status with breast cancer risk. JAMA 2004; 291(20):2433–40.
198. Zhang Y, Coogan PF, Palmer JR, et al. Use of nonsteroidal antiinflammatory drugs and risk of breast cancer: the Case-Control Surveillance Study revisited. Am J Epidemiol 2005;162(2):165–70.
199. Garcia Rodriguez LA, Gonzalez-Perez A. Risk of breast cancer among users of aspirin and other anti-inflammatory drugs. Br J Cancer 2004;91(3):525–9.
200. DuBois RN. Aspirin and breast cancer prevention: the estrogen connection. JAMA 2004;291(20):2488–9.
201. Harvie M, Howell A. Energy balance adiposity and breast cancer—energy restriction strategies for breast cancer prevention. Obes Rev 2006;7(1):33–47.

Postmenopausal Hormone Therapy and Breast Cancer Risk: Current Status and Unanswered Questions

Wendy Y. Chen, MD, MPH[a,b,*]

KEYWORDS

• Menopause • Hormone therapy • Breast cancer • Estrogen

In 2002, the use of postmenopausal hormone therapy (HT) declined dramatically world-wide with the first publication of results from the Women's Health Initiative (WHI), the landmark randomized clinical trial that showed an increased risk of breast cancer among women randomized to combination estrogen and progesterone therapy (EPT) compared with placebo.[1–3] Although use of HT dropped significantly after 2002, millions of women still take HT for menopausal symptom control, so it is crucial to understand the data on HT and breast cancer risk and the unanswered questions.

MAIN RESULTS FOR BREAST CANCER: WOMEN'S HEALTH INITIATIVE

The largest randomized placebo-controlled trial evaluating the overall health effects of HT was the WHI. The WHI was a large, multicenter trial conducted in the United States that randomized 27,347 postmenopausal women depending on their hysterectomy status: 16,608 women with a uterus were randomized to either the combination of 0.625 mg conjugated equine estrogen and 2.5 mg medroxyprogesterone acetate (EPT)[4] daily or placebo and 10,739 women without a uterus were randomized to either 0.625 mg of conjugated equine estrogen therapy (ET) daily or placebo.[5] After mean follow-up of 5.2 years, the study was unblinded for the EPT arms when event rates for breast cancer and a global index for overall harm exceeded predetermined

[a] Channing Laboratory, Brigham and Women's Hospital, Harvard Medical School, 181 Longwood Avenue, Boston, MA 02115, USA
[b] Department of Medical Oncology, Dana Farber Cancer Institute, Harvard Medical School, 450 Brookline Avenue, Boston, MA 02215, USA
* Channing Laboratory, Brigham and Women's Hospital, Harvard Medical School, 181 Longwood Avenue, Boston, MA 02115.
E-mail address: wendy.chen@channing.harvard.edu

Endocrinol Metab Clin N Am 40 (2011) 509–518
doi:10.1016/j.ecl.2011.05.006
0889-8529/11/$ – see front matter © 2011 Elsevier Inc. All rights reserved.

endo.theclinics.com

stopping rules.[4] With mean follow-up of 5.6 years, there was a 24% increase in the risk of invasive breast cancer with EPT compared with placebo (95% confidence interval [CI] 1.10–1.54; P = .003) with the risk becoming apparent in the third year of use among women who had previously used HT and by the fourth year of use among women who had never used HT.[6] The increased breast cancer risk was seen in all subgroups when stratified by Gail risk score, prior HT use, or body mass index (BMI). Compared with placebo, EPT was associated with higher risk of an abnormal mammogram and increased breast density.[7] In addition, the use of EPT was associated with significantly poorer diagnostic accuracy for mammography,[8] a finding that has also been described in observational studies.[9] After discontinuation of HT, breast cancer risk fell rapidly.[10]

In contrast, there was no increased breast cancer risk in the ET arm compared with placebo after an average of 7.1 years of follow-up. There was a nonsignificant decrease in invasive breast cancer risk (hazard ratio [HR] 0.80; 95% CI 0.62–1.04).[11] However, ET was also associated with a significant increase in mammographic density compared with placebo, although the magnitude of increase was less than that seen with EPT.[12] Similar to EPT, there was an increased risk of an abnormal mammogram for women using ET. However, unlike EPT, there was no increase in risk of more serious findings and there was only a short-term impact on diagnostic accuracy of mammography.[13]

CURRENT GUIDELINES FROM PROFESSIONAL SOCIETIES ON HT USE

Based on the WHI data and multiple observational studies,[14,15] most professional societies do not currently recommend HT for cardiovascular disease prevention and they recommend minimizing duration and dose when HT is used for treatment of menopausal symptoms.[16–19] However, some characteristics of the WHI participants have called into question the generalizability of the results to women taking HT in the United States. Additional unanswered questions regarding HT and breast cancer risk, including the effects of age at initiation of HT, longer-term ET therapy, the effects of different doses and formulations of HT besides those evaluated in the WHI, the characteristics of breast cancers that develop on HT, and identification of lower risk groups for HT use.

Age of Initiation of HT

In the WHI, the mean age at randomization in both the EPT and ET arms was 63 to 64 years, with only about one-third of subjects aged 50 to 59 years, which is generally older than women who take HT for menopausal symptoms in clinical practice.[4,5] Because of this concern, subgroup analyses by age at initiation were performed within the WHI randomized trial.[20] To increase statistical power, the EPT and ET arms were combined for this subgroup analysis. For women aged 50 to 59 years, there was a lower risk of mortality for those taking HT (HR 0.70; 95% CI 0.51–0.96) that was not seen in women aged 60 to 69 years or 70 to 79 years, although for trend across age groups, P = .06. For coronary heart disease (CHD), lower risks were also seen for women less than 10 years since menopause at randomization, compared with women more than 10 years since menopause (HR 0.76; 95% CI 0.50–1.16; trend by years since menopause, P = .02). Most of the benefit appeared to be in the ET arm. Relative risk for stroke was similar across age groups, but the absolute risks were much lower in women younger than 50 years.

To further evaluate gap time (defined as the time from menopause to first use of HT) and the effects of age at initiation of menopause as well as control for prior

HT use, a later analysis pooled data from the WHI randomized trial with data from the parallel WHI observational study, which consisted of 93,676 postmenopausal women in the same age range as participants in the WHI randomized trial. This subgroup analysis pooled participants from the WHI randomized trial with a known age at menopause and known age at first HT use (9129 from the ET trial, ie, ~85% of the original participants, and 15188 from the EPT trial, ie, 90%–93% of original participants) and from the WHI observational study who would have met criteria for entry onto the randomized trial and also had known ages at menopause and first HT use (20,117 who had hysterectomy, 10,582 taking ET and 9535 not on ET, and 24,186 with an intact uterus, 6756 who used EPT and 24,186 who were not using HT). There did not seem to be a significant effect of gap time for most of the outcomes evaluated. However, for breast cancer, women who began EPT within 5 years of menopause had a higher breast cancer risk than those who started EPT 5 or more years after menopause. It should be noted that gap time was closely correlated with both age and duration of HT use, so there may have still been some residual confounding. In addition, the relative risks were sensitive to the modeling parameters and assumptions, suggesting that the findings were not robust and may not represent a true biologic effect.

Only 1 other observational study also evaluated the impact of gap time drawing on a prospective cohort of 98,995 French women. They seemed to show similar results with a higher risk of breast cancer among women who began HT within the 3-year period after menopause onset (HR 1.54; 95% CI 1.28–1.86), compared with those who started it after 3 years (HR 1.00; 95% CI 0.68–1.47) (P = .04 for heterogeneity). However, this was only seen in a specific subgroup of short-term (≤2 years) recent EPT users and in no other subgroup, calling into question whether this may represent a chance finding or lack of power to detect an effect among women with gap time greater than 3 years given the smaller number of cases in that strata (786 cases with ≤3 years' gap time versus only 151 cases with >3 years' gap time among recent EPT users).[21] Overall, the randomized WHI trial data would still be considered the strongest data and these clearly show an increased risk of breast cancer across all age subgroups.[6]

Nevertheless, interest remains about a possible window of opportunity for HT in the prevention of cardiovascular disease among recently premenopausal women but, at this point, the data remain speculative and more definitive results are awaited. The Kronos Early Estrogen Prevention Study (KEEPS) has completed enrollment and should provide important additional data on the effects of HT closer to menopause.[22] KEEPS randomized 728 postmenopausal women aged 42 to 58 years (mean 52.7 years) who were 6 to 36 months within their last menses to 1 of 3 arms: (1) daily oral conjugated equine estrogen plus oral progesterone 12 d/mo, (2) transdermal 17β-estradiol patch plus oral progesterone 12 d/mo, or (3) placebo. Primary endpoints include surrogates for cardiovascular disease, including changes in carotid intima-medial thickness and coronary artery calcification.

Characteristics of Breast Cancer that Develop on HT

In a recently published update on breast cancer incidence and mortality comprising 678 breast cancer cases in the WHI clinical trial, cancers that developed in women taking EPT were generally similar to those on placebo in terms of tumor size, histology, and HER2 and hormone receptor status, but did have a greater chance of being node-positive (23.9% on EPT vs 16.2% on placebo, P = .03).[23] More women died of breast cancer in the EPT arm (n = 25 deaths) compared with placebo (n = 12 deaths) (P = .049). Reconsent was required after 2005 and approximately 17% of participants did not reconsent, so were censored in 2005 for both the incidence and mortality analyses.

In contrast, the observational studies have shown different results in terms of the characteristics of the breast cancers that develop in women on HT. Most notably, although the WHI did not observe differences in the ER (estrogen receptor) and progesterone receptor (PR) status of the tumors between the placebo and the EPT arms, this is contrary to what was reported by most observational studies and what physiologically would be most plausible.[24] Medications that block the estrogen receptor, such as tamoxifen, or lower estrogen levels, such as the aromatase inhibitors, only affect the growth of cancers that are hormone receptor positive, but not cancers that are hormone receptor negative.[25] Therefore, it could be hypothesized that HT would preferentially stimulate the growth of cancers that are hormone receptor positive, as was seen in multiple observational studies.[24] Part of the discrepancy may be that the WHI study only had a limited number of breast cancer cases with known ER status (356 on EPT and 264 on placebo), compared with the larger observational studies. Therefore, although no difference was seen in the distribution of tumors by hormone receptor status in the WHI, given the biologic mechanism and the additional power of the observational studies to evaluate differences by receptor status, it is still possible that HT is more strongly associated with cancers that are hormone receptor positive than cancers that are negative.

In terms of the increased breast cancer mortality reported by WHI, this recent analysis combined both incidence and mortality.[23] Given the higher incidence of breast cancer in the EPT arm, it would be expected that there would be more breast cancer deaths. Currently, there are not enough events to compare survival after breast cancer between the 2 groups, which would be the more relevant comparison to understand whether the biology of breast cancers that develop on HT differ from sporadic ones. In addition, breast cancer treatment was not controlled for in the analyses, because data were not available, and this could have been an important confounder.

Longer Duration of Unopposed Estrogen

Although the WHI did not see an association between unopposed estrogen alone and breast cancer risk with an average follow-up of 7.1 years, the effect of longer-term use of unopposed estrogen and breast cancer risk still needs to be considered. In both the combined analysis of 51 epidemiologic studies led by the Oxford group and in the large observational Nurses' Health Study cohort (which was included in the Oxford pooled analysis), no increase in breast cancer risk was seen with less than 5 years of unopposed estrogen. However, with more than 5 years' use of current estrogen alone, the Oxford group reported a pooled relative risk (RR) of 1.34 (standard error 0.09).[14] In the Nurses' Health Study, when we analyzed only women older than 50 years who had undergone a hysterectomy so that the population would be comparable with the WHI, we did not observe an increased risk of breast cancer with shorter periods of use. However, with much longer durations of use, we did observe an increased risk of breast cancer (RR 1.42; 95% CI 1.13–1.77 for 20+ years of use). When limited to ER+/PR+ cancers, we observed an increase in breast cancer after 15 years of current use of unopposed estrogen (RR 1.48; 95% CI 1.05–2.07).[26] Although ET was not associated with an increased risk of breast cancer in the WHI trial, there was an increased risk of benign proliferative breast lesions (HR 2.11; 95% CI 1.58–2.81).[27] If the sojourn time required for tissue to progress from proliferative lesions to atypia to invasive breast cancer is considered, this finding would be consistent with the association of longer-term ET with breast cancer risk. Therefore, for durations of unopposed estrogen use similar to that in the WHI (ie, less than 7 years), there does not seem to be an increased breast cancer risk. However, the impact for longer-term users is less clear.

Other Forms of HT

In the United States, the most common form of prescription HT remains conjugated equine estrogens alone or given with medroxyprogesterone acetate. However, in Europe, many other formulations of estrogens and progestins are used and their effects on breast cancer have not been as well quantified. None of these studies were randomized and many only had limited numbers of users of the other types of hormones.

Estrogen

The predominant form of estrogen used in the United States is oral conjugated equine estrogen, the same formulation used in the WHI clinical trial.[2] However, in Europe, more variation exists in terms of the type of estrogen used. The single largest prospective study of HT conducted in Europe was the Million Women's Study (MWS) in the United Kingdom. They did not observe any variation in risk between conjugated estrogens and ethinylestradiol. In addition, they also reported an increased risk of breast cancer with tibolone, a progestin analogue that is considered a selective estrogen enzyme modulator.[15] Other large prospective studies in Denmark and France, in which the predominant estrogen used was estradiol, rather than conjugated estrogens, also observed an increased risk with estrogen-only and combination estrogen plus progesterone regimens and tibolone.[28–30] The risk of breast cancer observed with estrogen only in some of the studies was higher than that seen in WHI. Both ethinylestradiol and estradiol would be considered medium-potency estrogens similar to conjugated estrogens.

Progesterone

Interest has also focused on the type of progesterone. The WHI used medroxyprogesterone acetate, a synthetic progesterone. In contrast, the prospective French E3N cohort did not see an increased breast cancer risk with natural progesterone or its isomer dydrogesterone,[28] nor did a Finnish study evaluating dydrogesterone; both studies only had a limited number of women taking these regimens.[30] However, studies that evaluated more androgenic progestins, such as norethisterone and norgestrel, still observed an increased breast cancer risk when given in combination with estrogens.[15,29,30] In sum, although limited data suggest that natural progesterone may be associated with less breast cancer risk then synthetic progesterone, further research needs to be done to confirm these differences and evaluate long-term safety of the natural progesterone.

Testosterone

Only a few studies have evaluated the use of testosterone-based HT and most studies have a small number of cases, so power has been limited. In the largest prospective study of oral testosterone given alone or in combination with oral estrogen to date (E+T), we observed a twofold increase risk of breast cancer within the Nurses' Health Study compared with never users (multivariate RR 1.77 for current users; 95% CI 1.22–2.56).[31] The WHI observational cohort reported similar findings with a nonsignificant increased risk of breast cancer for users of any type of E+T (RR 1.42; 95% CI 0.95–2.11) and a significantly increased risk associated with Estratest, the most common E+T preparation (HR 1.78; 95% CUI 1.05–3.11), compared with never users. Paradoxically, they observed higher risk with shorter-term, rather than longer-term, use.[32] An increased risk was also seen in a Danish study evaluating injectable estrogen and testosterone.[33] In addition, higher endogenous testosterone levels have been consistently associated with increased breast cancer risk in both premenopausal and postmenopausal women.[34,35] Therefore, although data are limited, caution should be used for testosterone-based HT among postmenopausal women.

Dose or route of administration of HT

All of the professional societies recommend using the lowest HT dose possible for menopausal symptom relief. However, there are no randomized trial data to determine whether a lower dose is associated with a more favorable risk/benefit ratio than the doses evaluated in the WHI (0.625 mg conjugated equine estrogen alone or with 2.5 mg medroxyprogesterone acetate). Although transdermal ET has become more popular since publication of the WHI results, again no randomized controlled data exist to determine whether the overall risk/benefit ratio would be more favorable than for standard oral HT. Observational studies suggest that risks are similar regardless of the route of administration (oral/transdermal/implanted).[15,30,36] In addition, for women with an intact uterus, transdermal ET would still need to be taken with oral progesterone for endometrial protection.[19]

Can Low-risk Groups be Identified for HT Use?

Because HT still remains the gold standard for menopausal symptom relief, besides minimizing dose and duration, clinicians have often wondered whether some women a priori could be classified as higher or lower risk for HT complications. In general, the effect of HT on breast cancer risk does not seem to be modified by many of the traditional breast cancer risk factors, such as family history. That is, both family history and HT are independently associated with breast cancer risk but do not seem to interact either negatively or positively.[37-39] However, there is an exception in that several studies have suggested that BMI may modify the effect of HT in that breast cancer risk was greater in women with lower BMI and attenuated in heavier women.[14,40-43] In addition, one study suggested that women with low breast density would not be at increased risk of breast cancer, regardless of HT use, but no detail was provided on type or duration of HT use or the distribution of ET compared with EPT users, so it is not known whether these findings pertain to short-term users or long-term users, or what type of HT.[44] As discussed previously, the relative risks for breast cancer observed in the WHI randomized trial were similar across a large variety of subgroups, although power was limited and the study was not designed to evaluate effect modifications by any of these risk factors.[6] Overall, the relative risk for breast cancer by HT should still be considered similar across subgroups, but absolute risks differ in that younger women without a family history of breast cancer have lower absolute risks than older women with a family history. Therefore, the absolute risks could vary considerably by individual, which could influence individual decision making, even if the relative risks were similar.

Use of HT in Breast Cancer Survivors

Many breast cancer survivors develop menopausal systems, whether as a consequence of treatment-induced menopause or side effects of treatment. Selective serotonin reuptake inhibitors and other nonhormonal interventions may provide some relief, but are still inferior to HT for treatment of menopausal symptoms. Two small prospective studies were closed early because of slow accrual and concerns regarding HT use in the breast cancer population, and did not observe an increased recurrence risk with HT, but were clearly underpowered.[45,46] However, the HABITS (hormonal replacement therapy after breast cancer – is it safe?) trial from Stockholm enrolled 447 breast cancer survivors beginning in 1997 and assigned them to either hormone therapy (health care provider's choice) or none, and was terminated in December 2003 when the event rate in the HT exceeded predetermined stopping rules. However, follow-up was continued and, at 4 years' median follow-up and 56 events, the HT group was found to have more than twice the risk of breast cancer recurrence compared with controls, with absolute differences in event rates at 2 and 4 years of 5.7% (95% CI 3.5–7.9) and 14.2% (95% CI 10.9–17.5%) respectively.[47] Results were similar regardless of ER status of the tumor and tamoxifen use, but power was limited for the subgroup analyses. Similar results were seen in a randomized trial of tibolone 2.5 mg daily compared with placebo (n = 3148 women randomized), with an increased risk of recurrence in the tibolone arm after median follow-up of 3.1 years (HR 1.40; 95% CI 1.16–1.79).[48] Therefore, among breast cancer survivors regardless of the ER status of the tumor, even short-term systemic HT use is not recommended.

SUMMARY

Although HT use declined significantly after publication of the WHI results, many women still continue taking HT for menopausal symptom relief. The breast cancer risk associated with EPT is greater than that with ET, but questions still remain about the safety of longer-term ET use. Studies since the WHI have tried to clarify whether various factors can modify the risk of HT, such as the age at initiation, dose, or type of HT, or characteristics of the individual, such as family history of BMI. At this point, the relative risks of breast cancer associated with HT across various subgroups of women should still be considered similar, but absolute risks can vary significantly among women and this may inform individual decision making. For breast cancer survivors, systemic HT should be discouraged.

REFERENCES

1. Faber A, Bouvy ML, Loskamp L, et al. Dramatic change in prescribing of hormone replacement therapy in The Netherlands after publication of the Million Women Study: a follow-up study. Br J Clin Pharmacol 2005;60:641–7.
2. Hersh AL, Stefanick ML, Stafford RS. National use of postmenopausal hormone therapy: annual trends and response to recent evidence. JAMA 2004;291:47–53.
3. Watson J, Wise L, Green J. Prescribing of hormone therapy for menopause, tibolone, and bisphosphonates in women in the UK between 1991 and 2005. Eur J Clin Pharmacol 2007;63:843–9.
4. Rossouw JE, Anderson GL, Prentice RL, et al. Risks and benefits of estrogen plus progestin in healthy postmenopausal women: principal results from the Women's Health Initiative randomized controlled trial. JAMA 2002;288:321–33.
5. Anderson GL, Limacher M, Assaf AR, et al. Effects of conjugated equine estrogen in postmenopausal women with hysterectomy: the Women's Health Initiative randomized controlled trial. JAMA 2004;291:1701–12.
6. Chlebowski RT, Hendrix SL, Langer RD, et al. Influence of estrogen plus progestin on breast cancer and mammography in healthy postmenopausal women: the Women's Health Initiative Randomized Trial. JAMA 2003;289:3243–53.
7. McTiernan A, Martin CF, Peck JD, et al. Estrogen-plus-progestin use and mammographic density in postmenopausal women: Women's Health Initiative randomized trial. J Natl Cancer Inst 2005;97:1366–76.

8. Chlebowski RT, Anderson G, Pettinger M, et al. Estrogen plus progestin and breast cancer detection by means of mammography and breast biopsy. Arch Intern Med 2008;168:370–7 [quiz: 345].

9. Banks E, Reeves G, Beral V, et al. Hormone replacement therapy and false positive recall in the Million Women Study: patterns of use, hormonal constituents and consistency of effect. Breast Cancer Res 2006;8:R8.

10. Chlebowski RT, Kuller LH, Prentice RL, et al. Breast cancer after use of estrogen plus progestin in postmenopausal women. N Engl J Med 2009;360:573–87.

11. Stefanick ML, Anderson GL, Margolis KL, et al. Effects of conjugated equine estrogens on breast cancer and mammography screening in postmenopausal women with hysterectomy. JAMA 2006;295:1647–57.

12. McTiernan A, Chlebowski RT, Martin C, et al. Conjugated equine estrogen influence on mammographic density in postmenopausal women in a substudy of the Women's Health Initiative randomized trial. J Clin Oncol 2009;27:6135–43.

13. Chlebowski RT, Anderson G, Manson JE, et al. Estrogen alone in postmenopausal women and breast cancer detection by means of mammography and breast biopsy. J Clin Oncol 2010;28:2690–7.

14. Breast cancer and hormone replacement therapy: collaborative reanalysis of data from 51 epidemiological studies of 52,705 women with breast cancer and 108,411 women without breast cancer. Collaborative Group on Hormonal Factors in Breast Cancer [see comments] [Erratum appears in Lancet 1997;350(9089):1484]. Lancet 1997;350:1047–59.

15. Beral V. Breast cancer and hormone-replacement therapy in the Million Women Study. Lancet 2003;362:419–27.

16. U.S. Preventive Services Task Force. Hormone therapy for the prevention of chronic conditions in postmenopausal women: recommendations from the U.S. Preventive Services Task Force. Ann Intern Med 2005;142:855–60.

17. American College of Obstetricians, Gynecologists Committee on Gynecologic Practice. ACOG Committee Opinion No. 420, November 2008: hormone therapy and heart disease. Obstet Gynecol 2008;112:1189–92.

18. Gompel A, Rozenberg S, Barlow DH, EMAS board members. The EMAS 2008 update on clinical recommendations on postmenopausal hormone replacement therapy. Maturitas 2008;61:227–32.

19. North American Menopause Society. Estrogen and progestogen use in postmenopausal women: 2010 position statement of The North American Menopause Society. Menopause 2010;17:242–55.

20. Rossouw J, Prentice R, Manson J, et al. Postmenopausal hormone therapy and risk of cardiovascular disease by age and years since menopause. JAMA 2007;297:1465–77.

21. Fournier A, Mesrine S, Boutron-Ruault MC, et al. Estrogen-progestagen menopausal hormone therapy and breast cancer: does delay from menopause onset to treatment initiation influence risks? J Clin Oncol 2009;27:5138–43.

22. Miller VM, Black DM, Brinton EA, et al. Using basic science to design a clinical trial: baseline characteristics of women enrolled in the Kronos Early Estrogen Prevention Study (KEEPS). J Cardiovasc Transl Res 2009;2:228–39.

23. Chlebowski RT, Anderson GL, Gass M, et al. Estrogen plus progestin and breast cancer incidence and mortality in postmenopausal women. JAMA 2010;304:1684–92.

24. Chen WY, Colditz GA. Risk factors and hormone-receptor status: epidemiology, risk-prediction models and treatment implications for breast cancer. Nat Clin Pract Oncol 2007;4:415–23.

25. Early Breast Cancer Trialists' Collaborative Group (EBCTCG). Effects of chemotherapy and hormonal therapy for early breast cancer on recurrence and 15-year survival: an overview of the randomised trials. Lancet 2005;365:1687–717.
26. Chen WY, Manson JE, Hankinson SE, et al. Unopposed estrogen therapy and the risk of invasive breast cancer. Arch Intern Med 2006;166:1027–32.
27. Rohan TE, Negassa A, Chlebowski RT, et al. Conjugated equine estrogen and risk of benign proliferative breast disease: a randomized controlled trial. J Natl Cancer Inst 2008;100:563–71.
28. Fournier A, Berrino F, Clavel-Chapelon F. Unequal risks for breast cancer associated with different hormone replacement therapies: results from the E3N cohort study. Breast Cancer Res Treat 2008;107:103–11.
29. Stahlberg C, Pedersen AT, Lynge E, et al. Increased risk of breast cancer following different regimens of hormone replacement therapy frequently used in Europe. Int J Cancer 2004;109:721–7.
30. Lyytinen H, Pukkala E, Ylikorkala O. Breast cancer risk in postmenopausal women using estradiol-progestogen therapy. Obstet Gynecol 2009;113:65–73.
31. Tamimi RM, Hankinson SE, Chen WY, et al. Combined estrogen and testosterone use and risk of breast cancer in postmenopausal women. Arch Intern Med 2006; 166:1483–9.
32. Ness RB, Albano JD, McTiernan A, et al. Influence of estrogen plus testosterone supplementation on breast cancer. Arch Intern Med 2009;169:41–6.
33. Ewertz M. Influence of non-contraceptive exogenous and endogenous sex hormones on breast cancer risk in Denmark. Int J Cancer 1988;42:832–8.
34. Kaaks R, Berrino F, Key T, et al. Serum sex steroids in premenopausal women and breast cancer risk within the European Prospective Investigation into Cancer and Nutrition (EPIC). J Natl Cancer Inst 2005;97:755–65.
35. Key T, Appleby P, Barnes I, et al. Endogenous sex hormones and breast cancer in postmenopausal women: reanalysis of nine prospective studies. J Natl Cancer Inst 2002;94:606–16.
36. Fournier A, Berrino F, Riboli E, et al. Breast cancer risk in relation to different types of hormone replacement therapy in the E3N-EPIC cohort. Int J Cancer 2005;114: 448–54.
37. Olsson H, Bladstrom A, Ingvar C, et al. A population-based cohort study of HRT use and breast cancer in southern Sweden. Br J Cancer 2001;85:674–7.
38. Sellers TA, Mind PJ, Cerhan JR, et al. The role of hormone replacement therapy in the risk for breast cancer and total mortality in women with a family history of breast cancer. Ann Intern Med 1997;127:973–80.
39. Gramling R, Eaton CB, Rothman KJ, et al. Hormone replacement therapy, family history, and breast cancer risk among postmenopausal women. Epidemiology 2009;20:752–6.
40. Magnusson C, Baron JA, Correia N, et al. Breast-cancer risk following long-term oestrogen- and oestrogen-progestin-replacement therapy. Int J Cancer 1999;81: 339–44.
41. Schairer C, Lubin J, Troisi R, et al. Menopausal estrogen and estrogen-progestin replacement therapy and breast cancer risk. JAMA 2000;283:485–91.
42. Brinton LA, Richesson D, Leitzmann MF, et al. Menopausal hormone therapy and breast cancer risk in the NIH-AARP Diet and Health Study Cohort. Cancer Epidemiol Biomarkers Prev 2008;17:3150–60.
43. Reeves GK, Beral V, Green J, et al. Million Women Study Collaborators. Hormonal therapy for menopause and breast-cancer risk by histological type: a cohort study and meta-analysis. Lancet Oncol 2006;7:910–8.

44. Kerlikowske K, Cook AJ, Buist DS, et al. Breast cancer risk by breast density, menopause, and postmenopausal hormone therapy use. J Clin Oncol 2010;28: 3830–7.
45. Vassilopoulou-Sellin R, Cohen DS, Hortobagyi GN, et al. Estrogen replacement therapy for menopausal women with a history of breast carcinoma: results of a 5-year, prospective study. Cancer 2002;95:1817–26.
46. von Schoultz E, Rutqvist LE. Menopausal hormone therapy after breast cancer: the Stockholm randomized trial. J Natl Cancer Inst 2005;97:533–5.
47. Holmberg L, Iversen OE, Rudenstam CM, et al. Increased risk of recurrence after hormone replacement therapy in breast cancer survivors. J Natl Cancer Inst 2008;100(7):475–82.
48. Kenemans P, Bundred NJ, Foidart JM, et al. Safety and efficacy of tibolone in breast-cancer patients with vasomotor symptoms: a double-blind, randomised, non-inferiority trial. Lancet Oncol 2009;10:135–46.

Hormonal Modulation in the Treatment of Breast Cancer

Kerin Adelson, MD[a],*, Doris Germain, PhD[b],
George Raptis, MD, MBA[a], Noa Biran, MD[c]

KEYWORDS

- Hormonal modulation • Breast cancer • Aromatase inhibitors
- Ovarian suppression • GnRH agonist • Antiestrogens
- SERM • SERD

BREAST CANCER EPIDEMIOLOGY

Breast cancer is the most commonly diagnosed malignancy in women worldwide. It is estimated that 207,090 women were diagnosed with and 39,840 women died of breast cancer in 2010. Surveillance, Epidemiology and End Results data predict that 12% of women born today, or 1 in 8 women, will be diagnosed with breast cancer in their lifetime. Long-term survival rates are closely linked to breast cancer stage at presentation. Sixty percent of women are diagnosed when the cancer is confined to the breast (without lymph node involvement), and these women have an excellent 5-year relative survival of 98%. Thirty-three percent of women with breast cancer present with disease that has spread to local/regional lymph nodes and for this group, 5-year relative survival is 83.6 %. Only 5% of women with breast cancer present with initial metastatic disease, and for this population 5-year relative survival is only 23.4% and close to none are cured of the cancer.[1]

Breast cancer can metastasize many years after the initial diagnosis and treatment. Thus, the 5-year relative survival statistics omit recurrences that occur after 5 years, which is more common in women treated with adjuvant chemotherapy, trastuzumab, or hormonal modulation than in most other cancers. Furthermore, most of these relapses are outside the breast, leading to incurable stage IV disease. Despite recent advances in breast cancer therapy and earlier diagnosis with screening, 24% to 30%

Disclosures: Dr Adelson has worked as a consultant for GTx pharmaceuticals
[a] Division of Hematology and Medical Oncology, Mount Sinai School of Medicine, One Gustave L. Levy Place, Box 1079, New York, NY 10029, USA
[b] Division of Hematology/Oncology, Department of Medicine, Tisch Cancer Insitute, Mount Sinai School of Medicine, One Gustave L. Levy Place, Box 1079, New York, NY 10029, USA
[c] Samuel Bronfman Department of Medicine, Mount Sinai Medical Center, One Gustave L. Levy Place, New York, NY 10029, USA
* Corresponding author.
E-mail address: kerin.adelson@mssm.edu

Endocrinol Metab Clin N Am 40 (2011) 519–532
doi:10.1016/j.ecl.2011.05.011
0889-8529/11/$ – see front matter © 2011 Elsevier Inc. All rights reserved.

of women with node-negative disease at diagnosis will eventually experience a disease recurrence, and 40% to 80% of women with node-positive disease will experience relapse. When distant metastases occur, the prognosis is poor, with a median survival of 18 to 36 months from time of recurrence.[2] Thus, an urgent need still exists to improve curative treatments for women with breast cancer and to improve efficacy of treatment for women with metastatic disease.

Metastatic relapse is generally explained by the theory that many women with primary breast cancer have subclinical metastases at presentation.[3] Surgery and radiotherapy are targeted at removing the primary tumor and preventing local relapse, while systemic treatments including chemotherapy, hormonal modulation, and Her-2 targeted immunotherapy, are directed at eliminating micrometastases. Systemic treatments given before surgery are called neoadjuvant therapy and those given after surgery are called adjuvant therapy.

In the United States and Canada, breast cancer incidence has recently leveled off and even decreased slightly in age groups older than 45 years.[4] One theory attributed the decline in incidence to the reduced use of hormone replacement therapy (HRT) after the Women's Health Initiative study showed HRT increased incidence of breast cancer and failure to prevent cardiac and thrombotic events.[5]

ESTROGEN RECEPTOR EXPRESSION AND HORMONAL MODULATION IN BREAST CANCER

Seventy percent of breast cancers express the estrogen receptor (ER) and usually have a lower-grade phenotype than ER-negative cancers. During the first several years after diagnosis, patients with ER-positive tumors tend to have a lower recurrence rate than those with ER-negative tumors. The recurrence rate of ER-positive tumors remains stable through years 6 or 7 and drops thereafter. Most importantly, ER status is an important predictor of the likelihood of response to endocrine therapies. In patients with localized disease, adjuvant hormonal modulation is used for 5 to 10 years to reduce the risk of distant recurrence. When metastases occur in women receiving an adjuvant therapy, tumors are likely to have primary or acquired resistance to that agent.

Although many laboratories have described mechanisms of resistance to endocrine therapies, none of these mechanisms have been clinically validated to guide treatment decisions. Thus, the choice of an adjuvant hormonal agent depends entirely on the patient's menopausal status; women with intact ovarian function receive selective estrogen receptor modulators (SERMs) and postmenopausal women receive aromatase inhibitors (AIs).

Women with metastatic breast cancer require treatment for the duration of their lives. In this setting, hormonal therapy is used to slow tumor progression. Hormonal modulation is highly effective and less toxic than chemotherapy. However, in this population a significant portion of ER-positive tumors will not respond to antiestrogen therapy initially, and most that do respond will ultimately develop resistance. Once the tumor becomes resistant to therapies to which it has been exposed, cytotoxic chemotherapy is required. Both primary and acquired resistance to endocrine therapy underscore the need to develop new treatments and to better tailor which treatments are chosen for which tumors.

This article explores the history of endocrine therapy for the treatment of breast cancer, the clinical evidence behind the current standards of care and controversies that may change these standards in the future.

Earlier Methods of Hormonal Modulation and Their Current Use

Ovarian suppression and ablation

Recognition of the relationship of ovarian function to breast cancer was first noted when Albert Schinzinger proposed surgical oophorectomy as a treatment for breast cancer in 1889.[6] He observed that the prognosis for breast cancer was better in older women than in younger women and reasoned that oophorectomy would make younger women prematurely old, causing atrophy of the breast and the cancer.[7] Despite Schinzinger's intellectual contribution, Beatson[8] was the first to use ovarian ablation to treat advanced breast cancer in 1896. The first randomized trials of ovarian ablation in the adjuvant setting began in 1948.[9]

Several methods of ovarian ablation or ovarian suppression are available. Surgical oophorectomy causes a permanent reduction in ovarian steroid production. In women with BRCA1 or BRCA2 mutations, surgical oophorectomy leads to a 50% reduction in breast cancer incidence and a 95% reduction in ovarian cancer. Radiation-induced ovarian ablation can be accomplished using a variety of fractionation schedules, ranging from 4.5 Gy in 1 fraction to 20 Gy in 10 fractions.[10]

Pharmacologic ovarian suppression is accomplished with gonadotropin releasing–hormone (GnRH) agonists, such as goserelin and leuprolide. Mechanistically, both of these agents mimic the hypothalamic hormone GnRH. In normal physiology, GnRH signals the pituitary gland to release luteinizing hormone (LH) and follicle-stimulating hormone (FSH), which in turn stimulate ovarian steroid hormone production. Unlike endogenous GnRH, synthetic GnRH agonists have substitutions in the sixth and ninth terminus amino acids, which increase lipophilicity and render them long-acting. When first given, GnRH agonists are stimulatory and can cause a flare phenomenon. However, after 10 to 14 days, the continuous action leads to downregulation of GnRH receptors, which ultimately decreases production of LH and FSH and medical castration. Menopausal side effects are reversible when the GnRH agonists are cleared.

The meta-analysis conducted by the Early Breast Cancer Trialists' Collaborative Group (EBCTCG) in 2005 compared treatment with and without ovarian suppression and ablation in nearly 8000 women younger than 50 years.[11] Results showed that ovarian ablation reduced the 15-year probability of breast cancer recurrence and mortality. The benefit was much larger in women who did not receive any additional adjuvant treatment. One possible reason for this is that women who undergo chemotherapy often develop ovarian failure, thus attenuating any additional benefit seen from ovarian suppression or ablation.

Although multiple studies have shown that ovarian suppression or ablation is preferable to no adjuvant treatment in premenopausal women with breast cancer, long-term follow-up from the four-arm prospective Swedish ZIPP trial (Zoladex in Premenopausal Patients), which randomized patients to: no hormonal modulation, ovarian suppression with goserelin alone, tamoxifen alone, or the combination of goserelin and tamoxifen, showed that, individually, goserelin and tamoxifen offered similar benefit to no adjuvant endocrine therapy, but the combination was not superior to either modality alone.[12]

AIs act by inhibiting the production of estrogen in peripheral tissues and thus are only active in postmenopausal women who do not have an ovarian source of estrogens. Since 2003, when adjuvant AIs were shown to be more effective than tamoxifen in postmenopausal women, the question of whether premenopausal women should receive ovarian suppression and an AI rather than tamoxifen alone has generated increasing debate. This question will be answered by the three-arm SOFT trial, which is comparing 5 years of tamoxifen alone, 5 years of ovarian suppression combined with tamoxifen, and 5 years of ovarian suppression with exemestane (a steroidal AI).[13] However, induction of menopause is accompanied by a host of side effects, including hot flashes, changes in sex drive, vaginal dryness, loss of vaginal elasticity, dyspareunia, osteoporosis, sleep-cycle disturbance, and sometimes depression and anxiety. Therefore, unless the SOFT trial shows a benefit for ovarian suppression, tamoxifen alone will remain the standard of care for premenopausal women.

High-dose estrogen High-dose estrogen was the preferred endocrine treatment in postmenopausal women with advanced breast cancer before the introduction of tamoxifen in the 1970s. In 1979, Smith and colleagues[14] concluded that high-dose estrogen in the form of Premarin improved survival in postmenopausal women with advanced breast cancer. In 1981, a trial performed by Ingle and colleagues[15] concluded that the response rates between tamoxifen and diethylstilbestrol were similar, but that tamoxifen had significantly lower rates of thromboembolic disease. Based on tamoxifen's improved toxicity profile, high-dose estrogen therapy was abandoned.

Use of high-dose estrogen is now being revisited. One hypothesis suggests that in patients who have been exposed to long-term estrogen deprivation as a result of AI therapy, the estrogen dose–response curve shifts to the left, with cancer cells showing increasing sensitivity to the toxic effects of estrogen. A recent phase II study showed a clinical benefit rate of 29% with 6 mg of daily estradiol in 66 patients with AI-refractory metastatic breast cancer.[16]

Megestrol acetate

The use of megestrol acetate (MA), an orally active synthetic derivative of progesterone, was first reported in breast cancer by Ansfield and colleagues[17] in 1974. Its mechanism in the treatment of advanced breast cancer is unclear. In the 1980s, several trials showed that the response rate to MA was comparable to that observed with tamoxifen in postmenopausal women with metastatic breast cancer[18,19] but was associated with an increased risk of thromboembolic events. Today, MA is only used in metastatic disease refractory to multiple lines of endocrine therapy.

SERMs

The SERMs, tamoxifen and toremifene are hormonal agents that compete with estradiol for binding to ERs. In breast tissue, this blocks the ability of ERs to act as transcription factors and inhibits estrogen-dependent cell proliferation and mammary tumor growth.[20] Although both of these drugs display estrogen antagonist activity in breast and on breast cancer cells, they have estrogenic agonist activity on the endometrium, bone, and coagulation system. Tamoxifen has been a critical component in the treatment of breast cancer for more than 30 years and has served as the gold standard against which newer endocrine therapies were compared. Although it is highly effective for prevention and treatment of breast cancer, it is accompanied by a small but definitive increased risk of endometrial cancer and thromboembolic disease.

TAMOXIFEN STUDIES

Tamoxifen was initially developed in 1966 in Great Britain as an infertility agent.[21,22] It was also found to suppress carcinogen-induced rat mammary tumors.[23] The first clinical trial of tamoxifen was published in 1971.[24] It was then studied in the United States, and was approved by the U.S. Food and Drug Administration (FDA) for the treatment of metastatic breast cancer in postmenopausal women in 1977.

The role of tamoxifen in the adjuvant setting has been widely established. Results from 15-year follow-up from the EBCTCG/Oxford Overview showed that tamoxifen reduced the annual recurrence rate by 41% and the overall mortality rate by 34% in women with ER-positive breast cancer.[11] Furthermore, adjuvant tamoxifen taken for 5 years after primary therapy also reduces the incidence of contralateral breast cancer by 47%.[25]

From the 1970s until 2002 when anastrozole was approved, tamoxifen was the first-line endocrine therapy for localized and metastatic breast cancer in both premenopausal and postmenopausal women. It remains the mainstay of treatment for premenopausal women in both the adjuvant and metastatic setting.

In 1998, the National Surgical Adjuvant Breast and Bowel Project (NSABP) P1 trial[26] showed that tamoxifen has a role in preventing breast cancer in women at increased risk for the disease. Among 13,388 women randomized to receive either tamoxifen or placebo, tamoxifen was shown to decrease the relative risk of invasive breast cancer by 49%. The benefit was especially strong for patients with a history of lobular carcinoma in situ (56% reduction) or atypical ductal hyperplasia (86% reduction). Very small but statistically significant increases were seen in the risk of endometrial cancer and thromboembolic events.

The following year, the NSABP B-24 study established the benefit of tamoxifen in the management of patients with preinvasive breast cancer, or ductal carcinoma in situ (DCIS).[27] Women who underwent surgical resection followed by radiation were then randomized to tamoxifen for 5 years or placebo. A reduction in new breast cancer events was seen (invasive and DCIS), from 13% in the placebo arm to 8% in the tamoxifen arm. These results were recently confirmed in long-term follow-up from the UK/ANZ trial,[28] which showed a reduction in the risk of ipsilateral recurrence by 22% and contralateral cancers by 56%.

TOREMIFENE

Toremifene, a SERM with a mechanism similar to that of tamoxifen, is used more commonly in Europe. Structurally, it has estrogenic and anti-estrogenic properties, but compared with tamoxifen, seems to exhibit less of a proliferative effect on the uterus.[29] In a phase III randomized clinical trial of 217 post-menopausal women with ER positive advanced breast cancer, toremifene was compared with tamoxifen.[30] A response rate of 64% was observed in the toremifene group as compared with 52% in the tamoxifen group.

Toremifene has also been studied in the adjuvant setting for perimenopausal and postmenopausal women with early-stage breast cancer, but is not FDA-approved for this indication. The combined analysis from the International Breast Cancer Study Group Trials 12-93 and 14-93 randomized 1035 perimenopausal and postmenopausal women with node-positive breast cancer to either toremifene or tamoxifen. Toremifene and tamoxifen yielded 5-year disease-free survival rates of 72% and 69%, respectively, and 5-year overall survival rates of 85% and 81%, respectively.[31] Although these data suggest that toremifene could have a role in the adjuvant setting, heterogeneity existed between the study populations in both trials, and the FDA did not allow combined analysis. Unfortunately, each individual study was underpowered to show efficacy.

RALOXIFENE

Raloxifene is a SERM that is approved for the treatment of osteoporosis and as prevention of invasive breast cancer in postmenopausal women. The MORE trial[32] was designed to examine the effect of raloxifene on osteoporosis fracture risk, with breast cancer incidence as a secondary end point. Raloxifene showed a 72% risk reduction in breast cancer incidence; 93 osteoporotic women would need to be treated with raloxifene for 4 years to prevent one case of invasive breast cancer.[33]

Subsequently, the STAR trial was designed to compare raloxifene with the gold standard tamoxifen for preventing breast cancer in postmenopausal women.[34] The study showed equivalent numbers of invasive breast cancers in both arms, suggesting equivalent chemoprevention benefit. Patients treated with raloxifene had fewer cases of endometrial carcinoma and fewer thromboembolic events than those treated with tamoxifen. Raloxifene has not been studied in premenopausal women or in women with a history of DCIS or invasive breast cancer, and therefore is not appropriate for these populations.

FULVESTRANT

The steroidal estrogen receptor downregulator fulvestrant is the first pure ER antagonist with no known agonist effects. It competitively and irreversibly binds the ER with an affinity 100 times stronger than tamoxifen, and leads to its rapid degradation.[35] As a result, the ER is sequestered away from DNA, blocking its function as a transcription factor and inhibiting the activation of downstream estrogen receptor–dependent genes. Fulvestrant is given through intramuscular injection once every 4 weeks and is FDA-approved for the treatment of postmenopausal women with metastatic, hormone receptor–positive, advanced breast cancer that has progressed on a prior hormonal therapy. Despite the FDA indication for second-line treatment, recent data shows that fulvestrant is more effective than the AI anastrozole as first-line therapy for metastatic breast cancer.

Two phase III trials (**Table 1**)[36–38] compared the time to disease progression for fulvestrant (250 mg intramuscular injection monthly) to anastrozole (1 mg orally daily) in 851 postmenopausal women with advanced breast cancer whose disease had progressed on adjuvant hormonal therapy or first-line endocrine therapy in the metastatic setting (96.5% of whom received tamoxifen). These studies showed that fulvestrant was equivalent to anastrozole in the second-line treatment of metastatic breast

Table 1
A comparison of fulvestrant to anastrozole in advanced breast cancer from two phase III trials

Treatment Group	European Trial[36]		North American Trial[37]	
	Fulvestrant	Anastrozole	Fulvestrant	Anastrozole
No. of Patients	222	229	206	194
Overall RR (%)	20.7	15.7	17.5	17.5
CR (%)	4.5	1.7	4.9	3.6
PR (%)	16.2	14.0	12.6	13.9
Clinical Benefit Rate (%)	44.6	45.0	42.2	36.1
SD for more than 24 wk (%)	23.9	29.3	24.8	18.6
Median TTP (mo)	5.5	5.1	5.4	3.4
Median Duration of Response (mo)	15.0	14.5	19.0	10.8
Median Follow-up (months)	14.4	—	16.8	—
Withdrawal Rate (%)	3.2	1.3	2.5	2.6
Overall Survival Combined Analysis at 27 mo[38]		Fulvestrant		Anastrozole
		27.4		27.7

Abbreviations: CR, complete response; PR, partial response; RR, relative risk; SD, stable disease; TTP, time to disease progression.

cancer. Fulvestrant was well tolerated and was associated with a significantly lower incidence of joint disorders.

Investigators in these early fulvestrant trials observed that a significant number of patients in the fulvestrant arm experienced early disease progression.[39] In addition, pharmacokinetic studies performed in early fulvestrant trials showed that it can take 3 to 6 months to achieve steady state blood levels.[40] Thus, investigators postulated that achieving steady state levels earlier might enhance the efficacy of fulvestrant. Loading and high-dose fulvestrant regimens were subsequently developed.[41]

The CONFIRM trial showed that 500 mg of fulvestrant given on day 1, 14, 28, and then every 28 days thereafter was superior to the FDA-approved 250-mg dose.[42] These findings led to FDA approval of the 500-mg fulvestrant dose in 2010. Later that year, updated results from the FIRST trial, which compared 500 mg of fulvestrant with anastrozole in the treatment of first-line metastatic disease, were presented at the 33rd annual San Antonio Breast Cancer Symposium.[43] Median time to disease progression was 23.4 months for fulvestrant versus 13.1 months for anastrozole, corresponding to a 35% reduction in risk of progression. Thus, when optimally dosed, fulvestrant seems to be superior to anastrozole in the treatment of first-line metastatic disease.

Although fulvestrant is not approved for use in premenopausal women, no mechanistic reason exists why it should not work in this population. One study randomized premenopausal women with ER-positive tumors to a single 750-mg intramuscular dose of fulvestrant or a daily 20-mg dose of tamoxifen for 14 to 16 days in the period between initial biopsy and surgery.[44] The drugs reduced the proliferative index (Ki-67) and downregulated ER expression equivalently, but only fulvestrant led to downregulation of the progesterone receptor (often used a marker to show downstream efficacy of ER inhibition). Although this study was not designed to show long-term clinical efficacy, results suggest that fulvestrant has biologic activity in this population. Phase I trials to find the optimal long-term dose in premenopausal women have not been performed.

RESISTANCE TO TAMOXIFEN

Multiple biologic factors predict resistance to tamoxifen, including overexpression of cyclin D1, underexpression of CDK10, and overexpression of coactivator AIB1, and possibly Her-2/neu overexpression (see the article by Doris Germain elsewhere in this issue for further exploration of this topic). Despite a large body of research enumerating mechanisms of tamoxifen resistance, none of these are used clinically because of the limited treatment options for women with preserved ovarian function. When adjuvant tamoxifen treatment fails and distant recurrences occur, the impact on quality and quantity of life is devastating. Thus, one must ask whether better treatment alternatives are available for premenopausal women whose tumors have characteristics that predict resistance to tamoxifen therapy. The SOFT trial will address whether premenopausal women with breast cancer should receive ovarian suppression and/or AIs. However, it will not address whether other non–menopause-inducing agents, such as fulvestrant, could be used in premenopausal women with tumor characteristics predictive of tamoxifen resistance. The authors of this article are actively pursuing this area of research.

The past several years has seen an intense interest in the role of hepatic CYP2D6 enzyme genetic variants and clinical outcome in women treated with tamoxifen. In the United States, 10% to 20% of the population have genetic variants of the CYP2D6 enzyme, which ineffectively metabolize tamoxifen to its active metabolite endoxifen. In 2005, a widely publicized study by Goetz and colleagues[45] correlated

CYP2D6 genotype with clinical outcome in 213 women treated with adjuvant tamoxifen, and concluded that those who were poor metabolizers had a hazard ratio for recurrence four times that of those who were extensive metabolizers. Since this publication, clinical testing of CYP2D6 spread rapidly before any clear data were available on how to integrate the results into clinical practice. Confounding the issue more, in late 2010, data correlating clinical outcome and CYP2D6 genotype in two large prospective studies on adjuvant hormone treatment were presented at the 33rd annual San Antonio Breast Cancer Symposium. Clinical outcomes from the ATAC trial[46] in 588 genotyped women and the BIG 1-98 trial[47] in 1243 genotyped women did not correlate with presence of the CYP2D6 variant in either the tamoxifen or the AI arms. These groups of women are the largest prospectively treated populations studied thus far. Thus, data currently do not support making clinical treatment decisions based on CYP2D6 genetic variants, and testing outside of research should not be routinely offered to the general population taking tamoxifen.

One possible exception is women taking potent CYP2D6 inhibiting medications, which have been shown to lead to lower levels of endoxifen. Fluoxetine, paroxetine, bupropion, and duloxetine are potent inhibitors of CYP2D6. Citalopram, escitalopram, desvenlafaxine, and sertraline are weaker inhibitors of CYP2D6. In patients who require these medications, it may be warranted to check the genotype. Another option is to use venlafaxine in patients treated with tamoxifen, because it does not interfere with CYP2D6 metabolism.

AIs

In postmenopausal women, the main source of estrogen production occurs in the peripheral tissues (adipose, liver, skin, muscle, and breast tissue), where androstenedione is converted into estrone and estradiol. The final step is catalyzed by the enzyme aromatase. The AIs anastrozole, letrozole, and exemestane inhibit the conversion of androstenedione into estrogens, and lower circulating estradiol levels. These drugs do not work in premenopausal women because of high levels of ovarian estrogen production.

AIs are now the mainstay of treatment in postmenopausal women in both the adjuvant and metastatic settings. Numerous trials have shown moderately improved efficacy over tamoxifen, with significantly lower rates of serious side effects, including endometrial carcinoma and thrombosis (deep vein thrombosis, pulmonary embolism, and cerebrovascular accident). A classwide effect of the AIs is higher incidence of osteoporotic fractures. Additionally, at least 5% of women develop diffuse joint pain. Two types of antiaromatase agents are available: the type I steroidal inhibitor exemestane and the type II nonsteroidal inhibitors anastrozole and letrozole. Thus far, all studies comparing one AI with another have shown them to be equivalent.

AIs IN PATIENTS WITH METASTATIC BREAST CANCER REFRACTORY TO TAMOXIFEN

AIs were first tested in postmenopausal women with metastatic breast cancer refractory to tamoxifen. Anastrozole was FDA-approved in 1996 based on two studies that showed it was more effective and less toxic than megestrol acetate.[48–50] The following year, letrozole was approved for the same second-line indication.[51,52] Exemestane was approved for patients refractory to tamoxifen in 2005.

AIs IN FIRST-LINE METASTATIC BREAST CANCER

In November of 2000, the *Journal of Clinical Oncology* published the results of two multinational randomized phase III trials comparing anastrozole with tamoxifen in the first-line treatment of metastatic breast cancer in postmenopausal women. The North American study showed a significant increase in time to disease progression in the anastrozole arm (11.1 vs 5.6 months).[53] Subsequent trials also showed that letrozole[54,55] and exemestane[56] were superior to tamoxifen in the first-line treatment of metastatic breast cancer.

Als in the Adjuvant Setting

Anastrozole was the first AI approved for the adjuvant treatment of breast cancer. The three-arm ATAC trial randomized more than 9000 women to 5 years of either tamoxifen, anastrozole or both.[57,58] The 100-month analysis showed that anastrozole is more effective than tamoxifen, with an absolute improvement in disease-free survival of 2.5% at 5 years and 4.1% at 9 years in patients with ER-positive disease, and with lower rates of thrombotic complications and endometrial cancer[59] (**Fig. 1**). A significant reduction in rates of contralateral breast cancer also occurred.

Letrozole was initially studied in the extended adjuvant setting. The MA 17 trial randomized more than 5000 women who had completed 5 years of treatment with tamoxifen to an additional 5 years of letrozole versus placebo.[60] At 4-year follow-up, the letrozole group showed a 4.6% absolute benefit in disease-free survival. Subsequently, the BIG 1-98 trial showed that up-front letrozole is superior to up-front tamoxifen in hormone therapy–naïve patients (**Fig. 2**).

Exemestane was first studied in the adjuvant setting in women who had received 2 to 3 years of tamoxifen. The Intergroup Exemestane Study randomized women either to an additional 2 to 3 years of tamoxifen or to change to 2 to 3 years of exemestane. At 8-year follow-up, the group that was switched from tamoxifen to exemestane had an

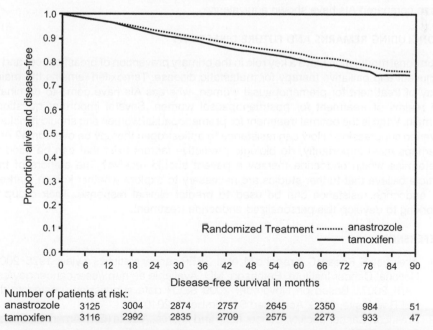

Fig. 1. Disease-free survival Kaplan-Meier curve for all patients randomized to anastrozole or tamoxifen monotherapy in the ATAC trial (intent to treat). (*From* DailyMed. Anastrozole tablet. Available at: http://dailymed.nlm.nih.gov/dailymed/drugInfo.cfm?id=19380.)

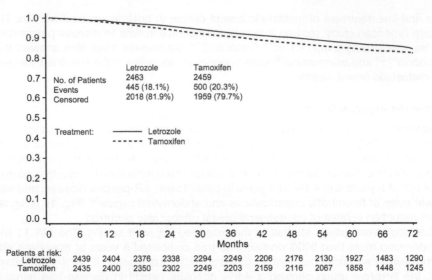

Fig. 2. Disease-free survival for patients treated with adjuvant letrozole versus tamoxifen. (*From* DailyMed. Femara (letrozole) tablet, film coated. Available at: http://dailymed.nlm. nih.gov/dailymed/drugInfo.cfm?id=19740.)

absolute overall survival benefit of 2.4% and absolute disease-free survival benefit of 4.4%.[61]

Overall, these studies show that AIs are the first choice in the adjuvant treatment of postmenopausal women with endocrine-sensitive tumors. Thus far, all studies that have compared AIs have shown equivalence.

CONCLUDING REMARKS AND FUTURE DIRECTIONS

Hormonal modulation plays a key role in the primary prevention of breast cancer and in adjuvant and palliative therapy for metastatic disease. Tamoxifen remains the mainstay of treatment for premenopausal women, whereas AIs have come to dominate all realms of treatment for postmenopausal women. Several important questions remain. What is the optimal treatment for premenopausal women and should it include ovarian suppression? How can resistance to antiestrogen therapy be overcome? And perhaps most importantly, do biologic predictive factors exist that can be used to determine which endocrine therapy a patient should receive? The authors of this article believe that further studies are necessary to explore whether known markers of endocrine resistance can be used to predict clinical response. Their group is working to develop this personalized endocrine treatment.

REFERENCES

1. Altekruse S, Kosary C, Krapcho M, et al. SEER cancer statistics review, 1975–2007, National Cancer Institute. Bethesda, MD. Available at: http://seer.cancer.gov/csr/ 1975_2007/. Based on November 2009 SEER data submission, posted to the SEER web site, 2010. Accessed September 1, 2010.
2. American Cancer Society. Cancer facts and figures. Atlanta (GA): American Cancer Society; 2002.
3. Fisher B. Biological and clinical considerations regarding the use of surgery and chemotherapy in the treatment of primary breast cancer. Cancer 1977;40:574.

 4. Jemal A, Ward E, Thun MJ. Recent trends in breast cancer incidence rates by age and tumor characteristics among U.S. women. Breast Cancer Res 2007;9:R28.
 5. Rossouw JE, Anderson GL, Prentice RL, et al. Risks and benefits of estrogen plus progestin in healthy postmenopausal women: principal results from the Women's Health Initiative randomized controlled trial. JAMA 2002;288:321.
 6. Love RR, Philips J. Oophorectomy for breast cancer: history revisited. J Natl Cancer Inst 2002;94:1433.
 7. Schinzinger A. Ueber carcinoma mammae [abstract]. 18th Congress of the German Society for Surgery, Beilage zum Centralblatt fur Chirurgie 1889;16: 55–6.
 8. Beatson G. On the treatment of inoperable cases of carcinoma of the mamma: suggestions for a new method of treatment. Lancet 1896;2:162.
 9. Dellapasqua S, Colleoni M, Gelber RD, et al. Adjuvant endocrine therapy for premenopausal women with early breast cancer. J Clin Oncol 2005;23:1736.
10. Hughes LL, Gray RJ, Solin LJ, et al. Efficacy of radiotherapy for ovarian ablation: results of a breast intergroup study. Cancer 2004;101:969.
11. (EBCTCG) EBCTG. Effects of chemotherapy and hormonal therapy for early breast cancer on recurrence and 15-year survival: an overview of the randomised trials. Lancet 2005;365:1687.
12. Sverrisdottir A, Johansson H, Johansson U, et al. Interaction between goserelin and tamoxifen in a controlled clinical trial of adjuvant endocrine therapy in premenopausal breast cancer. Presented at the 33rd Annual San Antonio Breast Cancer Symposium. San Antonio (TX), December 9, 2010.
13. Phase III randomized study of adjuvant therapy comprising tamoxifen citrate alone versus ovarian function suppression and tamoxifen citrate versus ovarian function suppression and exemestane in premenopausal women who have undergone surgery for hormone receptor-positive breast cancer (SOFT). Available at: http://clinicaltrials.gov/ct2/show/NCT00917969?term=premenopausal+breast+cancer&type=Intr&phase=2&rank=15. Accessed June 23, 2011.
14. Smith IE, Ford HT, Gazet JC, et al. Premarin in the management of metastatic breast carcinoma in post-menopausal patients. Clin Oncol 1979;5:159.
15. Ingle JN, Ahmann DL, Green SJ, et al. Randomized clinical trial of diethylstilbestrol versus tamoxifen in postmenopausal women with advanced breast cancer. N Engl J Med 1981;304:16.
16. Ellis MJ, Gao F, Dehdashti F, et al. Lower-dose vs high-dose oral estradiol therapy of hormone receptor-positive, aromatase inhibitor-resistant advanced breast cancer: a phase 2 randomized study. JAMA 2009;302:774.
17. Ansfield FJ, Davis HL Jr, Ellerby RA, et al. A clinical trial of megestrol acetate in advanced breast cancer. Cancer 1974;33:907.
18. Morgan LR. Megestrol acetate v tamoxifen in advanced breast cancer in post-menopausal patients. Semin Oncol 1985;12:43.
19. Muss HB, Paschold EH, Black WR, et al. Megestrol acetate v tamoxifen in advanced breast cancer: a phase III trial of the Piedmont Oncology Association (POA). Semin Oncol 1985;12:55.
20. Pritchard K. Should tamoxifen be used to treat premenopausal women with breast cancer? Cancer Invest 2000;18:685.
21. Harper MJ, Walpole AL. Contrasting endocrine activities of cis and trans isomers in a series of substituted triphenylethylenes. Nature 1966;212:87.
22. Klopper A, Hall M. New synthetic agent for the induction of ovulation: preliminary trials in women. Br Med J 1971;1:152.

23. Jordan VC. Antitumor activity of the antiestrogen ICI 46,474 (tamoxifen) in the dimethylbenzanthracene (DMBA)-induced rat mammary carcinoma model. J Steroid Biochem 1974;5:354.
24. Cole MP, Jones CT, Todd ID. A new anti-oestrogenic agent in late breast cancer. An early clinical appraisal of ICI46474. Br J Cancer 1971;25:270.
25. (EBCTCG) EBCTCG. Ovarian ablation in early breast cancer: overview of the randomised trials. Early Breast Cancer Trialists' Collaborative Group. Lancet 1996;348:1189.
26. Fisher B, Costantino JP, Wickerham DL, et al. Tamoxifen for prevention of breast cancer: report of the National Surgical Adjuvant Breast and Bowel Project P-1 Study. J Natl Cancer Inst 1998;90:1371.
27. Fisher B, Dignam J, Wolmark N, et al. Tamoxifen in treatment of intraductal breast cancer: National Surgical Adjuvant Breast and Bowel Project B-24 randomised controlled trial. Lancet 1993;353:1999.
28. Cuzick J, Sestak I, Pinder S, et al. Beneficial effect of tamoxifen for women with DCIS: long-term benefits from the UK/ANZ DCIS trial in women with locally excised DCIS. Presented at the 32nd Annual San Antonio Breast Cancer Symposium. San Antonio, December 10–13, 2009.
29. Tomas E, Kauppila A, Blanco G, et al. Comparison between the effects of tamoxifen and toremifene on the uterus in postmenopausal breast cancer patients. Gynecol Oncol 1995;59:261.
30. Milla-Santos A, Milla L, Rallo L, et al. Phase III randomized trial of toremifene vs tamoxifen in hormonodependant advanced breast cancer. Breast Cancer Res Treat 2001;65:119.
31. Pagani O, Gelber S, Price K, et al. Toremifene and tamoxifen are equally effective for early-stage breast cancer: first results of International Breast Cancer Study Group Trials 12-93 and 14-93. Ann Oncol 2004;15:1749.
32. Cummings SR, Eckert S, Krueger KA, et al. The effect of raloxifene on risk of breast cancer in postmenopausal women: results from the MORE randomized trial. Multiple Outcomes of Raloxifene Evaluation. JAMA 1999;281:2189.
33. Cauley JA, Norton L, Lippman ME, et al. Continued breast cancer risk reduction in postmenopausal women treated with raloxifene: 4-year results from the MORE trial. Multiple outcomes of raloxifene evaluation. Breast Cancer Res Treat 2001; 65:125.
34. Vogel VG, Costantino JP, Wickerham DL, et al. Update of the National Surgical Adjuvant Breast and Bowel Project Study of Tamoxifen and Raloxifene (STAR) P-2 Trial: preventing breast cancer. Cancer Prev Res (Phila) 2010;3:696.
35. Long X, Nephew KP. Fulvestrant (ICI 182,780)-dependent interacting proteins mediate immobilization and degradation of estrogen receptor-alpha. J Biol Chem 2006;281:9607.
36. Howell A, Robertson JF, Quaresma Albano J, et al. Fulvestrant, formerly ICI 182,780, is as effective as anastrozole in postmenopausal women with advanced breast cancer progressing after prior endocrine treatment. J Clin Oncol 2002;20: 3396.
37. Osborne CK, Pippen J, Jones SE, et al. Double-blind, randomized trial comparing the efficacy and tolerability of fulvestrant versus anastrozole in postmenopausal women with advanced breast cancer progressing on prior endocrine therapy: results of a North American trial. J Clin Oncol 2002;20:3386.
38. Howell A, Pippen J, Elledge RM, et al. Fulvestrant versus anastrozole for the treatment of advanced breast carcinoma: a prospectively planned combined survival analysis of two multicenter trials. Cancer 2005;104:236.

39. McCormack P, Sapunar F. Pharmacokinetic profile of the fulvestrant loading dose regimen in postmenopausal women with hormone receptor-positive advanced breast cancer. Clin Breast Cancer 2008;8:347.
40. Robertson JF, Harrison M. Fulvestrant: pharmacokinetics and pharmacology. Br J Cancer 2004;90(Suppl 1):S7.
41. Robertson JF. Fulvestrant (Faslodex)—how to make a good drug better. Oncologist 2007;12:774.
42. Di Leo A, Jerusalem G, Petruzelka L, et al. CONFIRM: a phase III randomized, parallel-group trial comparing fulvestrant 250 mg vs fulvestrant 500 mg in postemenopausal women with estrogen receptor-positive advanced breast cancer. Cancer Res 2009;69:491S.
43. Robertson J, Lindemann J, Llombart-Cussac A, et al. A comparison of fulvestrant 500 mg with anastrozole as first-line treatment for advanced breast cancer: followup analysis from the FIRST study. Presented at the 33rd Annual San Antonio Breast Cancer Symposium. San Antonio, December 8–12, 2010.
44. Young OE, Renshaw L, Macaskill EJ, et al. Effects of fulvestrant 750mg in premenopausal women with oestrogen-receptor-positive primary breast cancer. Eur J Cancer 2008;44:391.
45. Goetz MP, Rae JM, Suman VJ, et al. Pharmacogenetics of tamoxifen biotransformation is associated with clinical outcomes of efficacy and hot flashes. J Clin Oncol 2005;23:9312.
46. Rae J, Drury S, Hayes D, et al. Lack of correlation between gene variants in tamoxifen metabolizing enzymes with primary endpoints in the ATAC trial. Presented at the 33rd Annual San Antonio Breast Conference. San Antonio (TX), December 9, 2010.
47. Leyland-Jones B, Regan M, Bouzyk M, et al. Outcome according to CYP2D6 Genotype among postmenopausal women with endocrine-responsive early invasive breast cancer randomized in the BIG 1–98 trial. Cancer Res 2010;70:78S.
48. Buzdar AU, Jonat W, Howell A, et al. Anastrozole versus megestrol acetate in the treatment of postmenopausal women with advanced breast carcinoma: results of a survival update based on a combined analysis of data from two mature phase III trials. Arimidex Study Group. Cancer 1998;83:1142.
49. Buzdar AU, Jones SE, Vogel CL, et al. A phase III trial comparing anastrozole (1 and 10 milligrams), a potent and selective aromatase inhibitor, with megestrol acetate in postmenopausal women with advanced breast carcinoma. Arimidex Study Group. Cancer 1997;79:730.
50. Jonat W, Howell A, Blomqvist C, et al. A randomised trial comparing two doses of the new selective aromatase inhibitor anastrozole (Arimidex) with megestrol acetate in postmenopausal patients with advanced breast cancer. Eur J Cancer Am 1996;32:404.
51. Buzdar A, Douma J, Davidson N, et al. Phase III, multicenter, double-blind, randomized study of letrozole, an aromatase inhibitor, for advanced breast cancer versus megestrol acetate. J Clin Oncol 2001;19:3357.
52. Dombernowsky P, Smith I, Falkson G, et al. Letrozole, a new oral aromatase inhibitor for advanced breast cancer: double-blind randomized trial showing a dose effect and improved efficacy and tolerability compared with megestrol acetate. J Clin Oncol 1998;16:453.
53. Nabholtz JM, Buzdar A, Pollak M, et al. Anastrozole is superior to tamoxifen as first-line therapy for advanced breast cancer in postmenopausal women: results of a North American multicenter randomized trial. Arimidex Study Group. J Clin Oncol 2000;18:3758.

54. Hoctin-Boes G, Yates R, Steinberg M. Letrozole for advanced breast cancer. J Clin Oncol 1998;16:2892.
55. Mouridsen H, Gershanovich M, Sun Y, et al. Superior efficacy of letrozole versus tamoxifen as first-line therapy for postmenopausal women with advanced breast cancer: results of a phase III study of the International Letrozole Breast Cancer Group. J Clin Oncol 2001;19:2596.
56. Paridaens RJ, Dirix LY, Beex LV, et al. Phase III study comparing exemestane with tamoxifen as first-line hormonal treatment of metastatic breast cancer in postmenopausal women: the European Organisation for Research and Treatment of Cancer Breast Cancer Cooperative Group. J Clin Oncol 2008;26:4883.
57. Baum M, Budzar AU, Cuzick J, et al. Anastrozole alone or in combination with tamoxifen versus tamoxifen alone for adjuvant treatment of postmenopausal women with early breast cancer: first results of the ATAC randomised trial. Lancet 2002;359:2131.
58. Buzdar AU. Anastrozole (Arimidex) in clinical practice versus the old 'gold standard', tamoxifen. Expert Rev Anticancer Ther 2002;2:623.
59. Forbes JF, Cuzick J, Buzdar A, et al. Effect of anastrozole and tamoxifen as adjuvant treatment for early-stage breast cancer: 100-month analysis of the ATAC trial. Lancet Oncol 2008;9:45.
60. Goss PE, Ingle JN, Martino S, et al. A randomized trial of letrozole in postmenopausal women after five years of tamoxifen therapy for early-stage breast cancer. N Engl J Med 2003;349:1793.
61. Bliss J, Kilburn L, Coleman R, et al. Disease related outcome with long term follow-up: an updated analysis of the Intergroup Exemestane Study (IES). Presented at the 32nd Annual San Antonio Breast Cancer Symposium. San Antonio (TX), December 10, 2009.

Androgens and Breast Cancer in Men and Women

Constantine Dimitrakakis, MD[a,b,]*

KEYWORDS

- Androgens • Testosterone • Breast cancer • Hormone therapy
- Menopause • Male breast cancer

There has been increasing focus recently on the importance of androgens in human physiology. Supplementation of testosterone in women with hypoactive sexual desire disorder is an area of great interest at present.[1] Testosterone treatment in physiologic doses seems to improve sexual desire, responsiveness, and frequency of sexual activity, while at the same time it exhibits favorable effects on bone in postmenopausal women.[2] However, the risk-benefit ratio for such treatment remains unclear.

Androgen receptors (AR) are found in virtually every tissue in women as well as in men, including breast, bone, and brain, indicating that androgens and their metabolites may play an important role in normal tissue homeostasis and possibly in pathologies, such as breast cancer, osteoporosis, decreased libido, and cognitive decline. A continuing area of concern is the notion that excess androgen exposure may increase the risk of breast cancer.[3]

Over the past decade, there have been major advances in our understanding of the sources of endogenous sex steroids acting on mammary epithelium with the identification of tissue-specific expression of steroidogenic enzymes capable of converting circulating prohormones, such as dehydroepiandrosterone (DHEA), into potent androgens or estrogens. In addition, there have been great strides in the genetic elucidation of these steroidogenic enzymes and the steroid receptors.

Diverse clinical and experimental observations indicate that androgens moderate estrogenic effects on mammary proliferation and growth. Experimental data suggest

The author has nothing to disclose.

[a] Developmental Endocrinology Branch, National Institute of Child Health and Human Development, National Institutes of Health, CRC, Room 1-3330, 10 Center Drive, MSC-1103 Bethesda, MD 20892-1103, USA

[b] 1st Department of Obstetrics/Gynecology, Athens University Medical School, Alexandra Hospital, 80 Vas. Sophias Street, 11528, Athens, Greece

* 1st Department of Obstetrics/Gynecology, Athens University Medical School, Alexandra Hospital, 80 Vas. Sophias Street, 11528, Athens, Greece.

E-mail address: dimitrac@mail.nih.gov

Endocrinol Metab Clin N Am 40 (2011) 533–547

doi:10.1016/j.ecl.2011.05.007

0889-8529/11/$ – see front matter © 2011 Elsevier Inc. All rights reserved.

endo.theclinics.com

that conventional estrogen treatment regimens, both as oral contraceptives (OCs) and hormone therapy (HT),[4] upset the normal estrogen/androgen balance and promote the unopposed estrogenic stimulation of mammary epithelial proliferation and, hence, potentially breast cancer risk.

The author compares literature evidence indicating that androgens augment the risk for breast cancer versus the evidence that androgens protect the mammary gland from hormone-induced stimulation, increased proliferation, and neoplasia.

ACTION OF ANDROGENS IN BREAST PHYSIOLOGY: CLINICAL OBSERVATIONS

Breast tissue is similar in prepubertal boys and girls, and steroid hormones begin to interact mainly through their specific receptors. It is generally accepted that estrogens stimulate and androgens inhibit breast development independently of genetic sex. Pubertal rises in estrogen levels cause breast growth in girls and frequently in boys (transiently). In girls with premature thelarche, estradiol levels are significantly higher than in normal prepubertal girls. A familial autosomal dominant syndrome of aromatase hyperactivity that increases estrone while decreasing testosterone levels presents as pubertal gynecomastia in boys.[5] Decreasing testosterone levels may also trigger early breast growth, documented in girls that express a high activity isoform of the testosterone-metabolizing enzyme CYP3A4.[6] Conversely, androgen excess caused by an adrenal tumor or hyperplasia suppresses normal breast development in girls, despite apparently adequate estrogen levels.[7] In castrated male-to-female transsexuals, feminizing estrogen therapy stimulates breast growth with full acinar and lobular formation and estrogen-treated genetically male breast tissue exhibits normal female histology. Estrogens taken to treat prostate cancer also lead to breast development in men with suppressed gonadal function and reduced testosterone levels. Conversely, androgen use by female athletes and female-to-male transsexuals leads to breast atrophy.

Supporting the normal inhibitory role of endogenous androgens on breast growth, AR blockade with flutamide causes gynecomastia and rarely breast adenocarcinoma.[8] In the androgen insensitivity syndrome, the inactive AR fails to counteract estrogenic stimulation, and genetic males with normal androgen levels eventuate with normal female breast development. Males may also develop gynecomastia when the estrogen/androgen ratio is increased because of decreased androgen production or increased aromatization.[9]

ENDOCRINE AND INTRACRINE MODES OF ACTION

Mammary cell proliferation in both normal and malignant tissues is critically regulated by the dynamic balance between stimulatory effects of the estrogens and inhibitory effects of the androgens.[10] A specific estrogen/androgen ratio, predictive of breast stimulation or inhibition, that would be safe for breast tissue has not been identified for several reasons. Estradiol and testosterone assays have been neither very sensitive nor accurate in the lower ranges because both hormones bind to SHBG and total values are not as informative as free or bioavailable hormones.[11] Moreover, single hormone measurements may not be very informative about tissue exposure over time. Steroid levels vary hourly in response to diurnal rhythm, diet, stress, and exercise, so a single value may be inadequate to assess true tissue exposure. In addition, estradiol and testosterone may be synthesized locally in peripheral tissues from circulating precursors, such as the sulfate of DHEA (DHEA-S) and androstenedione. According to intracrinology, breast tissue has the ability and the enzymatic background to produce estrogens, to metabolize androgens precursors to active forms, and to respond to minimum hormonal concentrations. In this way, the breast controls steroid concentrations and homeostasis independently of circulating estrogen and androgen levels.[12] The conjugated products of steroid metabolism find their way into the circulation after peripheral action and provide evidence as to the proportion of the precursor pools of steroids used as androgen or estrogen. Analysis of these metabolites by Labrie and colleagues[13] and Sasano and colleagues[14] suggested that the major proportion of androgen effectors in women derive from such an endocrine mode of action, which will not be detected by assays of circulating testosterone or dihydrotestosterone (DHT). Although circulating levels of testosterone and DHT are 5- to 10-fold higher in men than in women, the abundance of androgen metabolites is less than 2-fold higher in men, suggesting that the local tissue production and the action of androgens in women may be more significant than historically suspected.

All the steroidogenic enzymes necessary for the formation of androgens and estrogens from steroid precursors (steroid sulfatase, 17β-hydroxysteroid dehydrogenases [17β-HSDs], 3β-HSDs, 5α-reductases, and aromatase) have been reported in normal mammary tissues, breast cancer specimens, or cell lines.[14] Androgens stimulate or inhibit the growth of breast cancer cells in vitro depending on the cell line and the clone under study according to former data.[15] Breast cancer cell lines and tissue specimens express the enzymes involved in DHT as well as estradiol synthesis. In a histochemical study, expression of 5α-reductase was significantly correlated with AR expression and 17β-HSD and 3β-HSD immunoreactivities, and the abundance of this androgenic molecular assembly was inversely correlated with tumor size, histologic grade, and proliferative index,[16] suggesting an inhibitory role for DHT in tumor growth.

ANDROGEN RECEPTOR: ASSOCIATIONS WITH BREAST CANCER RISK

The cellular response to steroid hormones requires their conjunction to a membrane-bound or to an intracellular receptor. The human AR is a member of the nuclear receptor superfamily that includes receptors for steroid hormones, vitamin D, rhodopsin, and other agents.[17] Normal mammary epithelium, but not stromal or myoepithelial cells, coexpress AR and estrogen and progesterone (PR) receptors.[18] The coexpression of estrogen receptors (ER) and AR in mammary epithelial cells suggests that the effects of estrogen and androgen on mammary epithelial proliferation are integrated within the mammary epithelial cell. AR expression is abundant in normal mammary epithelium and in the majority of breast cancer specimens and cell lines. There is emerging evidence that the androgen-signaling pathway plays a critical role in breast carcinogenesis.

Binding of testosterone or DHT triggers a cascade of signaling events, including phosphorylation and conformational changes in the receptor, which dissociates from cytoplasmic proteins and migrates to the cell nucleus. Ligand-activated AR regulates gene expression through binding to AR elements located in a gene's enhancer or promoter region. As with other similar receptors, the AR functions in transcriptional regulation in concert with a host of nuclear proteins, which may serve as coactivators or corepressors. Interestingly, the BRCA1 gene product has been identified as an AR coactivator.[19] The BRCA1 protein binds to the AR and potentates AR-mediated effects, suggesting that BRCA1 mutations may blunt androgen effects. However, other studies have not confirmed these findings.[20]

The AR gene is located on the X chromosome with no corresponding allele on the Y, so it functions solely as a single copy gene, as shown by the complete loss of androgen effect in XY individuals with an inactivating mutation of the AR.[21] AR has a highly polymorphic CAG repeat in exon 1 that encodes a polyglutamine stretch. The CAG polymorphisms have become the point of interest to a series of studies with various results. There is evidence that longer CAG repeats are associated with breast cancer onset earlier in life,[20] especially among women using oral contraceptives or menopausal hormone therapy[22] and probably among male patients with breast cancer.[23] However, another study found no association with breast cancer risk.[24] In a study nested within the Nurses' Health Study cohort,[25] no relation was found between AR genotype and breast cancer risk among postmenopausal Caucasian women overall, but an increased risk was observed when analysis was limited to those individuals with a first-degree family history of breast cancer. Another study[26] provides evidence that the association of breast cancer with the long AR-CAG was observed only in postmenopausal and not in premenopausal women, which may explain the insignificant results in studies restricted to young women. In other studies, reduced risk was observed with another trinucleotide repeat, GGC, in young women. AR-CAG repeat length was inversely associated with testosterone levels in both premenopausal and postmenopausal normal women.[27] On the level of AR-protein expression, some germline mutations in the AR gene confer variable degrees of androgen insensitivity and have been associated with the occurrence of breast cancer in men.[28]

Emphasis should be given to the fact that none of these studies had sufficient statistical power to implicate or exclude specific AR defects in breast cancer risk. A recent epidemiologic meta-analysis concludes that there is no association between AR genetic variations and breast cancer risk among Caucasian women.[24]

Mammographic density is a potent risk factor for breast cancer. It has been reported that postmenopausal carriers of a less active AR treated with estrogen/progesterone therapy, presented with a higher mammographic density than carriers of the more active AR.[29] This finding means that AR genotype modifies hormone-induced proliferation as reflected in mammographic density and may explain the mechanism by which estrogen/progesterone use increases breast cancer risk. However, the exact mechanisms and metabolic paths in which AR participates in normal tissues are still obscure. The role of AR in oncogenesis or breast tumor proliferation remains unclear. Experimental data suggest that breast cancer growth is inhibited primarily directly through AR stimulation or indirectly via downregulation of other receptors, such as PR or ER. It seems that AR presence is sometimes adequate to block ERα-related growth stimulation of breast cancer cells,[30] and overexpression of AR decreases ERα-related transcriptional activity.[31] Other preclinical data indicate that androgens, like antiestrogens, may act by promoting apoptosis in human breast cancer cell lines.[32] However, it is possible that the steroid receptor contributes differently in healthy compared with cancerous breast tissue; thus, several unanswered questions remain, and further studies are needed before safe conclusions are drawn.

The hypothesis that androgens are directly involved in breast carcinogenesis is based on the presence of ARs in the majority of breast cancers. It is proposed that androgens, through binding to their receptors, act independently to produce tumors with specific clinical behaviors.[33] A significant number of poorly differentiated breast carcinomas are ER negative and PR negative but AR-positive. On the other hand, hormone-dependent tumors with poor AR expression are connected to an increased risk of cancer-related-death.[30] Tumors classified as AR negative are usually characterized by poor prognosis, associated to larger tumor size, higher grade, and frequent lymph node metastasis. Some investigators have proposed that AR expression may be lost during the development process of more aggressive and larger tumors and that AR expression in both ER-positive and ER-negative tumors is an independent prognostic factor associated with improved recurrence-free survival.[34] These associations constitute important clinical and pathologic prognostic information. Recently, AR expression in a tumor is considered as an indicator of lower malignancy potential; this provides a new range of therapeutic targets for poorly differentiated cancers.[35]

EPIDEMIOLOGIC DATA

Long-term treatment with estrogens increases the risk of breast cancer in both men and women primarily through estrogenic stimulation of mammary epithelial proliferation, although additional carcinogenic effects by estrogen metabolites have been proposed.[36] The most widely accepted risk factor for breast cancer is the cumulative dose of estrogens that breast epithelium is exposed to over time. However, it has been difficult to correlate breast cancer risk with isolated serum estrogen levels in epidemiologic studies, probably secondary to problems using single random hormone levels for the evaluation of tissue-specific exposure as previously discussed.

Correlation of adrenal precursor steroids with breast cancer incidence has been consistent, perhaps reflecting the importance of local tissue conversion. Interest in a potential role for adrenal androgens in breast carcinogenesis began in the late 1950s, with the demonstration of reduced 17-ketosteroid excretion in the urine of premenopausal women with breast cancer. This observation has been repeatedly confirmed in subsequent studies showing reduced DHEA-S in the serum of premenopausal patients with breast cancer. In the first prospective study in this field, levels of androgen metabolites in urine were found to be abnormally reduced in premenopausal women who subsequently developed breast cancer,[37] indicating a protective role of androgens on the breast. In contrast, in more recent prospective studies of premenopausal women,[38,39] no association was found between plasma adrenal androgen levels and the risk of breast cancer. Interestingly, in the Nurses' Health Study II, among premenopausal women there was a positive association, especially for tumors that express both ERs and PRs.[39] Also, among premenopausal women, higher levels of testosterone and androstenedione were associated with the increased risk of invasive ER+/PR+ tumors, although with a nonstatistically significant increase in the overall risk of breast cancer.[39] In a recent study,[40] levels of testosterone and DHEA-S in saliva (where the unbound fraction of hormones is measured) were statistically significantly lower in patients with breast cancer compared with controls and these differences were more profound in postmenopausal women. Patients with breast cancer, when compared with controls, presented with an androgen insufficiency and a relative imbalance of sex steroid hormones in favor of estrogens.

In recent years, several epidemiologic studies have examined the correlation between circulating androgens, such as testosterone, and breast cancer risk. A major limitation of such studies is that the androgen assays used were developed primarily to measure the higher levels found in men and lack reliability in the low ranges found in normal women.[11] Moreover, testosterone and androstenedione levels demonstrate substantial variability from day to day and even from hour to hour, influenced by diurnal rhythms, diet, exercise, and stress; however, most of the epidemiologic data are based on a single blood sample collected at nonstandard times. Another problem using serum testosterone levels to gauge androgenic effects at the tissue level is that most of the circulating testosterone is tightly bound to SHBG although only the free hormone is bioactive. SHBG, and thus total testosterone levels, vary widely based on genetic, metabolic, and endocrine influences, and it is now accepted that measurement of free or bioavailable testosterone predicts androgenic effects more accurately than total testosterone levels.[11] Finally, as discussed previously, the major proportion of androgenic activity in women originates from the peripheral conversion of precursors, such as DHEA, into androgens within the cells of target tissues, and this activity will not be detected by the measurement of circulating androgens.

Several studies have revealed, however, that adrenal androgens are increased in postmenopausal women with breast cancer.[41] A possible explanation regarding the divergence between premenopausal and postmenopausal findings is that one adrenal androgen, androstenediol (also known as hermaphroditol), is a weak ER agonist. In the presence of high estrogen levels in premenopausal women, androstenediol could exhibit antiestrogenic effects, while in the hypoestrogenic postmenopausal milieu, the agonist effect may predominate. This view remains speculative and other possibilities still exist. It is possible that the high-estrogen environment in premenopausal women promotes androgenic enzyme and AR expression in mammary tissue, allowing androgenic effects by DHEA metabolites, whereas in postmenopausal women, an estrogen-deficient tissue microenvironment may favor estrogenic effects. Also, genetic variation in CYP19 and SHBG genes was found to contribute to the variance in circulating hormone levels in postmenopausal women, but none was statistically significantly associated with breast cancer risk.[42]

In some prospective epidemiologic studies, age-adjusted mean values of total and free testosterone and estradiol were significantly higher prediagnostically in postmenopausal breast cancer cases compared with controls, and estradiol and total testosterone were elevated in other case-control studies of postmenopausal breast cancer. It was observed that elevated serum levels of both estrogens and androgens contribute to a greater risk of breast cancer,[39] and a meta-analysis of 9 prospective studies revealed that breast cancer risk increases with increasing concentrations of almost all sex hormones.[43]

None of these studies, however, adjust for estrogen levels and this constitutes a serious bias.[44] As a result, they do not manage to disconnect the risk associated with increased estradiol levels from the androgen component, and because androgens are the obligate precursors for estradiol synthesis, this is a major confounding factor in assessing the role of androgen independently of the known cancer-promoting estrogen effect. Some epidemiologic data indicate that serum concentrations of estrogens, but not of androgens or sex-hormone binding globulin, are associated with breast hyperplasia in postmenopausal women, suggesting that estrogens may be implicated early in the pathologic process toward breast cancer.[45] In line with these observations, a recent study[46] concluded that increased breast cancer risk with increasing body mass index among postmenopausal women is largely the result of the associated increase in estrogens. The association of androgens with breast cancer risk did not persist after adjustment for estrone, the estrogen most strongly associated with the risk. Other investigators conclude that conversion of DHEA to estrogens, particularly estradiol, is required to exert a mitogenic response.[47] These results suggest that the contribution of androgens to breast cancer risk is largely through their role as substrates for estrogen production. Other studies have found no association between androgens and breast cancer.[48,49]

The previous observations indicate the difficulty in separating potential direct effects of circulating testosterone from its potential to be aromatized into estradiol. It would be more interesting to investigate levels of testosterone and DHT metabolites in these studies to more directly assess tissue exposure to androgens.

As previously noted, a single serum hormone measurement seems unlikely to be informative about a woman's true long-term exposure to that hormone or her specific risk of developing breast cancer; nor does it seem to be a biologically plausible mechanism that androgens acting as androgens could promote breast cancer because virtually all clinical data suggest just the opposite. If elevated androgen levels directly contribute to breast cancer, then women with clinically evident long-term hyperandrogenism (for example, polycystic ovary syndrome and congenital adrenal hyperplasia) should experience increased rates of breast cancer, but this is not the case.[50] Moreover, androgen levels are chronically elevated in men, who have a breast cancer risk less than 1% of that of women. Male breast cancer is a rare disease, but genetic syndromes explanation is not sufficient for the majority of the cases and other risk factors with hormonal impact have been implicated. In Klinefelter syndrome, a 50-fold increase of breast cancer risk has been observed,[51,52] and other hypogonadal situations share a percentage of new cases of male breast cancer. In these conditions, the patients have normal estrogen levels in the lower percentage, but they lack the protective androgenic effect of testosterone.[53] Bone fractures in men, in contrast to women, are associated with an elevated risk for breast cancer. The interpretation for that fact also implicates testosterone deficiency advancing the age, which may be the causal factor for reduced bone density and strength.[54] Conditions, such as obesity or liver cirrhosis, that increase estrogen conversion and metabolic maintenance while reducing androgens bioavailability alter the estrogen/androgen ratio and are also correlated to increased breast cancer risk in men, as in women.[54,55] Epidemiologic studies in men indicate that low urinary androsterone and serum-free testosterone levels are related to the early onset of breast cancer, a much higher relapse rate, and a worse response to endocrine therapy.[56]

HORMONE THERAPY, ANDROGENS, AND BREAST CANCER

Both endogenous and exogenous estrogen exposure is thought to contribute to increased breast cancer risk. Since the introduction of combined OCs, many changes in doses and their biochemical structures have taken place; however, the impact of OCs on breast cancer remains controversial. Epidemiologic studies provide inconclusive results,[57,58] whereas a recent meta-analysis reports increased premenopausal breast cancer risk with the use of OCs.[59] However, because pill users are young, this represents a very small increase in absolute risk. It is not yet known if lower dose and variable OC formulations are associated with a similar increase in risk, making comparisons very difficult.

There are many lines of evidence supporting a causal relationship between the use of HT and breast cancer. Recent and long-term users of HT are associated with higher risk. The effect of concurrent progestin use appears to further increase risk greater than that with estrogens alone. The most important randomized clinical trial providing information about this issue is the Women's Health Initiative (WHI) study.[60,61] The results from observational studies are generally consistent with those of the WHI trial, reporting increased but no significant variation in the risk of breast cancer with use of different estrogens, progestins, doses, or routes of administration. A group of postmenopausal participants in the WHI study used testosterone combined with estrogens. In this group, the testosterone addition for a period of 1 year had no statistically significant effect on breast cancer occurrence, suggesting at least that androgen induction did not increase the number of breast cancer cases in this trial.[62] In the same study, rates of breast cancer were lower in longer-term compared with shorter-term users of estrogen plus testosterone. On the other hand, in a prospective study of more than 1 million person-years with 24 years of follow-up within the Nurses' Health Study, current users of estrogen plus testosterone have shown a 2.5-fold increased risk of developing breast cancer compared with menopausal women who used estrogen-only therapy or to women who never used postmenopausal hormone formulations.[63] However, in a recent study, adrenal androgens, such as DHEA and its sulfate, combined with an aromatase inhibitor to ensure that the androgenic maintenance has shown an inhibitory effect on human breast ER-negative breast cancer cell lines with a strong AR expression. Specifically, DHEA acting as an AR agonist presented apoptotic action on these cell lines augmenting the cell death rate.[64]

Suppression of normal endogenous androgen may be an adverse consequence of pharmacologic estrogen therapy, if androgens are indeed protective against estrogen-induced mammary proliferation. Conventional HT and OCs may promote breast cancer not only by increasing estrogen exposure but also by decreasing endogenous androgen activity. Oral estrogen therapy reduces free androgens by stimulating hepatic production of SHBG and by suppressing LH, thus inhibiting ovarian androgen production.[11] Testosterone levels are normally maintained at high levels throughout a woman's lifespan by uninterrupted ovarian and adrenal production. This continuous androgenic action may serve as a protective antiproliferative factor for breast tissue. Thus, institution of pharmacologic estrogen therapy at menopause may result in a drastic reduction in the testosterone/estradiol ratio, and increased risk for breast cancer (**Fig. 1**). Studies in ovariectomized rhesus monkeys have shown that the addition of low physiologic doses of testosterone (producing serum levels in the mid-normal range for women as well as rhesus monkeys) to estrogen therapy significantly inhibits HT-induced mammary epithelial proliferation (**Fig. 2**).[4] Additionally, testosterone treatment significantly reduced mammary epithelial ER expression, thus, suggesting a potential mechanism for the growth inhibitory effect. Moreover, treatment of intact cycling monkeys with the AR antagonist flutamide resulted in a significant increase in mammary epithelial proliferation,[4] adding to the burden of evidence that endogenous androgens normally limit mammary proliferation and, hence, cancer risk. Other studies on primates also suggest that inclusion of testosterone with estrogen/progesterone use may counteract breast cell proliferation.[65] In a recent randomized, double-blind, placebo-controlled study, testosterone use inhibited exogenous estrogen-induced breast tissue proliferation in postmenopausal women. There is also evidence that

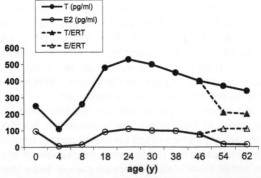

Fig. 1. Average estradiol (E2) and testosterone (T) levels across the female lifespan. Dash lines represent changes in T and E2 levels resulting from hormone therapy beginning at menopause.

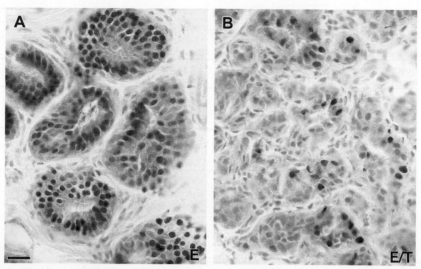

Fig. 2. Mammary epithelial proliferation shown by Ki67 immunoreactivity (*brown dots*) in ovariectomized monkeys treated with estradiol (*A*), and estradiol and testosterone (*B*). Proliferation is increased with estradiol, although this increase is attenuated by the addition of testosterone to estradiol.

testosterone does not influence mammographic breast density like conventional HT, a risk factor for breast cancer.[66,67]

Pertinent to these observations, a prospective study in 508 postmenopausal women in Australia receiving testosterone in addition to usual HT regimen[68] provides important information on this topic. The incidence of breast cancer in testosterone users was substantially less than in women receiving estrogen/progestin in the WHI study and in the Million Woman Study.[69] Breast cancer rates in the testosterone users was closer to that reported for HT never users, and their age-standardization rate was the same as for the general population in South Australia. These observations suggest that the addition of physiologic doses of androgen to OCs and HT could protect the breast from unopposed estrogenic effects.

Men with prostate cancer receiving antiandrogenic treatment present with gynecomastia and are at higher risk for male breast cancer. In the limited population of males-to-female castrated transsexuals that use estrogen/progesterone regiments, several cases of breast cancer have been documented.[70,71] These breast tumor cases presented after relatively short periods after exposure (5–10 years) and at an earlier age at diagnosis.[23] In contrast, no case of hormone-dependent cancer is documented at present for the female-to-male transsexual population.[72]

Women, and particularly postmenopausal women, have been treated with testosterone for female sexual dysfunction for decades. The main safety concern for women who have undergone years of this therapy has been the breast and endometrial cancer risk related to androgens. In a recent trial of 814 sexually hypoactive women, the results for breast cancer risk were inconclusive.[1] Nevertheless, current experience does not confirm a positive correlation between testosterone use and breast cancer occurrence (**Table 1**); thus, androgens can have a place in female sexual dysfunction treatment.

Table 1
Data supporting a protective role of androgens

Androgenic Conditions	Breast-Specific Action
Pubertal androgen excess caused by adrenal tumor or hyperplasia	Suppression of normal breast development
Treatment with exogenous androgens in female athletes and female-to-male transsexuals	Breast atrophy
Normal male androgenic status	Pronounced decrease in breast cancer risk compared with the mean risk of a normal woman (1% of female risk)
Hypoandrogenic status in men 1. Hypogonadism of men with Klinefelter syndrome 2. Antiandrogenic therapy with flutamide in men with prostate cancer 3. Male-to-female castrated transsexuals on estrogen replacement	Increased risk of male breast cancer[53] Gynecomastia (and rarely breast cancer) Breast cancer cases after a short time of exposure to estrogen therapy[70,71]
AR expression in breast cancer tumors	Independent prognostic factor of improved recurrence-free survival[34]
Breast tumors that do not express AR (poor testosterone action on the tumor)	Increased risk of cancer-related death (compared with tumors that express AR); poor prognosis, larger tumor size, and more frequent lymph node metastasis[30,35]
Salivary androgen levels	Statistically significantly decreased in patients with breast cancer compared with controls[40]
Androgen supplementation in estrogen/progesterone therapy in postmenopausal women	1. Inhibition of HT-induced breast tissue proliferation[66,67] 2. Decreased breast cancer incidence in androgen users compared with the established risk ratio of HT[68]
Experimental and Preclinical Observations	
Direct inhibition of breast cancer growth has been observed by AR stimulation[30]	
Indirect inhibition of breast cancer growth via ERα suppression and its related transcriptional activity by AR stimulation[31]	
Androgens may act as promoters of apoptosis[32,64]	
Administration of physiologic doses of androgens to ovariectomized rhesus monkeys, inhibited HT-induced mammary epithelial proliferation[4]	

SUMMARY

Measurement of circulating sex steroids and their metabolites demonstrates that androgen activity is normally abundant in healthy men and women throughout their entire lifetime. Epidemiologic studies investigating testosterone levels and breast cancer risk have major theoretical and methodological limitations and do not provide consensus. The molecular epidemiology of defects in pathways involved in androgen synthesis and activity in breast cancer hold great promise, but investigation of these is still in the early stages. Clinical observations and experimental data indicate that androgens inhibit mammary growth and neoplasia, and they have been used in the past with success to treat breast cancer. It is of concern that current forms of estrogen treatment in OCs and for ovarian failure result in suppression of endogenous androgen activity considering that the addition of testosterone to the HT regimen ameliorates the stimulating effects of estrogen/progestin on the breast. Further research is needed to address the role of androgens in breast cancer prevention and the efficacy and safety of hormonal supplementation.

Mammary gland growth and differentiation is under hormonal regulation, and it is now accepted that estrogens stimulate and androgens inhibit breast growth and proliferation independently of genetic sex. Experimental and molecular data, clinical observations, and epidemiologic studies, although not conclusive, indicate a breast cancer protective effect of androgens. Exposure to exogenous estrogens upsets the normal estrogen/androgen balance and promotes unopposed estrogenic stimulation of proliferation and, hence, breast cancer risk. Further research is needed for the potential preventive role of androgens in breast cancer and the safety of testosterone supplementation.

ACKNOWLEDGMENTS

Thanks to Carolyn Bondy, Aris Antsaklis, Alexandra Tsigginou, and Rebecca Glaser for their support.

REFERENCES

1. Davis SR, Moreau M, Kroll R, et al. Testosterone for low libido in postmenopausal women not taking estrogen. N Engl J Med 2008;359(19):2005–17.
2. North American Menopause Society. The role of testosterone therapy in postmenopausal women: position statement of The North American Menopause Society. Menopause 2005;12(5):496–511 [quiz: 649].
3. Schover LR. Androgen therapy for loss of desire in women: is the benefit worth the breast cancer risk? Fertil Steril 2008;90(1):129–40.
4. Dimitrakakis C, Zhou J, Wang J, et al. A physiologic role for testosterone in limiting estrogenic stimulation of the breast. Menopause 2003;10(4):292–8.
5. Binder G, Iliev DI, Dufke A, et al. Dominant transmission of prepubertal gynecomastia due to serum estrone excess: hormonal, biochemical, and genetic analysis in a large kindred. J Clin Endocrinol Metab 2005;90(1):484–92.
6. Kadlubar F, Berkowitz G, Delongchamp R, et al. The CYP3A4*1B variant is related to the onset of puberty, a known risk factor for the development of breast cancer. Cancer Epidemiol Biomarkers Prev 2003;12(4):327–31.
7. Forsbach G, Guitron-Cantu A, Vazquez-Lara J, et al. Virilizing adrenal adenoma and primary amenorrhea in a girl with adrenal hyperplasia. Arch Gynecol Obstet 2000;263(3):134–6.
8. Karamanakos P, Mitsiades CS, Lembessis P, et al. Male breast adenocarcinoma in a prostate cancer patient following prolonged anti-androgen monotherapy. Anticancer Res 2004;24(2C):1077–81.
9. Braunstein GD. Clinical practice. Gynecomastia. N Engl J Med 2007;357(12): 1229–37.
10. Labrie F. Dehydroepiandrosterone, androgens and the mammary gland. Gynecol Endocrinol 2006;22(3):118–30.
11. Lobo RA. Androgens in postmenopausal women: production, possible role, and replacement options. Obstet Gynecol Surv 2001;56(6):361–76.
12. Labrie F, Belanger A, Simard J, et al. DHEA and peripheral androgen and estrogen formation: intracrinology. Ann N Y Acad Sci 1995;774:16–28.

13. Labrie F, Luu-The V, Lin SX, et al. Intracrinology: role of the family of 17 beta-hydroxysteroid dehydrogenases in human physiology and disease. J Mol Endocrinol 2000;25(1):1–16.
14. Sasano H, Suzuki T, Nakata T, et al. New development in intracrinology of breast carcinoma. Breast Cancer 2006;13(2):129–36.
15. Birrell SN, Bentel JM, Hickey TE, et al. Androgens induce divergent proliferative responses in human breast cancer cell lines. J Steroid Biochem Mol Biol 1995; 52(5):459–67.
16. Suzuki M, Ishida H, Shiotsu Y, et al. Expression level of enzymes related to in situ estrogen synthesis and clinicopathological parameters in breast cancer patients. J Steroid Biochem Mol Biol 2009;113(3–5):195–201.
17. Federman DD. The biology of human sex differences. N Engl J Med 2006; 354(14):1507–14.
18. Zhou J, Anderson K, Bievre M, et al. Primate mammary gland insulin-like growth factor system: cellular localization and regulation by sex steroids. J Investig Med 2001;49(1):47–55.
19. Park JJ, Irvine RA, Buchanan G, et al. Breast cancer susceptibility gene 1 (BRCAI) is a coactivator of the androgen receptor. Cancer Res 2000;60(21): 5946–9.
20. Spurdle AB, Antoniou AC, Duffy DL, et al. The androgen receptor CAG repeat polymorphism and modification of breast cancer risk in BRCA1 and BRCA2 mutation carriers. Breast Cancer Res 2005;7(2):R176–83.
21. Avila DM, Zoppi S, McPhaul MJ. The androgen receptor (AR) in syndromes of androgen insensitivity and in prostate cancer. J Steroid Biochem Mol Biol 2001; 76(1–5):135–42.
22. MARIE-GENICA Consortium on Genetic Susceptibility for Menopausal Hormone Therapy Related Breast Cancer Risk. Polymorphisms in genes of the steroid receptor superfamily modify postmenopausal breast cancer risk associated with menopausal hormone therapy. Int J Cancer 2010;126(12): 2935–46.
23. Weiss JR, Moysich KB, Swede H. Epidemiology of male breast cancer. Cancer Epidemiol Biomarkers Prev 2005;14(1):20–6.
24. Cox DG, Blanche H, Pearce CL, et al. A comprehensive analysis of the androgen receptor gene and risk of breast cancer: results from the National Cancer Institute Breast and Prostate Cancer Cohort Consortium (BPC3). Breast Cancer Res 2006; 8(5):R54.
25. Haiman CA, Brown M, Hankinson SE, et al. The androgen receptor CAG repeat polymorphism and risk of breast cancer in the Nurses' Health Study. Cancer Res 2002;62(4):1045–9.
26. Giguere Y, Dewailly E, Brisson J, et al. Short polyglutamine tracts in the androgen receptor are protective against breast cancer in the general population. Cancer Res 2001;61(15):5869–74.
27. Westberg L, Baghaei F, Rosmond R, et al. Polymorphisms of the androgen receptor gene and the estrogen receptor beta gene are associated with androgen levels in women. J Clin Endocrinol Metab 2001;86(6):2562–8.
28. MacLean HE, Brown RW, Beilin J, et al. Increased frequency of long androgen receptor CAG repeats in male breast cancers. Breast Cancer Res Treat 2004; 88(3):239–46.
29. Lillie EO, Bernstein L, Ingles SA, et al. Polymorphism in the androgen receptor and mammographic density in women taking and not taking estrogen and progestin therapy. Cancer Res 2004;64(4):1237–41.

30. Peters AA, Buchanan G, Ricciardelli C, et al. Androgen receptor inhibits estrogen receptor-alpha activity and is prognostic in breast cancer. Cancer Res 2009; 69(15):6131–40.
31. Lanzino M, De Amicis F, McPhaul MJ, et al. Endogenous coactivator ARA70 interacts with estrogen receptor alpha (ERalpha) and modulates the functional ERalpha/androgen receptor interplay in MCF-7 cells. J Biol Chem 2005;280(21): 20421–30.
32. Kandouz M, Lombet A, Perrot JY, et al. Proapoptotic effects of antiestrogens, progestins and androgen in breast cancer cells. J Steroid Biochem Mol Biol 1999;69(1–6):463–71.
33. Nicolas Diaz-Chico B, German Rodriguez F, Gonzalez A, et al. Androgens and androgen receptors in breast cancer. J Steroid Biochem Mol Biol 2007; 105(1–5):1–15.
34. Niemeier LA, Dabbs DJ, Beriwal S, et al. Androgen receptor in breast cancer: expression in estrogen receptor-positive tumors and in estrogen receptor-negative tumors with apocrine differentiation. Mod Pathol 2010;23(2):205–12.
35. Ogawa Y, Hai E, Matsumoto K, et al. Androgen receptor expression in breast cancer: relationship with clinicopathological factors and biomarkers. Int J Clin Oncol 2008;13(5):431–5.
36. Yager JD, Davidson NE. Estrogen carcinogenesis in breast cancer. N Engl J Med 2006;354(3):270–82.
37. Bulbrook RD, Thomas BS, Utsunomiya J, et al. The urinary excretion of 11-deoxy-17-oxosteroids and 17-hydroxycorticosteroids by normal Japanese and British women. J Endocrinol 1967;38(4):401–6.
38. Page JH, Colditz GA, Rifai N, et al. Plasma adrenal androgens and risk of breast cancer in premenopausal women. Cancer Epidemiol Biomarkers Prev 2004; 13(6):1032–6.
39. Eliassen AH, Missmer SA, Tworoger SS, et al. Endogenous steroid hormone concentrations and risk of breast cancer among premenopausal women. J Natl Cancer Inst 2006;98(19):1406–15.
40. Dimitrakakis C, Zava D, Marinopoulos S, et al. Low salivary testosterone levels in patients with breast cancer. BMC Cancer 2010;10:57.
41. Tworoger SS, Missmer SA, Eliassen AH, et al. The association of plasma DHEA and DHEA sulfate with breast cancer risk in predominantly premenopausal women. Cancer Epidemiol Biomarkers Prev 2006;15(5):967–71.
42. Olson JE, Ingle JN, Ma CX, et al. A comprehensive examination of CYP19 variation and risk of breast cancer using two haplotype-tagging approaches. Breast Cancer Res Treat 2007;102(2):237–47.
43. Key T, Appleby P, Barnes I, et al. Endogenous sex hormones and breast cancer in postmenopausal women: reanalysis of nine prospective studies. J Natl Cancer Inst 2002;94(8):606–16.
44. Rosner W, Auchus RJ, Azziz R, et al. Position statement: utility, limitations, and pitfalls in measuring testosterone: an Endocrine Society position statement. J Clin Endocrinol Metab 2007;92(2):405–13.
45. Schairer C, Hill D, Sturgeon SR, et al. Serum concentrations of estrogens, sex hormone binding globulin, and androgens and risk of breast hyperplasia in postmenopausal women. Cancer Epidemiol Biomarkers Prev 2005;14(7): 1660–5.
46. Key TJ, Appleby PN, Reeves GK, et al. Body mass index, serum sex hormones, and breast cancer risk in postmenopausal women. J Natl Cancer Inst 2003; 95(16):1218–26.

47. Schmitt M, Klinga K, Schnarr B, et al. Dehydroepiandrosterone stimulates proliferation and gene expression in MCF-7 cells after conversion to estradiol. Mol Cell Endocrinol 2001;173(1–2):1–13.
48. Adly L, Hill D, Sherman ME, et al. Serum concentrations of estrogens, sex hormone-binding globulin, and androgens and risk of breast cancer in postmenopausal women. Int J Cancer 2006;119(10):2402–7.
49. Beattie MS, Costantino JP, Cummings SR, et al. Endogenous sex hormones, breast cancer risk, and tamoxifen response: an ancillary study in the NSABP Breast Cancer Prevention Trial (P-1). J Natl Cancer Inst 2006;98(2):110–5.
50. Gadducci A, Gargini A, Palla E, et al. Polycystic ovary syndrome and gynecological cancers: is there a link? Gynecol Endocrinol 2005;20(4):200–8.
51. Swerdlow AJ, Schoemaker MJ, Higgins CD, et al. Cancer incidence and mortality in men with Klinefelter syndrome: a cohort study. J Natl Cancer Inst 2005;97(16): 1204–10.
52. Hultborn R, Hanson C, Kopf I, et al. Prevalence of Klinefelter's syndrome in male breast cancer patients. Anticancer Res 1997;17(6D):4293–7.
53. Giordano SH, Buzdar AU, Hortobagyi GN. Breast cancer in men. Ann Intern Med 2002;137(8):678–87.
54. Brinton LA, Richesson DA, Gierach GL, et al. Prospective evaluation of risk factors for male breast cancer. J Natl Cancer Inst 2008;100(20):1477–81.
55. Johnson KC, Pan S, Mao Y. Risk factors for male breast cancer in Canada, 1994-1998. Eur J Cancer Prev 2002;11(3):253–63.
56. Bulbrook RD, Thomas BS. Hormones are ambiguous risk factors for breast cancer. Acta Oncol 1989;28(6):841–7.
57. Breast cancer and hormonal contraceptives: collaborative reanalysis of individual data on 53 297 women with breast cancer and 100 239 women without breast cancer from 54 epidemiological studies. Collaborative Group on Hormonal Factors in Breast Cancer. Lancet 1996;347(9017):1713–27.
58. Marchbanks PA, McDonald JA, Wilson HG, et al. Oral contraceptives and the risk of breast cancer. N Engl J Med 2002;346(26):2025–32.
59. Kahlenborn C, Modugno F, Potter DM, et al. Oral contraceptive use as a risk factor for premenopausal breast cancer: a meta-analysis. Mayo Clin Proc 2006; 81(10):1290–302.
60. Rossouw JE, Anderson GL, Prentice RL, et al. Risks and benefits of estrogen plus progestin in healthy postmenopausal women: principal results From the Women's Health Initiative randomized controlled trial. JAMA 2002;288(3):321–33.
61. Anderson GL, Limacher M, Assaf AR, et al. Effects of conjugated equine estrogen in postmenopausal women with hysterectomy: the Women's Health Initiative randomized controlled trial. JAMA 2004;291(14):1701–12.
62. Ness RB, Albano JD, McTiernan A, et al. Influence of estrogen plus testosterone supplementation on breast cancer. Arch Intern Med 2009;169(1):41–6.
63. Tamimi RM, Hankinson SE, Chen WY, et al. Combined estrogen and testosterone use and risk of breast cancer in postmenopausal women. Arch Intern Med 2006; 166(14):1483–9.
64. Nahleh Z. Androgen receptor as a target for the treatment of hormone receptor-negative breast cancer: an unchartered territory. Future Oncol 2008;4(1):15–21.
65. Somboonporn W, Davis SR. Testosterone effects on the breast: implications for testosterone therapy for women. Endocr Rev 2004;25(3):374–88.
66. Hofling M, Hirschberg AL, Skoog L, et al. Testosterone inhibits estrogen/progestogen-induced breast cell proliferation in postmenopausal women. Menopause 2007;14(2):183–90.

67. Conner P. Breast response to menopausal hormone therapy–aspects on proliferation, apoptosis and mammographic density. Ann Med 2007;39(1):28–41.
68. Dimitrakakis C, Jones RA, Liu A, et al. Breast cancer incidence in postmenopausal women using testosterone in addition to usual hormone therapy. Menopause 2004;11(5):531–5.
69. Beral V. Breast cancer and hormone-replacement therapy in the Million Women Study. Lancet 2003;362(9382):419–27.
70. Pritchard TJ, Pankowsky DA, Crowe JP, ct al. Breast cancer in a male-to-female transsexual. A case report. JAMA 1988;259(15):2278–80.
71. Ganly I, Taylor EW. Breast cancer in a trans-sexual man receiving hormone replacement therapy. Br J Surg 1995;82(3):341.
72. Mueller A, Gooren L. Hormone-related tumors in transsexuals receiving treatment with cross-sex hormones. Eur J Endocrinol 2008;159(3):197–202.

Management of Bone Disease in Patients Undergoing Hormonal Therapy for Breast Cancer

Faryal Sardar Ali Mirza, MD

KEYWORDS

- Aromatase inhibitors • Breast cancer • Bone • Osteoporosis
- Bisphosphonates

Estrogen deficiency at menopause is associated with increased risk of bone loss and osteoporosis. Tamoxifen had been the mainstay of treatment for hormone-sensitive breast cancer in postmenopausal women for many years. Aromatase inhibitors (AIs) are increasingly being used for the treatment of postmenopausal hormone-sensitive breast cancer because of better disease-free survival compared with tamoxifen seen in clinical trials with AIs. AIs cause a significant decline in circulating estradiol levels and further exacerbate the risk of osteoporosis in postmenopausal women.

The purpose of this article is to review the effect of endocrine therapies of breast cancer on bone, and the management of bone disease with these endocrine therapies. In view of space limitations, the effect of these therapies on bone mineral density (BMD) and bone turnover along with possible interventions are discussed. AIs in particular are also associated with skeletal-related events, which are not discussed here.

TAMOXIFEN AND BONE

Tamoxifen is a selective estrogen receptor (ER) modulator that has estrogen-antagonistic effects on the breast tissue and has estrogen-agonistic effects at most of the other sites including bone.[1,2] Tamoxifen treatment causes a decrease in bone resorption in postmenopausal women with low endogenous estrogen levels, acting as an estrogen agonist. In premenopausal women with higher estrogen levels, it competes with the more potent 17β-estradiol for the ER and results in bone loss.[3]

Financial disclosures: None.

Division of Endocrinology, University of Connecticut Health Center, 263 Farmington Avenue, Mc5456, Farmington, CT 06030, USA

E-mail address: fmirza@uchc.edu

Endocrinol Metab Clin N Am 40 (2011) 549–562

doi:10.1016/j.ecl.2011.05.008

The effect of tamoxifen based on the menstrual status was evaluated by Vehmanen and colleagues,[4] who followed premenopausal women with breast cancer, treated with chemotherapy. These investigators compared ER-positive women on tamoxifen after chemotherapy with ER-negative women who received only chemotherapy. They found a significant bone loss of −4.6% in the lumbar spine (LS) BMD (P<.0001) in tamoxifen-treated patients who continued to menstruate after chemotherapy at 3 years of follow-up, compared with a modest gain of +0.6% in the control group. In contrast, tamoxifen-treated women who developed chemotherapy-induced early menopause had less bone loss at the LS than amennorheic controls (−6.8% and −9.5%, respectively), although both of these groups had a greater decline in BMD compared with menstruating women.

In a review of 27 peer-reviewed articles to evaluate the relationship between tamoxifen and bone health, Ding and colleagues[5] reported that most studies found a protective effect of tamoxifen therapy on BMD at spine and hip compared with no treatment in postmenopausal women with early-stage breast cancer. In the bone substudy of the Anastrozole, Tamoxifen, Alone or in Combination (ATAC) trial, the tamoxifen group showed an increase in median BMD over the 5-year period (LS, +2.77%; total hip [TH], +0.74%), which occurred in the first 2 years; no additional increase was seen in years 2 to 5.[6] When given in combination with chemotherapy, tamoxifen partially prevented or reversed the bone loss resulting from chemotherapy. These investigators did not find a protective effect of tamoxifen on fracture incidence. In a large randomized controlled trial (N = 1716) directly investigating femoral fractures in postmenopausal patients with breast cancer treated with tamoxifen for 1 year, Kristensen and colleagues[7] found a higher incidence of fractures in the tamoxifen group compared with patients not receiving tamoxifen. Overall, in postmenopausal women with early stage breast cancer, tamoxifen use has been associated with an increase in BMD.

AIs AND BONE

Aromatase is a cytochrome p450 enzyme that catalyzes the conversion of androgens to estrogens. It is the rate-limiting step for estrogen production in postmenopausal women. The aromatase enzyme is expressed in adipose tissue, muscle, brain, breast, and bone, and the estradiol made at these sites contributes to the circulating estradiol in postmenopausal women. The AIs may affect bone metabolism via systemic estrogen suppression as well as inhibition of local estrogen production in the bone microenvironment, resulting in bone loss.

The third-generation inhibitors anastrozole, letrozole, and exemestane are specific for the aromatase enzyme and are 100-fold to 10,000-fold more potent compared with the first-generation nonselective inhibitor aminoglutethimide. Based on their mechanism of action, AIs are described as nonsteroidal or competitive inhibitors (letrozole and anastrozole) or inactivators or steroidal inhibitors (exemestane, formestane). The competitive inhibitors are imidizole-based compounds that reversibly bind to the active moiety of the cytochrome P450 enzyme aromatase and block estradiol formation. The inactivators bind covalently and irreversibly to the active site of the enzyme, causing loss of enzymatic activity and requiring more enzyme to be synthesized to resume estradiol synthesis. Three third-generation AIs (anastrozole, letrozole, and exemestane) are currently approved by the US Food and Drug Administration for treatment of breast cancer and are comparable in their suppression of the aromatase enzyme, with letrozole being the most potent. These agents are therefore being used for endocrine therapy for ER-positive breast cancer.

EFFECT OF AIs ON BONE
Studies of Healthy Women

Few studies have evaluated the effects of AIs on bone in healthy postmenopausal women. In a randomized, single-blind, placebo-controlled exploratory study, Goss and colleagues[8] evaluated the effect of AIs (anastrozole, letrozole, exemestane, or placebo) on markers of bone turnover in healthy postmenopausal women over 24 weeks. These investigators found a comparable reduction in plasma estrogen levels and increase in bone-resorption markers with all AIs. McCloskey and colleagues[9] also compared the 3 AIs in healthy postmenopausal women and found that serum β C-terminal cross-linking telopeptide of type I collagen (CTX) increased significantly after 24 weeks of all AIs, with statistically similar changes observed in all 3 groups. Heshmati and colleagues[10] compared the effect of letrozole with placebo on bone turnover markers in healthy postmenopausal women and found that letrozole reduced serum estrone and estradiol to near undetectable levels ($P<.0001$). It also caused a significant increase in bone resorption markers (urine pyridinoline and deoxypyridinoline) and significantly decreased serum parathyroid hormone levels. There were no significant changes in the bone formation markers.

There are 2 large, ongoing randomized trials evaluating the use of AIs for prevention of breast cancer in healthy postmenopausal women. The Second International Breast Cancer Intervention Study (IBIS-II) is comparing anastrozole with placebo in postmenopausal women at increased risk for breast cancer and women with ductal carcinoma in situ.[11] It has a bone substudy in which 400 women with a T score between −2.5 and −1.5 will be randomized to take a bisphosphonate (BP) or placebo. The National Cancer Institute of Canada Clinical Trials Group MAP3 study (Mammary Prevention 3) (ExCeL) is comparing exemestane with placebo in reducing the incidence of invasive breast cancer in postmenopausal women at an increased risk for developing breast cancer.[12] BMD will be followed in this study to help provide information regarding the true effects of AIs on bone health in otherwise healthy postmenopausal women.

Data on Postmenopausal Women

Because of concerns about increased risk for osteoporosis associated with endocrine therapy for breast cancer in postmenopausal women, most of the clinical trials of AIs and tamoxifen have had subprotocols evaluating their effects on BMD. The data on the changes in BMD are usually easy to interpret when AIs are used as monotherapy and compared with tamoxifen, but are difficult to interpret when the 2 agents are used as sequential therapy.

AIs AS FIRST-LINE THERAPY FOR BREAST CANCER COMPARED WITH TAMOXIFEN
Anastrozole

Anastrozole was evaluated for its efficacy in breast cancer compared with tamoxifen in the ATAC trial, which randomized 9366 postmenopausal women with early stage breast cancer to receive anastrozole, tamoxifen, or a combination of the two. The combination arm was terminated at 33 months. A bone subprotocol within the main trial assessed and quantified the changes in BMD among 308 women receiving anastrozole compared with tamoxifen for the duration of trial. In the anastrozole group, there was a decrease in median BMD over 5 years both at LS and TH (−6.08% and −7.24%), whereas the tamoxifen group showed an increase in LS and TH (+2.77% and +0.74%). This increase occurred in the first 2 years and no additional increase was seen in years 2 to 5.[6] The differences between treatment groups were highly significant at both sites (P<.0001). The control group had a median change in BMD of +1.35% at the LS and −2.97% at the TH over 5 years. Anastrozole was associated with a significantly higher frequency of musculoskeletal symptoms and fractures.[13] The overall incidence of fractures in the anastrozole group was 11% compared with 7.7% with tamoxifen (P<.0001). There were significantly more vertebral fractures in the anastrozole group (1.5% vs 0.9%, P = .03), with no significant increase in the incidence of hip fractures.[14]

Letrozole

Letrozole is being compared with tamoxifen in the Breast International Group (BIG) 1-98 study, which is a randomized, phase 3, double-blind trial comparing 5 years of treatment with letrozole with tamoxifen as letrozole alone, tamoxifen alone, letrozole followed by tamoxifen, and tamoxifen followed by letrozole.[15] The incidence of bone fractures has been reported and was higher among patients treated with letrozole compared with tamoxifen (9.3% vs 6.5%), although the difference did not reach statistical significance. The incidence of multiple fractures while on treatment was also higher among patients treated with letrozole compared with tamoxifen (0.9% vs 0.4%). Statistically significant risk factors that contributed to fractures during treatment included age, smoking history, osteoporosis at baseline, prior fracture history, and previous hormone replacement therapy.

Exemestane

The Tamoxifen Exemestane Adjuvant Multicenter trial[16] is a phase III, randomized, parallel-group, multicenter trial designed to compare the disease-free survival after 5 years of adjuvant exemestane versus 2.5 years of tamoxifen followed by 2.5 years of exemestane among postmenopausal women with early breast cancer. Results of the bone substudy evaluating BMD[17] in 167 patients who have completed baseline, 12 and 24 months of the study have been reported. After 12 and 24 months of treatment, patients treated with exemestane showed significantly more bone loss at the spine (P = .002 and P = .02, respectively) compared with patients treated with tamoxifen.

Lonning and colleagues[18] evaluated the effect of exemestane on BMD compared with placebo in 147 postmenopausal women with early breast cancer in a randomized double-blind trial. At 2 years, their results show that exemestane significantly increased the mean annual rate of BMD loss at the hip (P = .024) but not at the spine. A total of 21% of patients with osteopenia of the spine at baseline and 11% with osteopenia of the hip became osteoporotic with exemestane treatment.

AIs AFTER 2 TO 3 YEARS OF TAMOXIFEN VERSUS TAMOXIFEN ALONE

Recently the third-generation AIs have proved their efficacy and tolerability compared with tamoxifen in the adjuvant treatment of women with hormone-responsive early breast cancer. Sequential therapies with AIs and tamoxifen are currently evaluating the best sequence of these medications for improved outcome. The effect of AIs on BMD and bone turnover markers may be influenced by previous tamoxifen treatment.

Anastrozole

The Austrian Breast and Colorectal Study Group (ABCSG) 8/Arimidex-Nolvadex (ARNO) 95 study[19] is a prospective combined analysis of 2 trials in which sequential treatment with anastrozole after 2 years of tamoxifen was compared with tamoxifen alone. After a median follow-up of 28 months, there were significantly more clinical fractures in patients who switched to anastrozole than in those who received only tamoxifen (2% vs 1% respectively; P = .015). The clinical fracture rate in the anastrozole group was lower than that seen at a similar point in the ATAC trial, suggesting that previous treatment with tamoxifen may have conferred some benefit.

Letrozole

In the BIG 1-98 trial,[15] the incidence of fractures was highest among women assigned to letrozole monotherapy and lowest among women assigned to tamoxifen monotherapy (P = .02). The incidence of fractures among women assigned to tamoxifen followed by letrozole was similar to that among women assigned to letrozole alone (9.4% and 9.8%, respectively), and the incidence of fractures in the group assigned to letrozole followed by tamoxifen was similar to that among women assigned to tamoxifen alone (7.5% and 7.3%, respectively). This protective effect of tamoxifen on bone when used after AI needs to be evaluated further in other studies.

Exemestane

Gonneli and colleagues[20] compared the effects of the steroidal aromatase inactivator exemestane on bone turnover markers and on BMD in 70 postmenopausal women (62.0 ± 8.9 years) with completely resected breast cancer and who were disease-free after 2 to 3 years on tamoxifen. The subjects were randomly assigned to continue tamoxifen or switch to exemestane. There was a progressive decline in BMD at the LS (−2.37%, P<.05 at 12 months and −2.99%, P<.01 at 24 months) and at the femoral neck (FN) (−1.24%, −1.61% and −1.92% at months 12, 18, and 24, respectively, P<.05 at months 18 and 24) in patients switched to exemestane, with no significant changes in the patients who continued tamoxifen. The bone turnover markers showed a significant increase in the exemestane group compared with tamoxifen at 6 and 9 months for CTX and bone specific alkaline phosphatase (B-ALP) respectively.

The Intergroup Exemestane Study (IES) compared tamoxifen for 5 years with tamoxifen for 2 to 3 years followed by exemestane for a total of 5 years (N = 4724) in postmenopausal women.[21] Results from 206 women in the bone substudy have been reported by Coleman and colleagues.[22] Within 6 months of switching to exemestane, there was a decline in the BMD by 2.7% (P<.0001) at the LS and 1.4% (P<.0001) at the TH compared with baseline and a further 1.0% (P = .002) in year 2 at the LS and 0.8% (0.3–1.4; P = .003) at the TH, respectively. Bone resorption and formation markers increased at all time points in women receiving exemestane (P<.001). At a median follow-up of 58 months in all IES participants (n = 4274) the reported fractures were 7% and 5% of patients in the exemestane and tamoxifen groups, respectively (odds ratio 1.45 [1.13–1.87]; P = .003).

AIs VERSUS PLACEBO AFTER TAMOXIFEN FOR 5 YEARS
Letrozole

The National Cancer Institute of Canada Clinical Trials Group (NCIC CTG) study (MA.17) compared letrozole with placebo after 5 years of standard adjuvant tamoxifen.[23,24] Eligible women had a baseline BMD T score of at least −2.0 in either the hip or L2 to L4 spine; all received calcium 500 mg and vitamin D 400 U daily. Change in BMD (L2–L4 spine and hip) at 12 and 24 months and in markers of bone formation (serum B-ALP) and resorption (serum CTX) and urine N-telopeptide (NTX) at 6, 12, and 24 months were compared.[24] Two hundred and twenty-six patients (122 letrozole, 104 placebo) were enrolled. Baseline characteristics were similar in the 2 groups, including BMD, median age of 60.7 years (81% <70 years), and median follow-up of 1.6 years. At 24 months, patients receiving letrozole had a significant decrease in TH BMD (−3.6% vs −0.71%; P = .044) and LS BMD (−5.35% vs −0.70%; P = .008). Letrozole increased urine NTX at 6, 12, and 24 months (P = .054, < .001, and .016, respectively). More women became osteoporotic by BMD while receiving letrozole (4.1% vs 0%; P = .064). There were also more clinical fractures in the letrozole group compared with placebo, although the difference was not significant (3.6% vs 2.9%, respectively; P = .24). MA.17B was the bone subprotocol in which a total of 226 patients were randomly assigned into the study (122 to letrozole and 104 to placebo). At 24 months, patients receiving letrozole had a significant decrease in TH (−3.6% vs −0.71%; P = .044) and LS BMD (−5.35% vs −0.70%; P = .008) and an increase in urine NTX at 6, 12, and 24 months (P = .054, <.001, and .016, respectively). At the LS (L2–L4), more women receiving letrozole became osteoporotic by BMD (4.1% vs 0%; P = .064).

These studies show that AIs, whether used in otherwise healthy women or for the treatment of breast cancer as first-line therapy, sequential therapy, or after 5 years of tamoxifen result in an increase in bone turnover markers and a decrease in BMD, likely related to lowering of estradiol levels. Hence they increase the risk for developing osteoporosis in a population already at increased risk of osteoporosis because of lower endogenous estradiol levels due to menopause.

BPs AND PREVENTION OF BONE LOSS WITH BREAST CANCER TREATMENT

BPs are potent inhibitors of osteoclasts. They act on the bone through several different mechanisms, including induction of osteoclast apoptosis, inhibition of osteoclast maturation and differentiation, and reduced osteoclast activity.[25] They are also used for prevention and treatment of metastatic bone disease.

Prevention and Treatment of Bone Loss in Breast Cancer

Estrogen has a positive influence on bone metabolism and mediates its effects via production of several cytokines that inhibit osteoclastogenesis and increase osteoclast apoptosis.[26,27] Endocrine therapy for breast cancer with AIs causes depletion of estrogen, resulting in increased bone resorption, increased risk for fractures, and osteoporosis.[28] Therefore, use of these therapies mandates increased vigilance for monitoring of BMD in this population. There are several studies that have evaluated the role of BPs in the prevention of AI-associated bone loss (AIBL).

Gasser and colleagues[29] evaluated the effects of the BP zoledronic acid (ZA) on BMD and bone strength in rats treated with the AI, letrozole. These investigators found that treatment of rats with daily letrozole (1 mg/kg) induced significant bone loss and cortical thinning compared with control animals (P<.01). Treatment with ZA protected against letrozole-induced bone loss and cortical thinning in a dose-dependent manner, with the highest dose group (20 μg/kg) having BMD values that were not significantly different from the controls over the 24-week study period.[29]

In humans, oral BPs (risedronate and ibandronate) and intravenous ZA have been evaluated for their efficacy in preventing AIBL. BPs are potent inhibitors of osteoclastic activity and therefore counteract the estrogen deficiency-induced osteoclastic stimulation seen with AI therapy. Both oral and intravenous BPs have been evaluated for their effectiveness in the prevention of AIBL.

Oral BPs and AI-induced Bone Loss

Several studies have evaluated oral risedronate and ibandronate as to their efficacy in the prevention of AIBL. The SABRE (Study of Anastrozole with the Bisphosphonate

RisedronatE) trial[30] assigned postmenopausal women with hormone receptor-positive early breast cancer receiving anastrozole to 1 of 3 treatment groups based on their risk of fragility fractures. The highest-risk group received risedronate 35 mg/wk orally, the moderate-risk group received risedronate or placebo in a double-blind manner, and the low-risk group did not receive risedronate. LS and TH BMD were assessed at baseline, 12 months, and 24 months. At 24 months, treatment with risedronate in the moderate-risk group resulted in a significant increase in BMD at the LS and TH compared with placebo (2.2% vs −1.8%; $P<.0001$; and 1.8% vs −1.1%; $P<.0001$, respectively). In the high-risk group, LS and TH BMD increased significantly (3.0%; $P = .0006$; and 2.0%; $P = .0104$, respectively). Patients in the low-risk group showed a significant decrease in LS BMD (−2.1%; $P = .01$) and a nonsignificant decrease in TH BMD (−0.4%; $P = .60$). These findings show that risedronate was effective in preventing and treating osteoporosis in postmenopausal women at risk of fragility fracture who were receiving adjuvant anastrozole for early breast cancer.

Markopoulos and colleagues[31] have also reported on the effect of risedronate on BMD in postmenopausal with early breast cancer receiving anastrozole in a similar study design with BMD assessment at 12 and 24 months. At 24 months, in the moderate-risk group, treatment with risedronate resulted in a significant increase in BMD at LS and TH compared with the nonrisedronate group (5.7% vs −1.5%, Wilcoxon test $P = .006$, and 1.6% vs −3.9% Wilcoxon test $P = .037$, respectively). In the high-risk group, a significant increase at LS was detected both at 12 and 24 months (6.3% and 6.6%, $P<.001$) but not at TH. In the low-risk group without risedronate, a significant decrease was seen at 12 months for LS and HP (−5.3% $P<.001$ and −2.4% $P<.001$, respectively,); at 24 months, a significant decrease of BMD was detected only for LS (−2.5%, $P<.001$). Twenty-two percent of patients became osteopenic and only 4% became osteoporotic.

Yonehara and colleagues[32] have also evaluated the prevention of AIBL by risedronate administration in postmenopausal women with breast cancer. These investigators compared 17 postmenopausal women with breast cancer receiving anastrozole 1 mg/d with 10 women receiving anastrozole and risedronate sodium, 2.5 mg daily for 6 months. They found that in the anastrozole-only group, BMD, T scores and Z scores significantly decreased from the baseline during the 6-month therapy period ($P<.05$), with a mean decrease of 2.5% in the L2 to L4 BMD. In the anastrozole + risedronate group, the BMD increased, with a mean increase of 4.5% at the LS ($P<.01$).

In a prospective open cohort study of 118 postmenopausal women treated with anastrozole for an early hormone-dependent breast cancer, Confavreux and colleagues[33] evaluated bone turnover markers and change in BMD. Women without osteoporosis were not treated and compared with an age-matched control group of 114 healthy women. Osteoporotic patients (T score ≤2.5 standard deviation) received weekly risedronate. BMD and the bone turnover markers including serum osteocaloin and serum CTX were measured at baseline and 1 year later. At 1 year, the anastrozole group had a decline in BMD by −3.3% at the spine and −2.8% at the hip compared with controls ($P<.0001$). There was a significant increase in osteocalcin (+36.6%, $P<.0001$) and CTX (+34%, $P<.0001$). In osteoporotic women treated simultaneously with anastrozole and risedronate, bone loss was prevented at the hip, and BMD increased significantly at the spine by 4.1 % ($P = .008$). Bone turnover marker showed a significant decrease for both osteocalcin and CTX, indicating that risedronate prevented the anastrozole-induced bone loss in this group.

Lester and colleagues[34] evaluated the effectiveness of oral ibandronate in preventing anastrozole-induced bone loss in the ARIBON (effect of oral ibandronate on anastrozole-induced bone loss) trial. This was a double-blind, randomized, placebo-controlled study in which 131 postmenopausal, surgically treated women with early breast cancer were initiated on anastrozole therapy, besides being started on calcium and vitamin D supplementation. Of these patients, 50 had osteopenia (T score −1.0 to −2.5) at either the hip or LS, who were randomized to receive either treatment with ibandronate 150 mg orally every month or placebo. After 2 years, osteopenic patients treated with ibandronate gained BMD at the LS and TH (+2.98% and +0.60% respectively). However, patients treated with placebo lost −3.22% at the LS and −3.90% at the TH. The differences between the 2 treatment arms were statistically significant at both sites ($P<.01$). These investigators also reported an increase in urinary NTX and serum CTX levels at 12 months in the placebo group (40.3%, 34.9%, and 37.0%, respectively) and decline in the ibandronate group (30.9%, 26.3%, and 22.8%, respectively). The investigators concluded that monthly oral ibandronate improves BMD and normalizes bone turnover in patients treated with anastrozole.

The Zometa-Femara Adjuvant Synergy Trial (Z-FAST)[35] was designed to evaluate if the addition of ZA to adjuvant letrozole therapy protects against AI-induced bone loss in postmenopausal women. This is a multicenter study in which postmenopausal women with early hormone receptor-positive breast cancer receiving adjuvant letrozole were randomized to receive upfront or delayed-start ZA (4 mg intravenously every 6 months) for 5 years. Delayed-start ZA was administered if the LS or TH T score decreased below −2.0 or a nontraumatic fracture occurred. The primary end point was to compare the change from baseline in LS BMD between groups at 12 months. Secondary end points, measured at other predetermined time points, included comparing changes in TH BMD, LS BMD, and markers of bone turnover, fracture incidence, and time to disease recurrence.[36] A total of 301 patients were randomized to each group. At 36 months, the absolute difference in mean LS and TH BMDs between the upfront and delayed groups was 6.7% and 5.2%, respectively ($P<.0001$ for both). Although this study was not designed to show antifracture efficacy, the incidence of fractures was slightly higher in the delayed group (17 [5.7%] vs 19 [6.3%] fractures in the upfront and delayed groups) but not statistically significant ($P = .86$). Pyrexia (27 [9%] vs 6 [2%]; $P = .0002$) and bone pain (39 [13%] vs 20 [6.7%]; $P = .01$) were more common in upfront patients; cough (13 [4.3%] vs 27 [9%]; $P = .03$) was more common in delayed patients. No severe renal dysfunction or confirmed cases of osteonecrosis of the jaw were reported. Disease recurrence was reported in 9 upfront (3.0%) and 16 delayed (5.3%) patients (Kaplan-Meier analysis, $P = .127$), with an absolute decrease of 2.3%. These investigators concluded that ZA effectively prevented AIBL in postmenopausal women with early breast cancer.

Bundred and colleagues[37] have also reported their results from the international ZO-FAST trial on the use of ZA as adjuvant endocrine therapy in postmenopausal women with breast cancer. These investigators randomized 1065 patients who were receiving adjuvant letrozole to immediate-start or delayed-start ZA (4 mg intravenously biannually for 5 years). The delayed group received ZA if LS or TH T score decreased less than −2.0 or when a nontraumatic fracture occurred. The primary end point was change in LS BMD at 12 months. Secondary end points included changes in TH BMD, serum bone turnover markers, and safety at 12 months. At 36 months, the mean change in LS BMD was +4.39% for immediate versus −4.9% for delayed ZA ($P<.0001$). Between-group differences for LS were 5.27% at 12 months, 7.94% at 24 months, and 9.29% at 36 months ($P<.0001$ for all).[38] Mean changes in TH BMD were smaller but similar ($P<.0001$ for each comparison). Among patients with baseline L2 to L4 T scores between −2.0 and −1.0, many immediate-ZA patients but relatively few delayed-ZA patients transitioned to normal BMD (T score >−1.0). Conversely, relatively few immediate-ZA patients ($\leq$1.4% at each time point) but more delayed-ZA patients ($\sim$14%) at month 36 had severe osteopenia/osteoporosis (T score <−2.0), despite ZA initiation in some delayed-ZA patients. Between-group differences were statistically significant (P<.001) at each postbaseline assessment. Similarly, among patients with normal baseline BMD, more maintained T scores greater than −1.0 at 36 months in the immediate-ZA versus delayed-ZA groups (61% vs 43.8%, respectively). Both regimens were well tolerated, with few serious adverse events. Bone pain was higher in the immediate group and some patients experienced acute-phase reactions after ZA infusion.

In an integrated analysis of pooled data from the Z-FAST and ZO-FAST trials that had similar study designs,[37] data on 1667 postmenopausal women were evaluated. The LS BMD increased by 5.2% in the upfront group than in the delayed group and TH BMD was 3.5% higher. NTX and BSAP decreased by 21.3% and 12.8% in the upfront group and increased by 21.7% and 24.9% in the delayed group, respectively (P<.0001). Fewer patients receiving upfront ZA experienced disease recurrence than patients in the delayed group (7 patients [0.84%] vs 17 patients [1.9%], P = .0401). Fracture rates were similar in the 2 groups. No confirmed osteonecrosis of the jaw was reported. The results of this analysis strengthen the statistical validity of the preliminary results of the Z-FAST and ZO-FAST studies, showing that upfront ZA prevents AIBL more effectively than delayed-start ZA in postmenopausal women with early-stage breast cancer receiving letrozole. In addition, disease recurrence seems to be lower with upfront ZA, but further follow-up is needed to confirm these interim results.

In another open-label study, Hines and colleagues[39] evaluated whether ZA prevents the AIBL expected when these patients initiate letrozole. These investigators administered 4 mg ZA every 6 months to postmenopausal women initiating letrozole for estrogen and/or progesterone receptor-positive breast cancer and a BMD T score less than −2.0 and assessed the BMD at baseline and 1 year. They found that after 1 year of treatment. LS BMD increased by 2.66% (P = .01), FN by 4.81% (P = .01), and any measured end point by 4.55% (P = .0052), leading them to conclude that ZA prevents AIBL in postmenopausal women with osteoporosis/osteopenia starting letrozole with improvements in BMD.

These studies examined the optimal time of starting the BP, either at the initiation of AI therapy or delayed until after patients had developed a T score of less than −2.0 or a fracture. However, the reported results primarily reflect treated versus untreated patients because only 20% of the delayed groups developed T scores of less than −2.0 or a fracture, the indications to initiate BP therapy.

A few studies have also evaluated the efficacy of ZA in preventing bone loss associated with adjuvant endocrine therapy in premenopausal women with breast cancer. The Austrian Breast and Colorectal Cancer Study Group[40] (ABCSG-12 trial) evaluated the role of ZA in preventing bone loss associated with adjuvant endocrine therapy in premenopausal patients in a randomized, open-label, phase III, 4-arm trial comparing tamoxifen (20 mg/d orally) and goserelin (3.6 mg every 28 days subcutaneously) ± ZA (4 mg intravenously every 6 months) versus anastrozole (1 mg/d orally) and goserelin ± ZA in premenopausal women with hormone-responsive breast cancer. In a bone substudy, serial BMD measurements were obtained at 0, 6, 12, 24, and 36 months on 404 patients. After 3 years of treatment, endocrine therapy alone caused significant loss of BMD at the LS (−11.3%, mean difference −0.119 g/cm2 [95% confidence interval −0.146−−0.091], P<.0001) and trochanter (−7.3%, mean difference −0.053 g/cm2 [−0.076−−0.030], P<.0001). In patients who did not receive ZA, anastrozole caused greater BMD loss than tamoxifen at 36 months at the LS (−13.6%, vs −9.0%,

P<.0001 for both). Two years after the completion of treatment (median follow-up 60 months), patients not receiving ZA still had decreased BMD at both sites compared with baseline (LS −6.3%, *P* = .001; trochanter −4.1%, *P* = .058). Patients who received ZA had stable BMD at 36 months (LS +0.4%, trochanter +0.8) and increased BMD at 60 months at both sites (LS +4.0, *P* = .02; trochanter +3.9%, *P* = .07) compared with baseline. Goserelin plus tamoxifen or anastrozole for 3 years without concomitant ZA caused significant bone loss. Although there was partial recovery 2 years after completing treatment, patients receiving endocrine therapy alone did not recover their baseline BMD levels. Concomitant ZA prevented bone loss during therapy and improved BMD at 5 years.

RANK Ligand Antibody

The recent approval of the RANK ligand antibody denosumab for treatment of osteoporosis presents an alternative option for the prevention of AIBL. Ellis and colleagues[41,42] have reported on the results of a 2-year, randomized, double-blind, placebo-controlled study comparing denosumab with placebo to prevent bone loss in AI-treated patients. At 12 months, LS BMD increased by 5.5% in the denosumab group versus the placebo group (4.8% vs −0.7%; *P*<.0001)[41] irrespective of the duration of AI treatment. At 24 months, the increase in the denosumab group was +6% versus −1.5% in the placebo group. Similar increases in LS BMD compared with placebo at 12 months were seen in patients treated with nonsteroidal (anastrozole or letrozole) and steroidal (exemestane) AI therapy (5.6% and 5.8%, respectively; *P*<.0001 vs placebo for both subgroups). Patients who had previous treatment with tamoxifen also had similar increases in LS BMD compared with placebo at 12 months to those with no previous experience with tamoxifen (5.3% and 5.8%, respectively; *P*<.0001 vs placebo for both subgroups). There was a significant decline in markers of bone turnover including serum CTX at 1 month, with a median 91% reduction from baseline compared with 9% reduction in the placebo group (*P*<.0001). Procollagen type 1 N-terminal propeptide (P1NP) declined similarly, with reductions of 71% to 73% at 6 and 24 months with 2% decline for placebo (*P*<.0001). There were no differences in the number of fractures in the denosumab versus the placebo groups.

Fracture Reduction

The risedronate, ibandronate, ZA, and denosumab clinical trials were not powered to show statistically significant reductions in the incidence of fractures. Valachis and colleagues[43] conducted a meta-analysis of AI trials and included 14 studies. These investigators found that adjuvant breast cancer treatment with BPs did not reduce the fracture rate compared with placebo or no use in these trials, leading them to conclude that treatment with BPs was not beneficial in postmenopausal patients receiving AIs, although some studies did show a trend toward lower fractures in the BP group as described earlier.

OSTEOPOROSIS PREVENTION AND TREATMENT IN PATIENTS WITH BREAST CANCER

Most women with newly diagnosed breast cancer are at risk of osteoporosis because of either their age or ongoing breast cancer treatment. Guidelines for management of bone health in women without bone metastases have been published by the Technology Committee of the American Society of Clinical Oncology,[44] National Comprehensive Cancer Network Task Force,[45] UK panel of experts[46] and the international ad hoc group.[47] All patients starting AIs should be evaluated for adequacy of calcium and vitamin D intake and started on supplements if needed, along with obtaining a baseline

BMD. Women with osteoporosis at the baseline BMD should be evaluated for secondary causes of osteoporosis. Because morbidity and mortality of osteoporotic hip fractures is significant, treatment of moderate osteopenia in patients with 1 or more risk factors or existing osteoporosis with either oral or intravenous BPs is recommended. Based on the data obtained from the bone substudies of AI clinical trials, women should be stratified into low-risk, intermediate-risk, and high-risk groups. Women with osteoporosis need to be started on BP therapy. Women with normal BMD do not need to be treated. BP treatment is recommended in women with T scores of −2.0 or less. Women with T scores between −1 and −2 can be followed with serial BMD every 12 to 24 months, with initiation of BP treatment if the annual rate of bone loss is more than 4% to 5%.

In terms of the BP of choice, the trials described earlier have been performed with risedronate 35 mg/wk and ibandronate 150 mgevery 28 days and ZA 4 mg every 6 months. ZA is currently approved for the treatment of osteoporosis in the United States at a dose of 5 mg annually, although it has not been evaluated at this dose in postmenopausal women with breast cancer in the absence of metastatic disease. ZA may also offer the additional benefit of a lower recurrence rate of breast cancer.[48] Denosumab has also been approved both for osteoporosis and for metastatic bone disease in the United States and may offer other options in the future.

SUMMARY

Use of AIs as adjuvant endocrine therapy for ER-positive breast cancer results in a lowering of estradiol levels and an increased risk for bone loss and osteoporosis, when used as initial therapy or when given after 2 to 3 years of tamoxifen treatment, with significant bone loss shown both in postmenopausal and premenopausal women. Tamoxifen may confer some protection against bone loss in postmenopausal women with breast cancer. BP therapy results in maintenance and improvement of BMD when used in women receiving AI treatment of breast cancer with moderately severe osteopenia as well as osteoporosis.

REFERENCES

1. Love RR, Wiebe DA, Newcomb PA, et al. Effects of tamoxifen on cardiovascular risk factors in postmenopausal women. Ann Intern Med 1991;115(11):860–4.
2. Love RR, Mazess RB, Barden HS, et al. Effects of tamoxifen on bone mineral density in postmenopausal women with breast cancer. N Engl J Med 1992; 326(13):852–6.
3. Powles TJ, Hickish T, Kanis JA, et al. Effect of tamoxifen on bone mineral density measured by dual-energy x-ray absorptiometry in healthy premenopausal and postmenopausal women. J Clin Oncol 1996;14(1):78–84.
4. Vehmanen L, Elomaa I, Blomqvist C, et al. Tamoxifen treatment after adjuvant chemotherapy has opposite effects on bone mineral density in premenopausal patients depending on menstrual status. J Clin Oncol 2006;24(4):675–80.
5. Ding H, Field TS. Bone health in postmenopausal women with early breast cancer: how protective is tamoxifen? Cancer Treat Rev 2007;33(6):506–13.
6. Eastell R, Adams JE, Coleman RE, et al. Effect of anastrozole on bone mineral density: 5-year results from the anastrozole, tamoxifen, alone or in combination trial 18233230. J Clin Oncol 2008;26(7):1051–7.
7. Kristensen B, Ejlertsen B, Mouridsen HT, et al. Femoral fractures in postmenopausal breast cancer patients treated with adjuvant tamoxifen. Breast Cancer Res Treat 1996;39(3):321–6.

8. Goss PE, Hadji P, Subar M, et al. Effects of steroidal and nonsteroidal aromatase inhibitors on markers of bone turnover in healthy postmenopausal women. Breast Cancer Res 2007;9(4):R52.

9. McCloskey EV, Hannon RA, Lakner G, et al. Effects of third generation aromatase inhibitors on bone health and other safety parameters: results of an open, randomised, multi-centre study of letrozole, exemestane and anastrozole in healthy postmenopausal women. Eur J Cancer 2007;43(17):2523–31.

10. Heshmati HM, Khosla S, Robins SP, et al. Role of low levels of endogenous estrogen in regulation of bone resorption in late postmenopausal women. J Bone Miner Res 2002;17(1):172–8.

11. Cuzick J. Aromatase inhibitors in prevention–data from the ATAC (arimidex, tamoxifen alone or in combination) trial and the design of IBIS-II (the second International Breast Cancer Intervention Study). Recent Results Cancer Res 2003;163:96–103 [discussion: 264–6].

12. Richardson H, Johnston D, Pater J, et al. The National Cancer Institute of Canada Clinical Trials Group MAP.3 trial: an international breast cancer prevention trial. Curr Oncol 2007;14(3):89–96.

13. Baum M, Buzdar A, Cuzick J, et al. Anastrozole alone or in combination with tamoxifen versus tamoxifen alone for adjuvant treatment of postmenopausal women with early-stage breast cancer: results of the ATAC (Arimidex, Tamoxifen Alone or in Combination) trial efficacy and safety update analyses. Cancer 2003; 98(9):1802–10.

14. Buzdar AU, Cuzick J. Anastrozole as an adjuvant endocrine treatment for postmenopausal patients with breast cancer: emerging data. Clin Cancer Res 2006;12(3 Pt 2):1037s–48s.

15. Rabaglio M, Sun Z, Price KN, et al. Bone fractures among postmenopausal patients with endocrine-responsive early breast cancer treated with 5 years of letrozole or tamoxifen in the BIG 1-98 trial. Ann Oncol 2009;20(9):1489–98.

16. Jones SE, Cantrell J, Vukelja S, et al. Comparison of menopausal symptoms during the first year of adjuvant therapy with either exemestane or tamoxifen in early breast cancer: report of a Tamoxifen Exemestane Adjuvant Multicenter trial substudy. J Clin Oncol 2007;25(30):4765–71.

17. Jones S, Stokoe C, Sborov M, et al. The effect of tamoxifen or exemestane on bone mineral density during the first 2 years of adjuvant treatment of postmenopausal women with early breast cancer. Clin Breast Cancer 2008;8(6):527–32.

18. Lonning PE, Geisler J, Krag LE, et al. Effects of exemestane administered for 2 years versus placebo on bone mineral density, bone biomarkers, and plasma lipids in patients with surgically resected early breast cancer. J Clin Oncol 2005;23(22):5126–37.

19. Jakesz R, Jonat W, Gnant M, et al. Switching of postmenopausal women with endocrine-responsive early breast cancer to anastrozole after 2 years' adjuvant tamoxifen: combined results of ABCSG trial 8 and ARNO 95 trial. Lancet 2005; 366(9484):455–62.

20. Gonnelli S, Cadirni A, Caffarelli C, et al. Changes in bone turnover and in bone mass in women with breast cancer switched from tamoxifen to exemestane. Bone 2007;40(1):205–10.

21. Coombes RC, Hall E, Gibson LJ, et al. A randomized trial of exemestane after two to three years of tamoxifen therapy in postmenopausal women with primary breast cancer. N Engl J Med 2004;350(11):1081–92.

22. Coleman RE, Banks LM, Girgis SI, et al. Skeletal effects of exemestane on bone-mineral density, bone biomarkers, and fracture incidence in postmenopausal

women with early breast cancer participating in the Intergroup Exemestane Study (IES): a randomised controlled study. Lancet Oncol 2007;8(2):119–27.
23. Goss PE, Ingle JN, Martino S, et al. A randomized trial of letrozole in postmenopausal women after five years of tamoxifen therapy for early-stage breast cancer. N Engl J Med 2003;349(19):1793–802.
24. Perez EA, Josse RG, Pritchard KI, et al. Effect of letrozole versus placebo on bone mineral density in women with primary breast cancer completing 5 or more years of adjuvant tamoxifen: a companion study to NCIC CTG MA.17. J Clin Oncol 2006;24(22):3629–35.
25. Dunstan CR, Felsenberg D, Seibel MJ. Therapy insight: the risks and benefits of bisphosphonates for the treatment of tumor-induced bone disease. Nat Clin Pract Oncol 2007;4(1):42–55.
26. Zheng SX, Vrindts Y, Lopez M, et al. Increase in cytokine production (IL-1 beta, IL-6, TNF-alpha but not IFN-gamma, GM-CSF or LIF) by stimulated whole blood cells in postmenopausal osteoporosis. Maturitas 1997;26(1):63–71.
27. Cenci S, Toraldo G, Weitzmann MN, et al. Estrogen deficiency induces bone loss by increasing T cell proliferation and lifespan through IFN-gamma-induced class II transactivator. Proc Natl Acad Sci U S A 2003;100(18):10405–10.
28. Tuck SP, Francis RM. Osteoporosis. Postgrad Med J 2002;78(923):526–32.
29. Gasser JA, Green JR, Shen V, et al. A single intravenous administration of zoledronic acid prevents the bone loss and mechanical compromise induced by aromatase inhibition in rats. Bone 2006;39(4):787–95.
30. Van Poznak C, Hannon RA, Mackey JR, et al. Prevention of aromatase inhibitor-induced bone loss using risedronate: the SABRE trial. J Clin Oncol 2010;28(6):967–75.
31. Markopoulos C, Tzoracoleftherakis E, Polychronis A, et al. Management of anastrozole-induced bone loss in breast cancer patients with oral risedronate: results from the ARBI prospective clinical trial. Breast Cancer Res 2010;12(2):R24.
32. Yonehara Y, Iwamoto I, Kosha S, et al. Aromatase inhibitor-induced bone mineral loss and its prevention by bisphosphonate administration in postmenopausal breast cancer patients. J Obstet Gynaecol Res 2007;33(5):696–9.
33. Confavreux CB, Fontana A, Guastalla JP, et al. Estrogen-dependent increase in bone turnover and bone loss in postmenopausal women with breast cancer treated with anastrozole. Prevention with bisphosphonates. Bone 2007;41(3):346–52.
34. Lester JE, Dodwell D, Purohit OP, et al. Prevention of anastrozole-induced bone loss with monthly oral ibandronate during adjuvant aromatase inhibitor therapy for breast cancer. Clin Cancer Res 2008;14(19):6336–42.
35. Brufsky A, Harker WG, Beck JT, et al. Zoledronic acid inhibits adjuvant letrozole-induced bone loss in postmenopausal women with early breast cancer. J Clin Oncol 2007;25(7):829–36.
36. Brufsky AM, Bosserman LD, Caradonna RR, et al. Zoledronic acid effectively prevents aromatase inhibitor-associated bone loss in postmenopausal women with early breast cancer receiving adjuvant letrozole: Z-FAST study 36-month follow-up results. Clin Breast Cancer 2009;9(2):77–85.
37. Bundred NJ, Campbell ID, Davidson N, et al. Effective inhibition of aromatase inhibitor-associated bone loss by zoledronic acid in postmenopausal women with early breast cancer receiving adjuvant letrozole: ZO-FAST Study results. Cancer 2008;112(5):1001–10.
38. Eidtmann H, de Boer R, Bundred N, et al. Efficacy of zoledronic acid in postmenopausal women with early breast cancer receiving adjuvant letrozole: 36-month results of the ZO-FAST Study. Ann Oncol 2010;21(11):2188–94.

39. Hines SL, Sloan JA, Atherton PJ, et al. Zoledronic acid for treatment of osteopenia and osteoporosis in women with primary breast cancer undergoing adjuvant aromatase inhibitor therapy. Breast 2010;19(2):92–6.
40. Gnant MF, Mlineritsch B, Luschin-Ebengreuth G, et al. Zoledronic acid prevents cancer treatment-induced bone loss in premenopausal women receiving adjuvant endocrine therapy for hormone-responsive breast cancer: a report from the Austrian Breast and Colorectal Cancer Study Group. J Clin Oncol 2007; 25(7):820–8.
41. Ellis GK, Bone HG, Chlebowski R, et al. Randomized trial of denosumab in patients receiving adjuvant aromatase inhibitors for nonmetastatic breast cancer. J Clin Oncol 2008;26(30):4875–82.
42. Ellis GK, Bone HG, Chlebowski R, et al. Effect of denosumab on bone mineral density in women receiving adjuvant aromatase inhibitors for non-metastatic breast cancer: subgroup analyses of a phase 3 study. Breast Cancer Res Treat 2009;118(1):81–7.
43. Valachis A, Polyzos NP, Georgoulias V, et al. Lack of evidence for fracture prevention in early breast cancer bisphosphonate trials: a meta-analysis. Gynecol Oncol 2010;117(1):139–45.
44. Hillner BE, Ingle JN, Chlebowski RT, et al. American Society of Clinical Oncology 2003 update on the role of bisphosphonates and bone health issues in women with breast cancer. J Clin Oncol 2003;21(21):4042–57.
45. Gralow JR, Biermann JS, Farooki A, et al. NCCN task force report: bone health in cancer care. J Natl Compr Canc Netw 2009;7(Suppl 3):S1–32 [quiz: S33–5].
46. Reid DM, Doughty J, Eastell R, et al. Guidance for the management of breast cancer treatment-induced bone loss: a consensus position statement from a UK Expert Group. Cancer Treat Rev 2008;34(Suppl 1):S3–18.
47. Hadji P, Body JJ, Aapro MS, et al. Practical guidance for the management of aromatase inhibitor-associated bone loss. Ann Oncol 2008;19(8):1407–16.
48. Brufsky A, Bundred N, Coleman R, et al. Integrated analysis of zoledronic acid for prevention of aromatase inhibitor-associated bone loss in postmenopausal women with early breast cancer receiving adjuvant letrozole. Oncologist 2008; 13(5):503–14.

PART 2:
Hormones and Prostate Cancer

Overview of Prostate Anatomy, Histology, and Pathology

Christine H. Lee, BA[a], Oluyemi Akin-Olugbade, MD[b],
Alexander Kirschenbaum, MD[c],*

KEYWORDS

- Prostate • Prostatic intraepithelial neoplasia • Adenocarcinoma
- Mouse model • Androgen receptor

The human prostate is the largest male accessory gland. It is the site of origin for the two most prevalent diseases of elderly men: benign prostatic hyperplasia (BPH) and prostate cancer (PCa). These two prostate diseases account for a significant proportion of the health care dollars spent on morbidity and mortality in the aging male population. BPH and PCa, although they both occur in the same population, are unrelated illnesses. PCa is thought to be many diseases with varied biological signatures and behavior. Moreover, even within one individual, there is a great heterogeneity of histologic and molecular features. Despite great strides in understanding the pathophysiology of these disorders, there remain many unanswered questions.

ANATOMY OF THE HUMAN PROSTATE

The prostate gland is located in the subperitoneal compartment between the pelvic diaphragm and the peritoneal cavity. It is located posterior to the symphysis pubis, anterior to the rectum, and inferior to the urinary bladder, thus allowing digital palpation for examination. Classically described as "walnut-shaped," it is conical in shape and surrounds the proximal urethra as it exits from the bladder.

The prostate gland is composed of a base, an apex, anterior, posterior, and inferior-lateral surfaces. The base is attached to the neck of the bladder and the prostatic urethra enters the middle of it near the anterior surface, which is narrow and convex. The apex rests on the superior surface of the urogenital diaphragm and contacts the

The authors have nothing to disclose.
[a] Department of Genetics and Genomic Sciences, Mount Sinai School of Medicine, 1452 Madison Avenue, New York, NY 10029, USA
[b] Department of Urology, Mount Sinai School of Medicine, 58A East 79th Street, 4th Floor, New York, NY 10075, USA
[c] Department of Urology, Mount Sinai School of Medicine, 229 East 79th Street, New York, NY 10075, USA
* Corresponding author.
E-mail address: akirschenb@aol.com

Endocrinol Metab Clin N Am 40 (2011) 565–575
doi:10.1016/j.ecl.2011.05.012
0889-8529/11/$ – see front matter © 2011 Elsevier Inc. All rights reserved.

medial surface of the levator ani muscles. The posterior surface is triangular and flat, and rests on the anterior wall of the rectum. The inferior-lateral surface joins the anterior surface and rests on the levator ani fascia above the urogenital diaphragm.

The human prostate is composed of glandular and stromal elements, tightly fused within a pseudocapsule. The inner layer of the prostate capsule is composed of smooth muscle with an outer layer covering of collagen. There are two anatomic defects in the prostatic capsule: at the apex (anterior and anterolaterally) and at the site of entry of the ejaculatory ducts. In these areas, it can be challenging to determine the pathologic stage of adenocarcinoma of the prostate.[1]

Nerve supply to the prostate is derived from prostatic plexus and arterial supply by the branches of the internal iliac artery. Lymphatics from the prostate drain predominantly into the internal iliac nodes.

The entire length of the prostatic urethra is encircled by sphincteric muscles (**Fig. 1**). The proximal urethra is surrounded by smooth muscle and maintains closure of the proximal urethra during ejaculation, thus preventing retrograde ejaculation. Damage to the preprostatic sphincter during transurethral resection (TURP) or treatment with α-blockers for BPH may cause retrograde ejaculation.[2] The distal urethral sphincter is composed of striated muscle fibers, is horse-shoe in shape, and is located distal to the apex of the prostate. This sphincter is incomplete posteriorly where its bundles anchor into the anterior surface of the peripheral zone. Damage to this sphincter during TURP, or more commonly during radical prostatectomy, may lead to urinary incontinence.

The prostate is divided into 3 zones: the central zone (CZ), transition zone (TZ), and peripheral zone (PZ) (see **Fig. 1**). These zones have different embryologic origins and

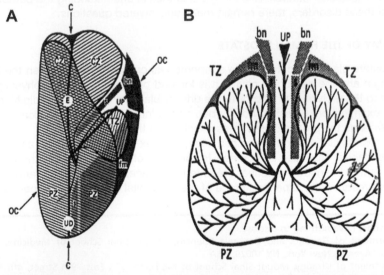

Fig. 1. Zonal anatomy of the human prostate. (*A*) Coronal view; (*B*) transverse view. The prostate is divided into 3 zones: central zone (CZ), transition zone (TZ), and peripheral zone (PZ). bn, bladder neck (located at the base of the prostate); C, the coronal plane; E, ejaculatory duct, which transverses the central zone and empties near the verumontanum (V); fm, fibromuscular layer, which is located anterior; OC, the oblique coronal plane; s, sphincteric muscle; UD, urethra distal; UP, urethra proximal. (*From* Bostwick DG. Pathology of the prostate. Contemporary issues in surgical pathology, vol. 15. Churchill Livingstone Inc; 1990. p. 2; with permission.)

can be distinguished by their histologies, anatomic landmarks, biological functions, and susceptibility to pathologic disorders. As indicated in **Table 1**, 70% of all prostate cancers arise from the PZ, which is primarily derived from the urogenital sinus. By contrast, the CZ, which is derived from the Wolfffian duct, has a very low incidence of prostate cancer, similar to another Wolffian-derived structure, the seminal vesicles. Given the unique embryologic origins of the CZ and the PZ, it is perhaps not surprising that they differ vastly in terms of their susceptibility to carcinogenesis. It is interesting that although the TZ has similar embryologic origins to the cancer-prone PZ, the percentage of PCa arising from the TZ is lower, on the order of 25% (vs 70% of all PCa arising from the PZ); this may be explained by differences in the stromal component of these two zones. The stroma of the TZ is more fibromuscular, and it has been postulated that BPH, which predominantly arises in the TZ, is a disease of the fibromuscular stroma.

ANATOMY OF THE MOUSE PROSTATE

Several transgenic mouse models of prostate cancer have been developed, which attempt to recapitulate the human disease. The mouse prostate consists of 4 distinct lobular structures, namely the ventral, dorsal, lateral, and anterior lobes. The dorsal and lateral lobes are often grouped together as the dorsolateral prostate. The 4 lobes surround the urinary bladder and the urethra, and rest against the urogenital diaphragm as the anterior lobe lies directly adjacent to the seminal vesicles (**Fig. 2**). The murine prostate is encapsulated in a thin mesothelial-lined connective tissue, allowing for a separation among all of the different lobes.[3] The stroma surrounding the glands of each lobe is composed of spindle cell layers, which are embedded in collagen fibers, and of nerve bundles along with their ganglia, typically along the dorsolateral lobes.[4]

The different lobes of the mouse prostate have various unique histologic characteristics and physiologic functions, while sharing a common grossly clear and gelatinous appearance. The ventral prostate is a leaf-like structure that incompletely surrounds the urethra dorsally and is surrounded by a thin stroma. The ventral lobe is composed of simple columnar epithelial cells, with basally located nuclei containing very small nucleoli (see **Fig. 2E**). This particular lobe does not present infolding or tufting that is typically observed in some of the other lobes. There is no anatomic and histologic counterpart to the ventral lobe of the mouse prostate in humans.

Table 1
Characteristics of the human prostate zones

	Central Zone (CZ)	Transition Zone (TZ)	Peripheral Zone (PZ)
Volume of normal prostate (%)	25	5	70
Proposed embryonic origin	Wolffian duct	Urogenital sinus	Urogenital sinus
Epithelium	Complex, large polygonal glands	Simple, small rounded glands	Simple, small rounded glands
Stroma	Compact	Compact	Loose
Origin of prostatic adenocarcinoma (%)	5	25	70
Benign prostatic hyperplasia (%)	—	100	—

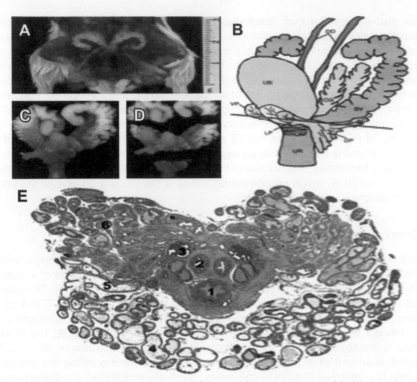

Fig. 2. Anatomy of the mouse prostate. (*A*) Exposed intact prostate, bladder, and seminal vesicles (genitourinary [GU] bloc) after linear ventral abdominal incision. The white curvilinear seminal vesicles are readily apparent. (*B*) Schematic of removed GU bloc (anterolateral view), after transection of the urethra (UR). CG, coagulating gland or anterior prostate; DD, ductus deferens; DP, dorsal prostate; LP, lateral prostate; SV, seminal vesicles; UB, urinary bladder; VP, ventral prostate. Horizontal black line indicates the level of transverse sectioning through the urethra to include both dorsolateral prostate and ventral prostate, at or near level of SV junction. (*C*) Removed GU bloc from animal in *A* corresponding to that illustrated schematically in *B*. The amputated segment of distal urethra is longitudinally oriented at the bottom. (*D*) Same bloc after transverse section through urethra as indicated in *B* generating the lower and middle portions of tissue shown. An additional transverse section through seminal vesicles and anterior prostate has been made (*top*). (*E*) Microscopic section illustrating the resulting tissue section, allowing typically adequate visualization of DP, LP, and ventral prostate, as well as other tissues that may have pathology (eg, ampullary glands, shown, and periurethral glands, not well visualized in section, but typically demonstrable in deeper sections). 1, urethra in cross section; 2, paired ductus deferens in cross section; 3, paired ampullary glands in cross section; 4, ventral prostate; 5, lateral prostate; 6, dorsal prostate. (*From* Shappell SB, Thomas GV, Roberts RL, et al. The consensus report from the Bar Harbor meeting of the Mouse Models of Human Cancer Consortium Prostate Pathology Committee. Cancer Res 2004;64:2301; with permission.)

The dorsal prostate is located dorsally and bilaterally to the base of the seminal vesicles. Surrounded by a very dense stroma, it consists of simple columnar epithelial cells with basophilic granular cytoplasm and centrally based nuclei (see **Fig. 2**E).[5] The lateral prostate, which is often functionally paired with the dorsal prostate, wraps around the urethra ventrally and bilaterally. Similar to the ventral prostate, the lateral lobe inherently exhibits very little infolding, and consists of a flat luminal surface with cuboidal to short columnar epithelial cells with basally located nuclei.[4] Granular and eosinophilic secretions are characteristic of this lobe (see **Fig. 2**E). Paired together with the dorsal lobe, the dorsolateral prostate is most analogous to the PZ of the human prostate.[5]

The anterior prostate, also known as the coagulating gland, is directly adjacent to the seminal vesicles bilaterally and follows its curvature (see **Fig. 2**B). It is lined by simple columnar epithelium with a natural papillary and cribriform growth pattern. The nuclei are centrally located in a granular cytoplasm. The anterior prostate is most analogous to the CZ of the human prostate.[5]

Although mice do not spontaneously develop prostate cancer, there are several transgenic mouse models that share some features with the human disease. The murine prostate has the ability and potential to present the full spectrum of prostate cancer, from preneoplastic lesions to metastatic disease. **Table 2** summarizes the molecular and histologic features of some of the transgenic models of high-grade prostatic intraepithelial neoplasia (HGPIN) and PCa. As predicted from the comparative zonal anatomies of the human and mouse prostate, the cancers that arise in the mouse models are generally detected in the dorsolateral lobes that most closely resemble the PZ of the human prostate.

HISTOLOGY OF THE PROSTATE AND PROSTATE ADENOCARCINOMA AND HIGH-GRADE INTRAEPITHELIAL NEOPLASIA

HGPIN is considered a precancerous lesion in humans and in the mouse model of prostate cancer.[3,6] HGPIN is characterized histologically by replacement of normal luminal cells with neoplastic cells and preservation of the basal cell layer. The neoplastic cells in HGPIN display large, hyperchromatic nuclei with prominent nucleoli. Chromatic margination is also frequently observed. On biopsies, HGPIN is often observed adjacent to cancer (**Fig. 3**A, B).

HGPIN can spread through prostatic ducts in different patterns.[7,8] The most common pattern is characterized by replacement of normal luminal cells with neoplastic cells. **Fig. 3**C and D demonstrate tufting versus a cribriform pattern, respectively.[9]

ADENOCARCINOMA OF THE PROSTATE

To confirm the histologic diagnosis of prostate cancer (PCa), the basal cell layer must be lost. The grade of PCa depends on the degree of differentiation and the architectural pattern. There is a strong correlation between histologic grade and biological behavior of the malignancy. The Gleason histologic grading system has been incorporated as a key prognostic factor in the 2010 TNM staging system for prostate cancer, and is solely based on the extent of glandular differentiation and pattern of growth of the tumor in the prostatic stroma (**Fig. 4**). Cytologic features of the cancer cells play no role in the Gleason grading system.[10] When evaluating the histology of prostatic tissue obtained from biopsy or radical prostatectomy, the 2 most abundant patterns of tumor are classified and graded Gleason 1 through 5, with 1 being the most and 5 being the least differentiated. The primary and secondary grades are then added to obtain the Gleason score. Gleason patterns 1 and 2 are predominantly located in the TZ and, for practical purposes, most biopsy and radical prostatectomy specimens are scored between 6 and 10.[11] **Fig. 5** shows Gleason patterns 3, 4, and 5 in radical prostatectomy specimens.

The Gleason grading system was modified in 2005 by the International Society of Urological Pathology Consensus Conference.[12] Contemporary pathologists believed that advances in immunohistochemical techniques and in the management of modern prostate cancer warranted a reassessment of the histologic grading of prostate

Table 2
Transgenic mouse models of prostate cancer[a]

Mouse Model	Transgene of Interest[a]	Phenotype	Reference(s)
LADY (LPB-Tag)	Overexpression of SV40 large T antigen	Develops murine prostatic intraepithelial neoplasm (mPIN) by 12 wk of age; invasive adenocarcinoma develops by as early as 24 wk; tumors are of neuroendocrine origin; metastasis occurs to regional lymph nodes, liver, and lungs as early as 6 mo	Kasper et al,[17] 1998 Masumori et al,[18] 2001
TRAMP	Overexpression of SV40 small and large T antigens	mPIN observed at ~8 wk; adenocarcinoma in dorsal prostate evident by 12 wk of age; develops hormone-refractory disease by 24 wk; tumors are of neuroendocrine origin; metastasis occurs to lungs, pelvic, and renal lymph nodes, and others	Greenberg et al,[19] 1995 Gingrich et al,[20] 1997 Kaplan-Lefko et al,[21] 2003
AR (PB-mAR)	Overexpression of the murine androgen receptor	Develops mPIN by ≥12 mo of age; no progression to overt adenocarcinoma	Stanbrough et al,[22] 2001
AKT (MPAKT)	Overexpression of Akt1	mPIN develops (age unspecified by investigators); no progression to overt adenocarcinoma	Majumder et al,[23] 2003
PTEN −/−	Homozygous deletion of PTEN	mPIN observed ~6 wk of age; invasive adenocarcinoma develops as early as 9 wk; signs of metastasis displayed at ~12 wk; tumors of epithelial origin, no neuroendocrine differentiation	Wang et al,[24] 2003

[a] All transgenes are driven by the prostate-specific promoter, probasin.

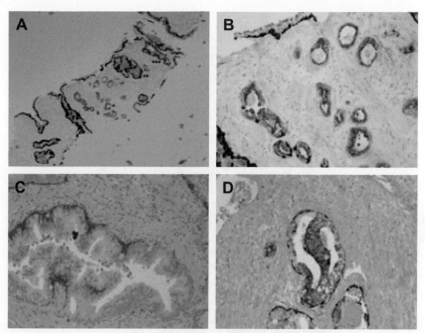

Fig. 3. High-grade prostatic intraepithelial neoplasia (HGPIN) in human specimens. Prostate biopsy specimens (core is represented, 1.2 cm × 0.2 cm). (*A, B*) The prostate biopsy tissue has been immunohistochemically stained for cytokeratin 14 to identify basal cells. Glands that do not stain for basal cells (cytokeratin 14 negative) are cancerous (*asterisk*). By contrast, glands that stain positively for cytokeratin 14 are characterized as either HGPIN (*double asterisk*) or histologically normal (*triple asterisk*) (original magnification: *A* ×50; *B* ×200). (*C, D*) Radical prostatectomy specimens. (*C*) HGPIN is present in the gland as evidenced by a partial loss of the basal cell layer, which expresses cytokeratin 14 along with a tufting pattern of the luminal cells (original magnification ×200). (*D*) Another depiction of HGPIN with positive immunohistochemical staining for cytokeratin 14, accompanied by a cribriform pattern (original magnification ×200). (*From* Epstein JI. An update of the Gleason grading system. J Urol 2010;183(2):433–40; with permission.)

cancer. The final article on histologic grading of PCa has not yet been written. As the molecular pathophysiology of PCa is further elucidated, the grading system will continue to be modified to define patterns and markers that predict the biological behavior of the disease.

ROLE OF ANDROGENS AND CELL OF ORIGIN IN THE DEVELOPMENT OF PROSTATE CANCER

Androgens are required for normal prostate development. The direct effect of androgens on prostate epithelial cells is to induce terminal differentiation. However, androgens also have profound indirect effects on prostate epithelium, via induction of secretory growth factors in adjacent stroma that stimulate epithelial cell proliferation.[13]

The role of androgens in prostate cancer development is not well defined. Prostate cancer is believed to arise from a minor population of slowly proliferating stem cells or the transit amplifying population (TAP) that are confined to the basal compartment.[13] During prostate development, the stem cell population differentiates into luminal cells in response to androgens.

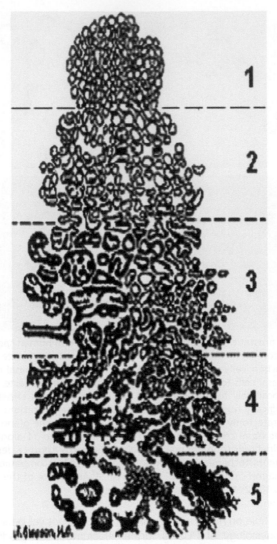

Fig. 4. Gleason patterns. Gleason pattern 3: Prostate cancer. These glands are single, rounded, and well circumscribed; they tend to infiltrate among nonneoplastic acini. These glands show a prominent variation in size, shape, and spacing of the acini. The acini remain isolated from each other and from surrounding stromal tissue. Gleason pattern 4: Prostate cancer consists of fused ill-defined microacinar glands or cribriform-patterned cells with poorly formed lumens. This grade can have a pattern consisting of ragged, infiltrating cords that form an anatomically sponge-like epithelium. This pattern is also described as being hypernephroid, as it may consist of cells with abundant clear cytoplasm. Gleason pattern 5: Cells are tightly packed together in sheets or nests and do not form glands. (*From* Epstein JI. An update of the Gleason grading system. J Urol 2010;183(2):433–40.)

It is established that the TAP expresses androgen receptor (AR). Moreover, androgens added to TAP cells in vitro promote differentiation by induction of markers of luminal cells, such as cytokeratin-18 (CK18), AR, prostate-specific acid phosphatase (PAP), and prostate-specific antigen (PSA). $\alpha_2\beta_1$ integrin expression is implicated in

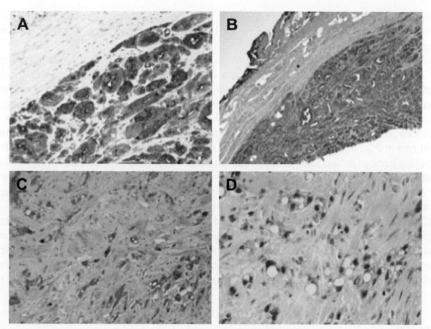

Fig. 5. Human radical prostatectomy specimens of Gleason patterns 3, 4, and 5. (*A*) Tissue that has positively stained for prostate-specific antigen (PSA); Gleason pattern 3 is displayed in the glands shown, and some areas are accentuated by the presence of cords (*asterisk*) (original magnification ×200). (*B*) The tissue has been stained for PSA, for which the surrounding prostatic capsule (*asterisk*) has stained negatively. Gleason pattern 4 is shown here (original magnification ×50). (*C*) Tissue that has stained positively for PSA; Gleason pattern 5 is present in the glands shown, which are extremely dedifferentiated (original magnification ×400). (*D*) Tissue that has stained positively for androgen receptor; very poorly differentiated tissue of the gland is shown and characterized as Gleason pattern 5 (original magnification ×400).

the maintenance of the immature basal cell phenotype, and androgens downregulate its expression.[14] Primary cultures of human basal cells derived from the PZ and TZ of radical prostatectomy specimens have been reported to express AR protein. The expression of AR increased in response to the potent androgen dihydrotestosterone in basal cells derived from the PZ, but not in basal cells derived from the TZ.[15]

A recent study also points to the basal cell as the cell of origin for human prostate cancer. These cells, in addition to expressing basal cell markers such as p63 and K5, also express AR. Basal cells infected with lentivirus carrying activated AKT and ERG developed HGPIN; a combination of AKT, ERG, and AR resulted in the development of adenocarcinoma in immunodeficient mice.[16]

In summary, the basal cell population, which encompasses stem and TAP cells, express low levels of functional AR and are androgen-independent for survival. This population of cells is reminiscent of the androgen-independent cell population in advanced castration-resistant prostate cancer.

SUMMARY

BPH and prostate adenocarcinoma are the leading causes of morbidity and mortality in the aging male population. In particular, prostate cancer is a histologically and clinically heterogeneous disorder for which the underlying genetic, epigenetic, and environmental processes responsible for initiating and driving the disease are only beginning to be elucidated.

Murine models of prostate cancer, although imperfect, serve as an invaluable tool for the study of this disease. As mice are easily genetically manipulated, this model system lends profound insight into the various molecular mechanisms that may initiate and drive PCa progression. In addition, novel therapies may be tested in genetically altered mice with different stages and varying molecular signatures of the disease.

Androgens and ARs have been well studied and have been found to play a significant role in PCa initiation and progression. A growing body of evidence suggests that prostate cancer arises from a stem cell population located in the basal layer. These cells are androgen sensitive in terms of their growth, but do not rely on androgens for survival. These putative prostate cancer stem cells are reminiscent of the majority of androgen-independent cells in castrate-resistant prostate cancer.

One of the greatest challenges in this field is to ascertain the biology of a given prostate cancer so as to render effective treatment decisions or even to recommend against any treatment. Through careful study of the histology of human PCa specimens and mouse models, a greater understanding of the molecular signatures that define the behavior of the disease will allow for personalized approaches to its management.

REFERENCES

1. McNeal JE, Bostwick DG, Kindrachuk RA, et al. Patterns of progression in prostate cancer. Lancet 1986;1:60.
2. McNeal JE. The prostate and prostatic urethra: a morphologic synthesis. J Urol 1972;107:1008.
3. Shappell SB, Thomas GV, Roberts RL, et al. Prostate pathology of genetically engineered mice: definitions and classification. The consensus report from the Bar Harbor meeting of the Mouse Models of Human Cancer Consortium Prostate Pathology Committee. Cancer Res 2004;64:2270–305.
4. Harmelin A, Danon T, Kela I, et al. Biopsy of the mouse prostate. Lab Anim 2005; 39(2):215–20.
5. Roy-Burman P, Wu H, Powell WC, et al. Genetically defined mouse models that mimic natural aspects of human prostate cancer development. Endocr Relat Cancer 2004;11:225–54.
6. McNeal JE. Origin and development of carcinoma in the prostate. Cancer 1969; 23(1):24–34.
7. Bostwick DG, Brawer MK. Prostatic intra-epithelial neoplasia and early invasion in prostate cancer. Cancer 1987;59(4):788–94.
8. Kovi J, Jackson MA, Heshmat MY. Ductal spread in prostatic carcinoma. Cancer 1985;56(7):1566–73.
9. McNeal JE, Reese JH, Redwine EA, et al. Cribiform adenocarcinoma of the prostate. Cancer 1986;58:1714.
10. Gleason DF. The Veterans Administration Cooperative Research Group: histologic grading and clinical staging of prostatic carcinoma. In: Tannenbaum M, editor. Urologic pathology: the prostate. Lee and Febiger: Philadelphia; 1977. p. 171–98.
11. Epstein JI, Allsbrook WC Jr, Amin MB, et al. The 2005 International Society of Urologic Pathology (ISUP) Consensus Conference on Gleason grading of prostatic carcinoma. Am J Surg Pathol 2000;24:477.
12. Epstein JI. An update of the Gleason grading system. J Urol 2010;183(2):433–40.

13. Isaacs JT, Coffey DS. Etiology and disease process of benign prostatic hyperplasia. Prostate Suppl 1989;2:33–50.
14. Heer R, Robson CN, Shenton BK, et al. The role of androgen in determining differentiation and regulation of androgen receptor expression in the human prostatic epithelium transient amplifying population. J Cell Physiol 2007;212(3):572–8.
15. Kirschenbaum A, Liu XH, Yao S, et al. Sex steroids have differential effects on growth and gene expression in primary human prostatic epithelial cell cultures derived from the peripheral versus transition zones. Carcinogenesis 2005; 27(2):216–24.
16. Goldstein AS, Huang J, Guo C, et al. Identification of a cell of origin for human prostate cancer. Science 2010;329(5991):568–71.
17. Kasper S, Sheppard PC, Yan Y, et al. Development, progression, and androgen-dependence of prostate tumors in probasin-large T antigen transgenic mice: a model for prostate cancer. Lab Invest 1998;78(6):i–xv.
18. Masumori N, Thomas TZ, Chaurand P, et al. A probasin-large T antigen transgenic mouse line develops prostate adenocarcinoma and neuroendocrine carcinoma with metastatic potential. Cancer Res 2001;61(5):2239–49.
19. Greenberg NM, DeMayo F, Finegold MJ, et al. Prostate cancer in a transgenic mouse. Proc Natl Acad Sci U S A 1995;92(8):3439–43.
20. Gingrich JR, Barrios RJ, Kattan MW, et al. Androgen-independent prostate cancer progression in the TRAMP model. Cancer Res 1997;57(21):4687–91.
21. Kaplan-Lefko PJ, Chen TM, Ittmann MM, et al. Pathobiology of autochthonous prostate cancer in a pre-clinical transgenic mouse model. Prostate 2003;55(3): 219–37.
22. Stanbrough M, Leav I, Kwan PW, et al. Prostatic intraepithelial neoplasia in mice expressing an androgen receptor transgene in prostate epithelium. Proc Natl Acad Sci U S A 2001;98(19):10823–8.
23. Majumder PK, Yeh JJ, George DJ, et al. Prostate intraepithelial neoplasia induced by prostate restricted Akt activation: the MPAKT model. Proc Natl Acad Sci U S A 2003;100(13):7841–6.
24. Wang S, Gao J, Lei Q, et al. Prostate-specific deletion of the murine Pten tumor suppressor gene leads to metastatic prostate cancer. Cancer Cell 2003;4(3): 209–21.

The Critical Role of Androgens in Prostate Development

Jean D. Wilson, MD

KEYWORDS

- Androgen • Testosterone • Dihydrotestosterone
- Androgen receptor • Leydig cell • Urogenital sinus

EMBRYOLOGY OF THE PROSTATE

In the male embryo, the prostate gland arises from multiple buds that grow out from the epithelium of the proximal urethra into the surrounding connective tissue. The buds (approximately 50 in number in men) can be identified histologically beginning at approximately the eighth week of gestation and by the eleventh week are grossly visible (illustrated in the wax reconstruction shown in **Fig. 1**).[1,2] These buds eventually arborize into a complex network of secretory units that after sexual maturation are responsible for formation of approximately 20% of the volume of the ejaculate.[3] Buds are also present in the remainder of the male urethra, where they give rise to the bulbourethral (Cowper) glands and the urethral glands of Littre. A puzzling feature of prostate embryogenesis in humans and most other mammals is why prostate formation is limited to the proximal urethra whereas androgen receptors and androgen-induced bud formation occur in all sections of the urethra. Cai[4] has presented evidence that the remnants of the caudal mullerian duct undergo epithelial-mesynchymal transition and incorporation into the urogenital sinus mesenchyme and may influence prostate development in this particular region of the urethra. The wolffian ducts also terminate in the proximal urethra in males and might also play a role in prostate development. Alternatively, Levine and colleagues[5] noted that in the human fetus, prostate development takes place in proximal urethral buds where steroid 5α-reductase 2 (discussed later) is expressed in epithelial cells. In some marsupial species, such as the American opossum, *Didelphis virginiana*, the prostate is a long tubular or carrot-shaped structure that encompasses a longer segment of the male urethra.[6]

ENDOCRINE CONTROL OF PROSTATE DEVELOPMENT

Demonstration that prostate development and prostate function are both controlled by testicular hormones goes back to the beginning of endocrinology as a discipline.

The author has nothing to disclose.
Department of Internal Medicine, University of Texas Southwestern Medical Center, 5323 Harry Hines Boulevard, Dallas, TX 75390-8857, USA
E-mail address: jean.wilson@utsouthwestern.edu

Endocrinol Metab Clin N Am 40 (2011) 577–590
doi:10.1016/j.ecl.2011.05.003
0889-8529/11/$ – see front matter © 2011 Elsevier Inc. All rights reserved.

endo.theclinics.com

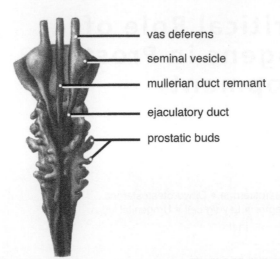

vas deferens

seminal vesicle

mullerian duct remnant

ejaculatory duct

prostatic buds

Fig. 1. Wax reconstruction of the neck of the urinary bladder and prostate in a week 11 human male embryo. (*Redrawn from* Losley OS. The development of the human prostate gland with reference to the other structures at the neck of the urinary bladder. Am J Anat 1912;8:526–41.)

In 1850 Frantz Leydig[7] described the cells situated between the seminiferous tubules of the testis that came to be termed, interstitial cells or Leydig cells. The function of these cells was unclear initially, but evidence (largely indirect) accumulated to suggest that the interstitial cells produce the male hormone (reviewed by Setchell[8]). In 1903 Bouin and Ancel[9] accumulated additional evidence that adult Leydig cells are the source of testicular hormone, and they subsequently noted that the interstitial cells of the pig embryo seem to elaborate a large amount of material at the time when male sexual differentiation is taking place.[10] The investigators went on to deduce that the internal secretion of the embryonic testis "imprints on the organism, from principle, its characteristic seal…and…procures (to the males) the essential characters of their sex that castration even practiced at birth will no more be able to suppress"[10] (translated by Alfred Jost).[11]

This remarkable deduction was confirmed by Jost and his colleagues in a series of articles published between 1947 and 1951 (summarized in Refs.[11–13]). Jost established that differentiation of the sexual phenotype is ultimately dependent on the type of gonad that develops. The paradigm that chromosomal (or genetic) sex determines gonadal sex and that gonadal sex, in turn, controls phenotypic sex is the central dogma of sexual differentiation (**Fig. 2**). This formulation was based on the observation that removing the gonads from embryos of either sex before the onset of phenotypic differentiation results in the development of a female anatomy. As a result of these castration studies as well as experiments involving transplantation of embryonic

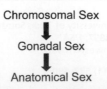

Fig. 2. Sequential events in mammalian sexual differentiation.

gonads or implantion of crystals of testosterone into the urogenital tracts, Jost concluded that the male phenotype is induced by testicular secretions whereas female development does not require hormones from the embryonic ovary. Jost went on to show that two products of the fetal testis are critical to development of the male urogenital tract. The first, mullerian-inhibiting hormone, causes regression of the mullerian ducts and thus prevents development of a uterus in males. The second is an androgenic steroid that is responsible for virilization of the wolffian ducts to form the epididymis, vas deferens, and seminal vesicles, for induction of prostate development in the urogenital sinus, and for conversion of the urogenital tubercle into the male external genitalia, including the penis and penile urethra and the scrotum. The fact that Jost also showed that grafting of fetal testes next to fetal ovaries causes virilization of the wolffian ducts and regression of the mullerian ducts whereas placement of a crystal of testosterone next to fetal ovaries causes virilization of the wolffian ducts but does not result in mullerian duct regression was powerful support for the validity of his formulation and for the formation of a mullerian inhibiting hormone by fetal testes.[11]

The validity of the Jost model has been confirmed and extended in subsequent years by a variety of types of evidence, including studies in men and animals with loss-of-function mutations that impair the formation or action of mullerian inhibiting hormone[13–15] or that impair androgen formation or androgen action.[16] Likewise, administration of androgens to female embryos in several species causes the formation of a male urogenital tract (but not suppression of the mullerian ducts),[17–19] and overproduction of androgens can virilize the urogenital tract in human female embryos, as in congenital adrenal hyperplasia secondary to steroid 21-hydroxylase deficiency.[20]

CONTROL OF PROSTATE GROWTH AT PUBERTY AND MAINTENANCE IN MATURITY

The human prostate weighs approximately 1 g at the time of birth, increases to approximately 4 g before puberty, and grows to approximately 20 g by age 20 under the control of testicular androgens, and there is usually no further change in weight for approximately 20 to 30 years.[21] Growth of the gland does not occur in prepubertal castrates.[22] Normal prostate growth encompasses stroma as well as epithelial elements and involves cell proliferation and transformation of the epithelial lining of the prostatic acini from cuboidal to columnar secretory cells.

The mature prostate requires continuing regulation by androgens. It was established in the nineteenth century that castration causes regression of the hyperplastic human prostate,[22,23] and lowering plasma testosterone levels in men with the use of luteinizing hormone-releasing hormone analogs has a similar effect on prostatic hyperplastia.[24,25] The prostate glands in eunuchs of the Ottoman and Chinese courts were reported to be prepubertal in size,[26–29] and castration in sexually mature male animals is followed by a wave of apoptosis in the prostate so that the total number of cells[3] and the amount of DNA in the gland[30] decrease, changes that are reversible with androgen replacement therapy at least after short-term castration. The report that 50 years after castration the prostate was completely impalpable in 21 of 26 Chinese eunuchs (and very small in the remaining 5)[28,29] was unexpected, however, and implies that the gland may atrophy completely in the long-term absence of androgen.[31]

MECHANISM OF ANDROGEN ACTION IN THE PROSTATE
Androgen Metabolism

As discussed previously, development, maturation, and maintenance of the prostate are all due to the action of androgen. Testosterone, the principal androgen secreted by the fetal and adult testes and the principal androgen in adult male plasma, enters target tissues down an activity gradient by a passive diffusion mechanism (reviewed by Wilson[32]).Testosterone is believed to exert few direct actions, however, but mainly serves as a prohormone for the formation of two potent metabolites in target tissues (**Fig. 3**).[32] Testosterone can undergo irreversible 5α-reduction to dihydrotestosterone, which mediates many of the differentiating, growth-promoting, and functional actions of androgens. Alternatively, circulating testosterone can be converted to estrogens in the peripheral tissues of both sexes. Estrogens in some instances act in concert with androgens to influence physiologic processes but may also exert independent effects and on occasion promote actions that are in opposition to those of androgens. Thus, the physiologic consequences of circulating testosterone constitute the sum of the combined actions of testosterone itself and of its estrogenic and 5α-reduced metabolites.

During embryogenesis, testosterone promotes virilization of the urogenital tract in two ways. It acts directly to stimulate the wolffian ducts and induce development of the epididymides, vasa deferentia, and seminal vesicles.[33] Whereas virilization of the wolffian ducts in the human embryo occurs before development of 5α-reductase in the tissue, testosterone acts as a prohormone for dihydrotestosterone in the urogenital sinus and urogenital tubercle.[33] As a consequence, dihydrotestosterone is the hormone that induces development of the male urethra and prostate and causes midline fusion of the urogenital folds and elongation and enlargement of the urogenital tubercle to form the penis and scrotum. The separate physiologic roles that testosterone and dihydrotestosterone play in male embryogenesis were deduced on the basis of time-sequence studies in the embryos of several species.

When it was established in the 1960s that dihydrotestosterone is the mediator of most androgen effects in male physiology, it was believed that the metabolite was

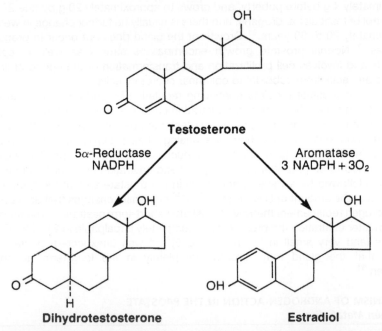

Fig. 3. Conversion of testosterone to other steroid hormones in extraglandular tissues and in the Leydig cells of the testis.

formed and acted intracellularly and that any circulating dihydrotestosterone is not physiologically significant. This concept was changed by two developments— discovery that there are two 5α-reductase enzymes and demonstration that circulating dihydrotestosterone does play a role in male physiology.

Recognition that two 5α-reductase enzymes exist occurred in 1991. These enzymes are membrane bound and have never been solubilized. Consequently, Andersson and coworkers[34] used expression cloning techniques to clone a 5α-reductase cDNA from a female rat liver cDNA library. That this was not the only such 5α-reductase that became apparent when the gene was sequenced and found to be normal in male subjects with an autosomal recessive disorder of sexual differentiation due to dihydro-testosterone deficiency.[35] Consequently, Andersson and colleagues[36] again used expression cloning techniques to clone a second 5α-reductase cDNA from a human prostate cDNA library and showed that subjects with 5α-reductase deficiency have loss-of-function mutations of isoenzyme 2.

Roles of the Two 5α-Reductases in Androgen Physiology

In humans, these two 5α-reductases are differentially expressed in that enzyme 2 is expressed early in embryogenesis in the urogenital tract of both sexes and throughout life in the male urogenital tract and genital skin. It is, therefore, logical that enzyme 2 plays a critical role in male sexual differentiation and in the maturation and sustenance of the mature male urogenital tissues. The expression of enzyme 1 is different anatom-ically and temporally. Enzyme 1 is not detectable in the human embryo, is transiently expressed in newborn skin, and is permanently expressed in skin and a few other tissues after the time of puberty.[37] Both isoenzymes are expressed in liver.

The fact that enzyme 1 plays a role in male physiology was deduced from studies of subjects with enzyme 2 deficiency. Such men have circulating levels of dihydrotestos-terone that are sometimes in the normal range. This circulating dihydrotestosterone could arise either from residual activity of the mutant enzyme 2 or from enzyme 1. Studies of two types of individuals with enzyme 2 deficiency indicate that enzyme 1 is the major source of dihydrotestosterone in the circulation. Subjects from New Guinea who have deletion of the entire coding sequence for enzyme 2 and who as a consequence make no enzyme 2 have measureable or normal levels of plasma dihy-drotestosterone and undergo considerable virilization at the time of puberty.[38] Like-wise, a subject with a splice-junction abnormality of the enzyme 2 gene and who also made no functional enzyme 2[39] virilized at puberty had serum dihydrotestoster-one levels that were in the low normal range and that rose even higher after he was given exogenous testosterone.[40] Because men with these two types of 5α-reductase 2 deficiency virilized considerably after puberty, it follows that dihydrotestosterone is a circulating hormone that is formed in large part if not exclusively by steroid 5α-reduc-tase 1 after puberty and contributes to virilization.

Why Does 5α-Reduction Matter?

At the structural level, 5α-reduction of the steroid molecule makes the molecule less polar and flatter (because of rearrangement of the A and B rings). Suggestions have been made that additional androgen metabolites may be active at the cellular level, including 5α-androstane-3α,17β-diol, which is the circulating androgen at the time of virilization of the male pouch young of an Australian marsupial, the tammar wallaby.[41] Bruchovsky[42] showed that all physiologically active 5α-reduced androgens exert their effects after conversion to dihydrotestosterone, and there is no compelling evidence that any naturally occurring steroids other than testosterone and dihydrotes-tosterone bind to the androgen receptor.

Several explanations have been proposed to explain the role of dihydrotestosterone in androgen physiology, including that 5α-reduction precludes the aromatization of androgen to estrogen and promotes intracellular accumulation of androgen. Most attention has focused on the androgen receptor, however. The genetic evidence is clear that testosterone and dihydrotestosterone act via a single androgen receptor,[17] and on the basis of structure-function correlations, Liao and Fang[43] deduced that the flatter dihydrotestosterone molecule fits more tightly into the hormone-binding domain of the androgen receptor. This enhanced binding affinity is due almost exclusively to a decreased rate of dissociation of the dihydrotestosterone-receptor complex. The net consequence of similar association rates but different dissociation rates is that dihydrotestosterone occupies most receptor sites in the steady state, even when testosterone is the predominant steroid in the cell.[44]

A fundamental question is whether the conversion of testosterone to dihydrotestosterone creates a different hormone or simply amplifies a hormonal signal (ie, whether the dihydrotestosterone-receptor complex is sufficiently different that it performs unique functions). The evidence is now clear that despite the differences in receptor-ligand interactions, testosterone at high concentrations promotes maximal transcription of reporter genes that are under the control of androgen-sensitive elements.[45]

Confirmation that the major consequence of 5α-reduction is to amplify the androgenic signal came from the finding that male mice with undetectable dihydrotestosterone as the result of targeted disruption of both steroid 5α-reductases 1 and 2 have normal male urogenital tracts and external genitalia and are fertile.[46] The reason for the difference in the effects of 5α-reductase deficiency in mice and men is that prostate testosterone levels in men change little after the administration of 5α-reductase inhibitors[47] whereas testosterone levels in prostate and seminal vesicles increase more than 100-fold after disruption of both 5α-reductase isoenzymes in the male mouse.[46] Thus, although dihydrotestosterone may exert some as yet unidentified unique functions, its fundamental effect is to amplify a weak hormonal signal.

Role of the Androgen Receptor (The Classical Pathway of Androgen Action)

Only one androgen receptor gene has been described in mammalian tissues, and severe loss-of-function mutations of this gene cause resistance both to testosterone and dihydrotestosterone.[17] Two different forms of the androgen receptor can be transcribed from this gene, depending on which of two sites in exon 1 is used to initiate transcription, but no evidence has accrued to date that these two androgen receptor forms (A and B) play different roles in androgen physiology.[48] Furthermore, although it has been proposed by Rosner and colleagues[49] that some androgen actions might be mediated by sex hormone–binding globulin, the fact that severe loss-of-function mutations of the androgen receptor gene preclude development of a prostate gland[50] suggests that the model of androgen action (shown schematically in **Fig. 4**) seems a valid formulation for androgen action in the human prostate.

The Nonclassical Pathway of Androgen Action

The term, nonclassical pathway of androgen action, refers to mechanisms that do not use the pathway (see **Fig. 4**) (ie, they do not involve binding of the androgen-androgen receptor complex to androgen regulatory elements in DNA). This concept may involve different mechanisms, including interaction of the androgen-androgen receptor complex with coregulators that do not require gene transcription, direct binding of androgen to target molecules in the absence of androgen receptor, cell surface transmembrane androgen receptor proteins, or alterations in membrane permeability.[51]

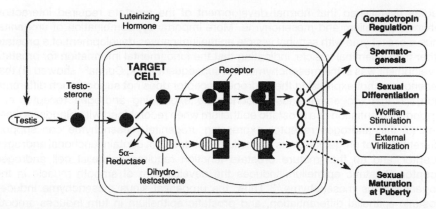

Fig. 4. Normal androgen physiology in males. Testosterone is secreted by the testes and binds to androgen receptors in target cells either directly or after conversion to dihydrotestosterone. The major actions of androgens, shown on the right, are mediated either by the testosterone-androgen receptor complex (*solid lines*) or the dihydrotestosterone-androgen receptor complex (*broken lines*). (*Reprinted from* Griffin JE. Androgen resistance—the clinical and molecular spectrum. N Engl J Med 1992;326:611–4. Copyright 1992 Massachusetts Medical Society. All rights reserved; with permission.)

Nonclassical androgen actions have been demonstrated in many tissues, including Sertoli cells.[52] The problem of interpreting the physiologic significance of the nonclassical pathways in the prostate is complicated by the fact that the prostate does not develop in the absence of functional androgen receptor. Consequently, vital androgen actions that function after the fundamental differentiation of the gland (and which is mediated by the androgen receptor) might go unrecognized. Clarification of this aspect of prostate physiology will require targeted disruption of each of the nonclassical mechanisms in turn to establish their effects on prostate function in the presence of normal androgen receptor.

HOW DOES THE ANDROGEN-ANDROGEN RECEPTOR COMPLEX CONTROL PROSTATE FUNCTION?
Androgen Action Begins in the Mesenchyme

Recognition that the fundamental action of androgen in the developing urogenital tract occurs in tissue mesenchyme was established in a pioneering series of studies by Gerald Cunha and colleagues (reviewed in Ref.[53]). Their studies were initiated on the background of principles that had been established in the understanding of mammalian tissue development.

1. Organogenesis requires an interaction between epithelium and mesenchyme.
2. Mesenchyme induces and patterns epithelial development.
3. Development of certain specialized epithelia occurs only in the presence of specific mesenchyme.
4. Mesenchymal-epithelial interactions are reciprocal in that mesenchyme induces epithelial development and epithelium induces mesenchymal differentiation.[54]

The fundamental design of Cunha and his colleagues approach was to dissect embryonic mouse tissues into epithelium and mesenchyme and to grow recombined tissues or individual components as implants in intact male adult hosts. The initial studies established that normal development of the prostate required interaction between epithelium and mesenchyme. More importantly, combination of urogenital sinus mesenchyme with seminal vesicle epithelium causes development of a prostate rather than a seminal vesicle, indicating that the fundamental information for prostate development was in the mesenchyme.[55] In subsequent work, Cunha[53] showed (1) that mesenchyme not expressing the androgen receptor does not support such differentiation, (2) that urogenital sinus mesenchyme expressing androgen receptor can support differentiation of a prostatic epithelium when recombined with bladder epithelium, (3) that androgen receptor expressing urogenital mesenchyme can support differentiation of urogenital sinus epithelium that does not contain functional androgen receptor, and (4) that mature prostate function requires epithelial cell androgen receptor. Prostatic epithelium induces the development of smooth muscle in the urogenital sinus mesenchyme.[56] Thus, the urogenital sinus mesenchyme induces prostatic epithelial differentiation, and prostatic epithelium in turn induces smooth muscle differentiation in the urogenital sinus mesenchyme.

Mechanisms of Androgen Action in Prostate Development

Because female embryos exposed to androgens develop prostates,[17–19] it follows that females possess the developmental programs required for prostate differentiation. As pointed out by Thomson,[57] there are at least 3 ways by which androgens might control these programs: (1) upregulation of factors that stimulate differentiation, (2) downregulation of constitutive factors that inhibit differentiation, or (3) a combination of upregulation and downregulation.

It is not entirely clear whether androgen action is involved in the initial appearance of buds in the embryonic urethra, but at the least, androgen controls the remaining phases of prostate development and function, including bud growth, branching morphogenesis, differentiation, and maturation. The proximal to distal outgrowth of all glandular structures, including the prostate, is controlled by time-specific and region- and/or cell-specific expression of master regulatory genes that are evolutionarily conserved throughout the animal kingdom.[58] The morphogenetic genes involved in androgen-induced prostate development have been reviewed by Prins and Putz[59] and include (1) nuclear transcription regulatory factors and (2) secreted signaling ligands that communicate paracrine and autocrine signals between mesynchymal and epithelial cells. Complications that affect unraveling the regulation of this system include the following: there are many redundancies; each of the morphogenetic proteins is under complex control by inhibitory and (probably) stimulatory factors in addition to androgens; the same molecules may have different effects at different stages of development; actions may differ with different local concentrations of protein; and the interaction of the various gene products is incompletely understood. Nevertheless, as a result of studies in many different laboratories, largely in rodent models, a tentative prostate morphogenetic code has been formulated.[59]

Homeobox genes and transcription regulatory factors

The homeobox gene superfamily of regulatory genes encodes transcription factors that contain highly conserved DNA-binding domains that recognize specific regulatory regions of target genes. Specific homeobox genes within developing prostate tissue are thought to control budding and morphogenesis. *Hoxa13* and *Hoxd13* are expressed primarily in prostate mesenchyme whereas *Hoxb13* localizes to the epithelial cells. All three are upregulated in the ventral lobe of the rat prostate by androgens, possibly constituting a fundamental mechanism by which androgens initiate prostate morphogenesis.[60] In addition, a novel member of the NK homeobox gene family,

NKX3.1, is expressed in the urogenital sinus epithelium at bud sites before bud development and throughout life, suggesting a critical role both in prostate formation and function.[59] In the developing prostate, *NKX3.1* is expressed in epithelial cells before expression of androgen receptor in the cells, but androgen administration later in development enhances *NKX3.1* expression.[61] Genes in a third family, the forkhead box genes (*Fox A1* and *A2*), are members of a widely distributed family of transcription regulatory factors. *Fox A1* is expressed early in prostate development and is maintained throughout adult life and is believed to interact with the androgen receptor on gene promoters.[62] *Fox A2* is only expressed in epithelial cells at the mesenchymal interface during early budding and declines thereafter.

The *Notch* signaling pathway is a highly conserved cell-cell signaling system involved in patterning developing tissues.[63] It consists of a transmembrane *Notch* receptor that interacts with *Jagged/Delta* membrane proteins on adjacent cells to cause proteolytic cleavage of *Notch*, releasing the intracellular domain, which translocates to the nucleus where it regulates gene expression. The protein is present early in the mouse urogenital sinus epithelium and in early prostate buds. Conditional deletion of the gene after prostate development was completed caused epithelial proliferation and reduced secretions, suggesting that *Notch* acts to inhibit expansion of prostate progenitor cells and to facilitate epithelial differentiation.[63]

Secreted signaling ligands

Branching morphogenesis is also controlled by a complex interplay between epithelial and mesenchymal cells that involves release of paracrine and autocrine signaling ligands, including *Sonic Hedgehog* (*Shh*), *fibroblast growth factor* (*Fgf-10*), *Bmps/ Tgfβ/activin*, and *Wnt*.[58] Each of these signaling ligands is peptide/protein in nature, and as a consequence they work via cell surface receptors as paracrine factors; the extent to which they may also serve autocrine functions is less easy to define. In general, they seem to fall into two broad categories. *Shh* and *Fgf-20* are enhanced by the addition of androgen, and their fundamental effect seems to be to upregulate factors that stimulate differentiation.[57] In contrast, signaling ligands of the *Bmps/Tgf β/activin* and *Wnt* families seem inhibited by androgen and retard differentiation in the absence of androgen.

The extent to which these various morphogenetic factors may be deranged in prostatic hyperplasia and prostatic cancer is a subject of intense interest.

ROLE OF DIHYDROTESTOSTERONE IN PROSTATIC HYPERPLASIA

In most mammals, prostate growth ceases and 5α-reductase expression in the prostate declines with the achievement of sexual maturation.[64] In a few species, however, exemplified by humans and dogs, 5α-reductase activity in the prostate remains high and continued growth of the prostate can result in prostatic hyperplasia with obstruction of urinary outflow (and in some species the rectum).[65] As a result of studies in the castrated dog administered various hormone regimens, the author proposed some years back that dihydrotestosterone is the androgen that mediates continued prostatic growth in the dog and that the growth is enhanced by estradiol (probably by enhancing the amount of androgen receptor in the gland).[66] The validity of this two-hormone model in the dog has been substantiated by studies of the effects of 5α-reductase inhibitors on natural and androgen-induced hyperplasia[67] and by studies of the effects of estrogen receptor antagonists and aromatase inhibitors that cause profound decrease in the size both of the normal and the hyperplastic dog prostates, despite an increase in plasma testosterone levels.[68]

In humans, several types of indirect evidence suggest that dihydrotestosterone is the androgen responsible for prostatic hyperplasia.[66] Not only does 5α-reductase remain high in the hyperplastic gland, but also, more importantly, administration of the 5α-reductase inhibitor finasteride causes approximately the same degree of shrinkage in the hyperplastic gland as surgical[69] or pharmacological[24,25] castration. In addition, long-term administration of finasteride profoundly decreases the incidence of obstructive complications of prostatic hyperplasia.[69] It has not been possible, however, to demonstrate that estrogen (generally elevated as men age) plays a synergistic role in the human disorder because in double-blind studies, treatment of men with prostatic hyperplastia with the aromatase inhibitor, atamestane, which lowers both serum and prostate levels of estradiol and estrone,[70] had no effect on prostate size, lower urinary tract symptoms, or urine flow.[71,72]

Because therapy with 5α-reductase inhibitors results in only a modest improvement in the size of the hyperplastic human prostate (in contrast to dogs, in which the prostate shrinks to normal size with 5α-reductase inhibitors), it is likely that the role of dihydrotestosterone in the human disorder is only one of several factors involved in the pathogenesis.

SUMMARY

Androgen plays a critical role in the prostate, from the beginning of differentiation of the gland toward the end of the second trimester of gestation to the growth of the gland at the time of male puberty, in promotion of the secretory function of the mature gland during adulthood, and in the hyperplasia of the prostate that is a common feature of male aging in men and dogs. Furthermore, androgen deprivation at any phase of life causes widespread apoptosis and decrease in cell number and DNA content of the gland. In one sense, a great deal is known about how androgen controls prostate function at different phases of life, but identification of the downstream genes and control mechanisms that translate hormonal information into complex cellular functions and structures is still in the process of being unraveled. Elucidation of the molecular biology of these various morphogenic factors can be predicted to provide therapeutic insight into prostate hyperplasia and prostate cancer.

REFERENCES

1. Lowsley OS. The development of the human prostate gland with reference to the development of other structures at the neck of the urinary bladder. Am J Anat 1912;8:526–41.
2. Johnson FP. The later development of the urethra in the male. J Urol 1920;4: 447–501.
3. Coffey DS. The molecular biology, endocrinology, and physiology of the prostate and seminal vesicles. In: Walsh PC, Retik AB, Stamey TA, et al, editors. Campbell's urology. 6th edition. Philadelphia: WB Saunders; 1991. p. 221–66.
4. Cai Y. Participation of caudal mullerian mesenchyma in prostate development. J Urol 2008;180:1898–903.
5. Levine A, Wang JP, Ren M, et al. Immunohistochemical localization of steroid 5α-reductase 2 in the human male fetal reproductive tract and adult prostate. J Clin Endocrinol Metab 1996;81:384–9.
6. Tyndale-Biscoe H, Renfree MB. Reproductive physiology of marsupials. London: Cambridge University Press; 1987. p. 147–9.
7. Leydig F. Zur anatomie der Mannlichen geschlechtorgane und analdrusen der saugetiere. Z Wiss Zool 1850;2:1–57 [in German].

8. Setchell BP. Male reproduction. New York: Van Nostrand Reinhold Inc; 1984. p. 219–20.
9. Bouin P, Ancel P. Rescherches sur les cellules interstititielles du testicule des mammiferes. Arch Zool Exp Gen Ser A 1903;1:437–523 [in French].
10. Bouin P, Ancel P. [Sur la signification de la glands interstitielle du testicule embryonnaire]. C R Seances Soc Biol Fil 1903;55:1682–4 [in French].
11. Jost A. Problems of fetal endocrinology: the gonadal and hypophyseal hormones. Recent Prog Horm Res 1953;8:379–413.
12. Jost A. The role of hormones in prenatal development. Harvey Lect 1961;55: 201–26.
13. Jost A. Hormonal factors in the sex differentiation of the mammalian foetus. Philos Trans R Soc Lond B Biol Sci 1970;259:119–30.
14. Josso N, Belville C, di Clemente N, et al. AMH and AMH receptor defects in persistent Mullerian duct syndrome. Hum Reprod Update 2005;11:351–6.
15. Josso N, Picard JY, Rey R, et al. Testicular anti-Mullerian hormone: history, genetics, regulation and clinical applications. Pediatr Endocrinol Rev 2006;3:347–58.
16. Griffin JE, McPhaul MJ, Russell DW, et al. The androgen resistance syndromes: steroid 5α-reductase 2 deficiency, testicular feminization, and related disorders. In: Scriver CR, Beaudet AL, Sly WS, et al, editors. The metabolic and molecular bases of interited disease. 8th edition. New York: McGraw-Hill; 2001. p. 4117–46.
17. Goldstein JL, Wilson JD. Studies on the pathogenesis of the pseudohermaphroditismin the mouse with testicular feminization. J Clin Invest 1972;51:1647–58.
18. Schultz FM, Wilson JD. Virilization of the wolffian duct in the rat fetus by various androgens. Endocrinology 1974;94:979–86.
19. Leihy MW, Shaw G, Wilson JD, et al. Virilisation of the urogenital sinus of the tammar wallaby is not unique to 5α-androstane-3α,17β-diol. Mol Cell Endocrinol 2001;181:111–5.
20. Nimkarn S, Lin-Su K, New MI. Steroid 21 hydroxylase deficiency congenital adrenal hyperplasia. Endocrinol Metab Clin North Am 2009;38:699–718.
21. Swyer GJ. Postnatal growth in the human prostate. J Anat 1944;78:130–45.
22. Huggins C. The etiology of benign prostatic hypertrophy. Bull N Y Acad Med 1947;23:1022–6.
23. Cabot AT. The question of castration for enlarged prostate. Ann Surg 1896;24: 265–309.
24. Peters CA, Walsh PC. The effect of nafarelin acetate, a luteinizing-hormone-releasing hormone agonist, on benign prostatic hyperplasia. N Engl J Med 1987;317:599–604.
25. Gabrilove JL, Levine AC, Kirchenbaum A, et al. Effect of a GnRH analogue (leuprolide) on benign prostatic hypertrophy. J Clin Endocrinol Metab 1987;64: 1331–3.
26. Hikmet, Regnault F. Les eunuchs de constantinople. Bull Mem Soc Anthropol Paris. 5th series 1901;12:232–40 [in French].
27. Wagenseil F. Bitrage zur Kenntnis der Kastrationsfolgen und des Eunuchoidismus beim Mann. Z Morphol Anthropol 1927;26:264–301 [in German].
28. Wu CP, Gu FL. The prostate 41–65 years post castration: an analysis of 26 eunuchs. Chin Med J (Engl) 1967;100:271–2.
29. Wu CP, Gu FL. The prostate in eunuchs. EORTC genitourinary group monograph 10. New York: Wiley-Liss; 1991. p. 249–55.
30. Moore RJ, Wilson JD. The effect of androgenic hormones on the reduced nicotinamide adenine dinuclotide phosphate: Δ^4-3-ketosteroid 5α-oxidoreductase of rat ventral prostate. Endocrinology 1973;93:581–92.

31. Wilson JD, Roehrborn C. Long term consequences of castration in men: lessons from the Skoptzy and the eunuchs of the Chinese and Ottoman courts. J Clin Endocrinol Metab 1999;84:4324–31.
32. Wilson JD. Metabolism of testicular androgens. In: Greep RO, Astwood EB, editors, Handbook of physiology, sect 7, vol. 5. Washington, DC: Ameican Physiological Society; 1975. p. 491–508.
33. Siiteri PK, Wilson JD. Testosterone formation and metabolism during male sexual differentiation in the human embryo. J Clin Endocrinol Metab 1974; 38:113–25.
34. Andersson S, Bishop KW, Russell DW. Expression cloning and regulation of steroid 5 alpha-reductase, an enzyme essential for male sexual differentiation. J Biol Chem 1989;264:16249–55.
35. Jenkins EP, Andersson S, Imperato-McGinley J, et al. Genetic and pharmacological evidence for more than one human steroid 5α-reductase. J Clin Invest 1992; 89:293–300.
36. Andersson S, Berman DM, Jenkins EP, et al. Deletion of steroid 5α-reductase 2 gene in male pseudohermaphroditism. Nature 1991;354:159–61.
37. Thigpen AE, Silver RI, Ruileyardo JM, et al. Tissue distribution and ontogeny of steroid 5α-reductase isoenzyme expression. J Clin Invest 1993;92:903–10.
38. Imperato-McGinley J, Miller M, Wilson JD, et al. A cluster of male pseudohermahroditism with 5α-reductase deficiency in Papua New Guinea. Clin Endocrinol (Oxf) 1991;34:293–8.
39. Thigpen AE, Davis DL, Milatovich A, et al. Molecular genetics of steroid 5α-reductase 2 deficiency. J Clin Invest 1992;90:799–809.
40. Price P, Wass JAH, Griffin JE, et al. High dose androgen therapy in male pseudoermaphroditism due to 5α-reductase deficiency and disorders of the androgen receptor. J Clin Invest 1984;74:1496–508.
41. Shaw G, Renfree MB, Leihy MW, et al. Prostate formation in a marsupial is mediated by the testicular androgen 5α-androstane-3α,17β-diol. Proc Natl Acad Sci U S A 2000;97:1236–9.
42. Bruchovsky N. Comparison of the metabolites formed in rat prostate following the in vivo administration of seven natural androgens. Endocrinology 1971;89: 1212–22.
43. Liao S, Fang S. Receptor-proteins for androgens and the mode of action of androgens on gene transcription in ventral prostate. Vitam Horm 1969;27:18–90.
44. Grino PB, Griffin JE, Wilson JD. Testosterone at high concentrations interacts with the human androgen receptor similarly to dihydrotestosterone. Endocrinology 1990;126:1165–72.
45. Deslypere J-P, Young M, Wilson JD, et al. Testosterone and 5α-dihydrotestosterone interact differently with the androgen receptor to enhance transcription of the MMTV-CAT reporter gene. Mol Cell Endocrinol 1992;88:15–22.
46. Mahendroo MS, Cala KM, Hess DL, et al. Unexpected virilization in male mice lacking steroid 5α-reductase enzymes. Endocrinology 2001;142:4652–62.
47. McConnell JD, Wilson JD, George FW, et al. Finasteride, an inhibitor of 5α-reductase, suppresses prostatic dihydrotestosterone in men with benign prostatic hyperplasia. J Clin Endocrinol Metab 1992;74:505–8.
48. Gao TS, McPhaul MJ. Functional activities of the A- and B-forms of the human androgen receptor in response to androgen receptor agonists and antagonists. Mol Endocrinol 1998;12:654–63.
49. Rosner W, Hryb DJ, Kahn SM, et al. Interaction of sex hormone-binding globulin with target cells. Mol Cell Endocrinol 2010;316:79–85.

50. Griffin JE. Androgen resistance—the clinical and molecular spectrum. N Engl J Med 1992;326:611–8.
51. Michels G, Hoppe UC. Rapid actions of androgens. Front Neuroendocrinol 2008; 29:182–98.
52. Rahman F, Christian HC. Non-classical actions of testosterone: an update. Trends Endocrinol Metab 2007;18:371–8.
53. Cunha GR. Mesenchymal-epithelial interactions: past, present, and future. Differentiation 2008;76:568–86.
54. Fleischmajer R, Billingham RE. Epithelial-mesenchyme interactions. Baltimore (MD): Williams & Wilkins; 1968.
55. Cunha GR. Epithelio-mesenchymal interactions in developing accessory sexual gland structures which become responsive to androgenic stimulation. Anat Rec 1972;172:179–96.
56. Cunha GR, Battle E, Young P, et al. Role of epithelial-mesenchymal interactions in the differentiation and spatial organization of visceral smooth muscle. Epithelial Cell Biol 1992;1:76–83.
57. Thomson AA. Mesenchymal mechanisms in prostate organogenesis. Differentiation 2008;76:587–98.
58. Hogan BL. Morphogenesis. Cell 1999;96:225–33.
59. Prins GS, Putz O. Molecular signaling pathways that regulate prostate gland development. Differentiation 2008;76:641–59.
60. Huang K, Pu Y, Birch L, et al. Posterior Hox gene expression and differential androgen regulation in the developing and adult rat prostate lobes. Endocrinology 2007;148:1235–45.
61. Pu Y, Huang L, Prins GS. Androgen regulation of prostate morphoregulatory gene expression: Fgf10-dependent and –independent pathways. Endocrinology 2007; 148:1697–706.
62. Gao N, Ishii K, Mirosevich J, et al. Forkhead box A1 regulates prostate ductal morphogenesis and promotes epithelial cell maturation. Development 2005; 132:4331–43.
63. Wang XD, Leow CC, Zha J, et al. Notch signaling is required for normal prostatic epithelial cell proliferation and differentiation. Dev Biol 2006;290:66–80.
64. Gloyna RE, Wilson JD. A comparative study of the conversion of testosterone to 17β-hydroxy-5α-androstane-3-one (dihydrotestosterone) by prostate and epididymis. J Clin Endocrinol Metab 1969;29:970–7.
65. Wilson JD, Gloyna RE. The intranuclear metabolism of testosterone in the accessory organs of reproduction. Recent Prog Horm Res 1970;26:309–36.
66. Wilson JD. The pathogenesis of prostatic hyperplasia. Am J Med 1980;68: 745–56.
67. Wenderoth UK, George FW, Wilson JD. The effect of a 5α reductase inhibitor on androgen-mediated growth of the dog prostate. Endocrinology 1983;113:569–73.
68. Gonzalez G, Guendulain C, Maffrand C, et al. Comparison of the effect of the aromatase inhibitor, anastrazole, to the antiestrogen, tamoxifen citrate, on canine prostate and semen. Reprod Domest Anim 2009;44(Suppl 2):316–9.
69. McConnell JD, Brushewitz R, Walsh P, et al, for the Finasteride Long-Term Efficacy and Safety Study Group. The effect of finasteride on the risk of acute urinary retention and the need for surgical treatment among men with benign prostatic hyperplasia. N Engl J Med 1998;338:557–63.
70. El Etreby MF, Nishing Y, Habenicht U, et al. Atamestane, a new aromatase inhibitor for the management of benign prostatic hyperplasia. J Androl 1991;12: 403–14.

71. Gingell JC, Knonagel H, Kurth KH, et al. Placebo controlled double-blind study to test the efficacy of the aromatase inhibitor atamestane in patients with benign prostatic hyperplasia not requiring operation. J Urol 1995;154:399–401.

72. Radlmaier A, Eickenberg HU, Fletcher MS, et al, for the atamestane study group. Estrogen reduction by aromatase inhibition for benign prostatic hyperplasia: results of a double-blind, placebo-controlled, randomized clinical trial using two doses of the aromatase-inhibitor atamestane. Prostate 1996;29:199–208.

Estrogens and Prostate Cancer: Etiology, Mediators, Prevention, and Management

Shuk-Mei Ho, PhD[a,b,*], Ming-Tsung Lee, MPhil[c],
Hung-Ming Lam, PhD[b,c], Yuet-Kin Leung, PhD[a]

KEYWORDS

- Estrogen receptor • Antiestrogens
- Selective estrogen receptor modulator (SERM) • Phytoestrogen
- Epigenetics • Chemoprevention • Prostate cancer risk
- Hormonal therapy

Androgens are traditionally recognized as the major hormone promoting normal and aberrant growth of the prostate. However, recent literature suggests that estrogen could also be an important mediator of these processes. Estrogen alone or in synergy with androgen is responsible for the pathogenesis of prostate cancer (PCa). More importantly, recent experimental data suggest that estrogen or its mimics could determine the risk of PCa development as early as the prenatal stage via a process known as estrogen imprinting. This article (1) reviews research findings that support a role for estrogens, estrogen mimics, and estrogen metabolites in prostate carcinogenesis; (2) discusses how different estrogen receptors (ER) mediate the action of estrogen in promoting the development and progression of PCa; and (3) evaluates the potentials

Funding support: NIH grants: DK061084, CA112532, CA015776, ES006096, ES015584, ES018758, ES018789 and ES019480 to Shuk-Mei Ho; Department of Defense Prostate Cancer Program (gs2) grant: PC030595 to Shuk-Mei Ho; Cincinnati Veterans Affairs Medical Center (gs4) Merit Award to Shuk-Mei Ho and Department of Defense Breast Cancer Program (gs3) grant: BC094017 to Ming-Tsung Lee.
Declaration of interest: The authors have nothing to disclose.
[a] Department of Environmental Health, Center for Environmental Genetics, Cancer Institute, College of Medicine, University of Cincinnati, 3223 Eden Avenue, Kettering Laboratory Complex, Cincinnati, OH 45267, USA
[b] Cincinnati Veterans Affairs Medical Center, 3200 Vine Street, Cincinnati, OH 45220, USA
[c] Department of Environmental Health, College of Medicine, University of Cincinnati, 3223 Eden Avenue, Kettering Laboratory Complex, Cincinnati, OH 45267, USA
* Corresponding author. Department of Environmental Health, College of Medicine, University of Cincinnati, Room 128, Kettering Complex, 3223 Eden Avenue, Cincinnati, OH 45267.
E-mail address: shuk-mei.ho@uc.edu

of estrogens, xenoestrogens, phytoestrogens, antiestrogens, and selective ER modulators (SERMs) for prevention and treatment of PCa.

EPIDEMIOLOGIC AND ANIMAL-MODEL STUDIES OF THE RELATIONSHIP BETWEEN ESTROGENS AND PATHOGENESIS OF PCa

Results from epidemiologic studies have suggested a role for estrogen in the pathogenesis of PCa. Racial/ethnic and geographic differences in the levels of estrogens provide a probable explanation for the disparity in the prevalence of PCa among various populations throughout the world.[1-3] Apropos to this view is the finding that levels of circulating estrogens in African American men, whose incidence of PCa is the highest in the United States, are higher than those in white Americans throughout their adult lives.[4-8] In contrast, Japanese men, whose incidence of PCa is low, have lower circulating levels of estrogen than do Dutch-European men.[9] A global study on 5003 men aged 65 years or older showed that black people (in the United States and in West Africa) had higher estrogen levels than white or Asian people (in the United States and in their homelands), with levels of total and free estradiol-17β (E2) 10% to 16% higher and levels of estrone (E1) 27% to 39% higher than in the Asian group.[10] Moreover, the ratios of total E2 to total testosterone (T) and E1 to androstenedione were higher in black people than in the other groups.[10] A comprehensive analysis of the levels of androgens, estrogens, and their metabolites in circulation led to the conclusion that 2 fundamental metabolic processes, increased aromatase activity and reduced androgen glucuronidation, are major factors governing the ratio of estrogen to androgen in elderly men.[10]

Age is also a key risk factor for PCa.[1] The prevalence of PCa increases dramatically as men age; this is paralleled by a significant increase in the ratio of circulating estrogen to androgen levels, which may increase by up to 40%.[11-17] This age-related hormonal change, often referred to as andropause, is caused by several endocrine events, including a decline in testicular function, and increases in adiposity, extragonadal aromatization, and the production of sex hormone–binding globulin (SHBG) as men age.[12,18-21] The level of 5α-dihydrotestosterone (DHT) was found to decrease, whereas those of estrogen (both E2 and E1) in the epithelial cells increase in the aging prostate (**Fig. 1**).[22] Because estrogens can be synthesized de novo via aromatase activity in the prostate,[23] tissue estrogen levels may be more important than circulating estrogen levels in promoting prostate carcinogenesis and progression. In this regard, recent studies using laser capture microdissection samples showed that stromal rather than epithelial aromatase activity may be important in upregulating the E2/T ratio in the tumor site via an alternative promoter activation mechanism during prostate carcinogenesis.[24,25] Furthermore, aromatase-knockout mice, which cannot produce E2 locally in the prostate, have increased levels of circulating T and DHT and, with age, are prone to the development of benign prostatic hyperplasia (BPH) but not PCa.[26] Collectively, increased estrogenic influences on the prostate caused by racial differences or andropause[27] may increase the risk of neoplastic transformation of the prostatic epithelium in men.[3,28,29]

Experimental models also support the suggestion that estrogens, alone or synergistically with androgens, are potent inducers of aberrant growth and neoplastic transformation in the prostate.[1,2,30-33] Prenatal exposure to maternal estrogens, or adult exposure to pharmacologic doses of estrogens, induces a benign lesion termed squamous metaplasia, which is derived from the basal-cell proliferation of the prostates of various species, including humans.[34] In a susceptible rat strain (Noble rats), chronic exposure to T plus E2 in adulthood promoted the evolution of a precancerous lesion similar to human prostatic intraepithelial neoplasia (PIN) and a high incidence of full-blown PCa[31,35–37] via the alteration of levels of estrogen to androgen in a manner mimicking that in aging men.[35–38] Paradoxically, dietary soy that is rich in phytoestrogens can mitigate the tumor-promoting effect of T plus E2 in this rat model.[39] Moreover, treatment of the nude mice with T plus E2 could promote the progression of PCa and metastasis at distant organs in the tissue recombinants composed of mouse mesenchyme and a human prostatic epithelial cell line.[40] Cellular and molecular changes implicated as the mechanisms leading to prostate carcinogenesis include (1) a dramatic increase in the proliferation of epithelial cells[37]; (2) upregulation of growth factor signaling pathways (eg, TGFα/EGF receptor signaling[41]; TGFβ,[42] insulin growth factor [IGF]-1, and vascular endothelial growth factor [VEGF] signaling,[43] and ER signaling)[44]; (3) prolactinemia or increased prolactin-receptor signaling[45]; (4) mitogen-activated protein kinase (MAPK) activation, possibly through Id-1[46,47]; (5) increased cell-survival potential through the overexpression of antiapoptotic mediators (eg, metallothionein[48] and TRPM-2/clusterin)[49,50]; (6) increase in oxidative stress-induced DNA damage[51–53]; (7) changes in gene expression profiles related to cell proliferation, DNA damage, activation of proto-oncogenes and transforming factors, interleukin (IL)-1B signaling, and TNF-α activation[54,55]; and (8) breakdown of epithelial basement membrane and stromal extracellular matrix caused by the increase in gelatinolytic proteinase activity and altered expression of glycoconjugates in smooth muscles and their associated extracellular matrix.[56–58] Another potential culprit associated with estrogen-induced/promoted PCa is hormone-induced chronic inflammation,[38,59–61] although this view is not uniformly supported by all studies.[62]

INFLUENCE OF ESTROGEN BIOACTIVATION AND DETOXIFICATION ON PCA RISK

The carcinogenic action of estrogen could be caused, in part, by metabolic activation of the natural estrogens E1 and E2 to genotoxic metabolites, such as 2-hydroxyl and 4-hydroxyl catechol estrogens, and their quinone/semiquinone intermediates that act as chemical carcinogens.[63] The bioactivation process is mediated principally by 2 cytochrome P450 enzymes, CYP1A1 and CYP1B1, whereas the enzyme catechol-O-methyltransferase (COMT) is responsible for the inactivation and removal of these genotoxic estrogen-derived intermediates.[63–66] Once formed, these genotoxic metabolites can cause genomic damage through processes such as the formation of DNA adducts.[67] Supporting the suggestion that the genotoxicity of estrogen metabolites is involved in prostate carcinogenesis is the observation of increased DNA strand breakage[52] and nuclear staining of 8-hydroxy-2′-deoxy-guanosine[60] in the prostates of rats treated with T plus E2. Conversely, increased expression or activity of COMT was shown to protect against estrogen-induced cancer by mediating the conversion of catechol estrogens into methoxyestrogens that have potent apoptotic activity against rapidly growing PCa cells,[68] prompting the testing of combinatory therapies involving methoxyestrogens and other standard therapies, such as hormone deprivation,[69] docetaxel,[70] and eugenol[71] against PCa growth in model systems.

Furthermore, the aforementioned estrogen metabolites and their intermediates induce oxidative stress and likely promote the generation of high levels of reactive oxygen species (ROS), with damaging effects on proteins, lipids, and DNA in target tissues.[29,66] Therefore, several isoforms of glutathione S-transferases (GSTs) have been reported to have protective effects against estrogen genotoxicity through the detoxification of ROS. Genetic polymorphisms that alter enzyme activity and epigenetics-mediated or mutation-mediated silencing of the cognate genes are expected to affect the PCa risk by modulating the extent of lifelong exposure to

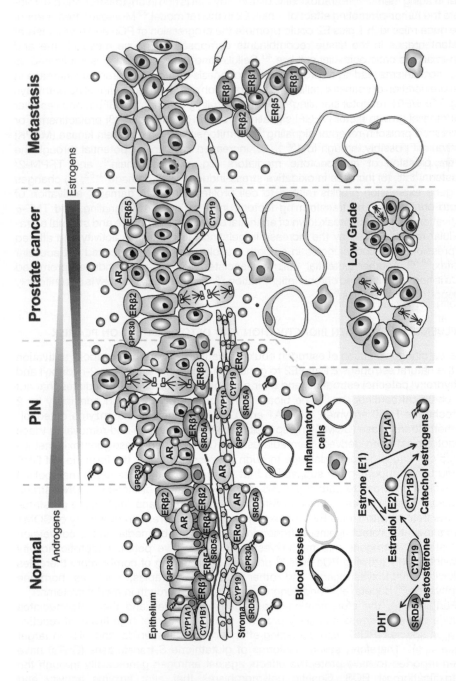

genotoxic estrogen metabolites.[29,72] Thus, polymorphisms of the *CYP1A1m1* allele, the *CYP1B1*-Leu432Val, *COMT* at codon 62 and 158, and the *GSTM1*-null genotype have been shown to modify PCa risk in certain populations.[73–80] In addition, a *CYP1A1* variant (*CYP1A1v*) that resides preferentially in the nucleus and mitochondria was found to confer higher carcinogenic potential than its wild-type cytosolic counterpart.[81] This finding is consistent with the hypothesis that genotoxic estrogen metabolites produced in nuclei are potent tumor initiators.

Another metabolic pathway of relevance to estrogen carcinogenicity in the prostate is the in situ production of estrogen from androgen via aromatase encoded by *CYP19*.[25] The enzyme and its activity have been shown in specimens of PCa and BPH.[25,82] Clinical trials designed to test the efficacy of aromatase inhibitors in treating BPH[83–85] and PCa[86–89] have been reported. Polymorphisms in *CYP19*, including intron 4[TTTA]n repeat[90] and C/T versus T/T genotype,[91] are associated with familial PCa. Continued investigation of the use of aromatase inhibitors as monotherapies or adjuvants for the treatment of PCa is warranted.[26,92]

DETERMINATION OF PCA RISK DURING EARLY LIFE

The risk of developing PCa as an adult could be determined by early-life exposure to natural or environmental estrogens through a mechanism known as estrogen imprinting.[93] Perinatal and neonatal exposure of rats[94–97] or mice[98–100] to estrogens or estrogen mimics induces inflammation, permanent changes in the levels of androgen and ERs, stromal hypertrophy, and increased proliferative potentials in the prostatic epithelium of the adult aged gland.[96,101–103] If the estrogenized adult glands are exposed to an increased estrogen challenge during adult life (the second hit), full-blown PIN develops in the affected glands.[104] An environmental estrogen, bisphenol A (BPA), is

---

Fig. 1. Expression of various hormone receptors and levels of hormones during the development and progression of PCa. In the normal human prostate (far left panel), androgen receptor (AR), ERα, different ERβ isoforms, and G protein–coupled receptor 30 (GPR30) are expressed differentially in the stroma and luminal and basal epithelium of the prostate. The epithelial cell compartment expresses only ERβ and AR, whereas the stromal compartment expresses both ERα and AR. GPR30 is expressed in both compartments. During tumor progression from high-grade prostatic intraepithelial neoplasia (PIN; second panel from the left) to prostate cancer (second panel from the right), expression of AR and ERα remains unchanged, whereas expression of the antiproliferative ERβ1 is lost in the basal epithelial cells along with the disruption of the basement membrane (*pink line*). Two ERβ isoforms, ERβ2 and ERβ5, which have been shown to have prometastatic potential, are expressed in the normal epithelium, but their coexpression in PCa specimens is associated with a poor prognosis and shorter metastasis-free survival. In prostate metastases (far right panel), ERβ1 is reexpressed at high levels. Other noncanonical ERs such as GPR30 and ERRs are differentially expressed in normal and malignant prostate tissues but their roles in prostate carcinogenesis remains to be elucidated. Throughout the development and progression of PCa, tissue estrogen levels (estradiol-17β [E2] and estrone [E1]) increase with concomitant decreases in levels of DHT. These changes are due in part to an increase in cytochrome P 19 (CYP19; aromatase) activity and a loss of SRD5A (5α-reductase) expression in the primary site (*inset*). SRD5A expression is completely lost in metastases. In addition, an age-related reduction in testicular testosterone (T) synthesis, an increase in levels of sex hormone–binding globulin, and increases in adiposity and peripheral aromatase activity collectively contribute to an increase in the estrogen/androgen ratio in circulation that further raises prostatic estrogen levels. In summary, a lifetime overexposure to estrogens and/or catecholestrogens could be an causal factor in prostate carcinogenesis. The localizations of these enzymes, as well as mediators of estrogen/androgen actions, are indicated.

equally effective in sensitizing the adult prostate to increased estrogenic influence during adulthood with regard to the induction of PIN. An unbiased screening has identified permanent alterations in the methylation status of a C-phosphate-G (CpG) island in the promoter of phosphodiesterase 4D4 (*Pde4e4*), an enzyme responsible for regulating cellular cAMP.[104] This finding suggests that estrogen imprinting may involve epigenetic reprogramming of prostatic transcription programs in early life. Whether analogous phenomena exist in humans is unclear. However, circulating E2 levels have been found to be higher in pregnant African American women than in pregnant white American women.[105,106] These data are consistent with the hypothesis that exposure to higher levels of E2 in utero may explain some of the differences in PCa risk among ethnic groups. Moreover, some indicators of high levels of estrogen during pregnancy, such as high birth weight and jaundice in the newborn, are associated with increased risk of PCa, whereas indicators of low estrogen levels, such as preeclampsia, are related to decreased risk.[107,108] The male offspring of women who took diethylstilbestrol (DES) during pregnancy may have a higher risk of PCa.[109] Taken together, these data indicate that PCa may be considered a fetal-based adult disease. In addition, the window of susceptibility for early-life reprogramming may extend to perinatal and peripubertal periods and exposures to environmental estrogens may have the same impact as natural estrogens. Of relevance to these hypotheses are studies reporting significant exposure of human fetuses to BPA, likely caused by maternal use of BPA-containing products.[110–116] Perinatal exposure to BPA has also been documented.[117–119] Paradoxically, concerns about developmental reprogramming of PCa risk by soy infant formulas containing high concentrations of phytoestrogens have seldom been raised.[120–122] However, the results of numerous human studies examining the risks and benefits of adult consumption of soy and phytoestrogens for prevention of PCa have been inconclusive.[123–127] In summary, if PCa risk can be reprogrammed in early life, cancer prevention strategies should be directed at the aforementioned early developmental stages.

ERα AND ERβ AS FUNCTIONALLY DIVERGENT MEDIATORS OF ESTROGEN ACTION IN THE PROSTATE

The actions of estrogens are now believed to be mediated primarily by 2 ER subtypes, ERα and ERβ, and their variant forms.[28,32,128,129] Both of the ERs have 6 common domains (A–F). They share a highly homologous DNA-binding domain (97% amino acid homology) but have a dissimilar N-terminal and C-terminal.[130] In addition, their ligand-binding domains are 56% homologous. These structural differences are the basis of the reported significant functional differences between the 2 receptor subtypes. Furthermore, it has been reported that the binding of the 2 receptors to the same ligand can initiate recruitments of different coregulators and trigger the use of different *cis*-regulatory elements, thus increasing the functional diversity of these 2 receptors.[130–135] The recent discovery of variant forms of ERα and ERβ (isoforms) caused by alternative splicing or mutations has added complexity to estrogen action because these variants clearly show distinct functional disparity and patterns of distribution specific to tissue/cell types.[129,132,136,137]

Many reports have shown differential expression patterns of the 2 receptors in the epithelial and stromal compartments of the normal and malignant human prostate (see **Fig. 1**).[33,137–144] In the normal human prostate, the wild-type ERβ (also known as ERβ1) is localized mainly in the basal epithelial compartment, where ERα is almost never found, whereas ERα, along with ERβ, is expressed in the stroma.[141] Both ER subtypes are absent in the luminal epithelial compartment.[137,141] A gradual loss of ERβ1 expression is apparent during the progression to high-grade PCa in the primary site.[115,139,140,145,146] The progressive silencing of ERβ is accompanied by hypermethylation of a CpG island in the proximal promoter of the gene.[147] Paradoxically, ERβ, but not ERα, is expressed at high levels in PCa metastasized to the bone and regional lymph nodes,[141] with a concomitant loss of methylation in the CpG island of ERβ.[147] Fine mapping of the CpG island revealed that this reversible silencing and reactivation of ERβ expression is attributable to cytosine methylation of an AP2 site within the CpG island of the ERβ promoter.[148] Moreover, antiestrogen-based therapies involving DES or PC-SPES lowered the level of ERβ1 expression in bone metastases of the treated patients.[149]

ERβ1 exerts an antiproliferative effect on the prostate epithelia[131,133] and inhibits epithelial-mesenchymal transition.[150] However, less is known about the biologic roles of its spliced variants. We recently showed that ERβ2 and ERβ5 promote metastasis and that their expression is associated with shorter metastasis-free survival in patients with PCa.[137] In support of a divergent functional role of various ERβ isoforms, when a pan-ERβ antibody was used, the retention of ERβ expression in primary PCa was associated with increased mortality.[139] The coexpression of ERβ with endothelial nitric oxide synthase (eNOS) and hypoxia-inducible factor 2α (HIF-2α) suggests that an estrogen-mediated NO-enriched environment may influence the aggressive phenotype of PCa significantly.[151] Thus, ERβ seems to play differential roles in human prostate carcinogenesis through differential expression of the various spliced variants and possibly alternative promoter use.[152] Differential binding of the receptor to different ligands and crosstalk with other transcriptional factor signaling cascades may also introduce additional divergence in ERβ action.[131,153,154]

Studies in animal models have provided strong evidence of the antiproliferative role of ERβ in the prostate gland. ERβ-knockout mice have been found to develop prostatic hyperplasia in old age, a phenomenon not seen in ERα-knockout mice.[155] Jiang and colleagues[156] observed an age-dependent decline in ERβ expression in the canine prostate. Chang and Prins[157] reported that neonatal exposure of rats to estrogen causes the downregulation of ERβ; the upregulation of ERα; and the development of hyperplastic, dysplastic, and neoplastic lesions in the adult ventral prostates. Consistent with the hypothesis of the antiproliferative role of ERβ, Risbriger and colleagues[158] showed that the administration of ERβ agonists, but not of an ERα agonist, to aromatase-knockout mice suppressed the prostate epithelial cell growth and promoted apoptosis, and that the action of the receptor is mediated via TNF-α signaling.[133]

Apart from ERβ expression, ERα, which is expressed primarily in the stromal compartment of the prostate, may contribute to the pathogenesis of PCa. Higher levels of ERα were observed in the prostatic stroma of Hispanic and Asian men than in that of white and African American men, who are at a higher risk for PCa.[159] In a genotyping and allelic frequency analysis of 6 different polymorphic loci of ERα in a Japanese population, polymorphism in codon 10 was found to be associated with a higher PCa risk.[160] These findings are in contrast with results from studies of genetic polymorphisms of ERβ[161–164] that reported no strong association of various polymorphic loci with PCa risk, with the exception of 1 promoter single-nucleotide polymorphism (SNP).[165,166]

During fetal development of the human prostate, ERβ is the first to appear in the prostate (by the seventh week of gestation) and is the only ER subtype expressed in the epithelial and stromal cells during the early ductal morphogenesis.[34,167] ERβ expression begins by week 15 of gestation and is strongly associated with the squamous metaplasia in the distal periurethral ducts and utricle.[167] These findings suggested that ERβ, perhaps in concert with the androgen receptor (AR), mediates the early stage of fetal prostate development, followed by the action of ERα. Thus, selective ERβ-activating compounds may play an important role in prenatal estrogen imprinting of PCa risk.

NONCANONICAL ACTIONS OF ESTROGEN AND A NEW THERAPEUTIC TARGET (G PROTEIN–COUPLED RECEPTOR 30)

Apart from acting as transcription factors, ERα and ERβ can trigger rapid nongenomic signal transduction at the cell membrane level through the activation of specific kinase activity or induction of a calcium influx.[168–170] These membrane ER-mediated events can activate gene-transcription activities with or without synergy with the classic genomic actions of nuclear ERs.[171] In this regard, membrane ERα has been shown to tether onto the epidermal growth factor receptor (EGFR) signaling pathway for the activation of the MAPK[172] and phosphoinositide 3-kinase (PI3K) signaling.[173] In addition, ERβ found localized in the mitochondria has been shown to act as a mitochondrial transcription factor that regulates mitochondrial gene expression.[174] ERβ has been reported to move from the mitochondria to the nucleus during neoplastic transformation.[175] However, the functions of cell membrane or mitochondrial ERα and ERβ in the prostate and PCa remain unknown and need further elucidation.

Estrogen has recently been found to be able to exert its action via the G protein-coupled receptor 30 (GPR30).[176] GPR30 has been localized in the cell membrane and endoplasmic reticulum of various estrogen-sensitive tissues and cell lines[176–178] and to mediate the nongenomic action of E2 in breast, endometrial, and ovarian cancer cells through the activation of Erk1/2 and cAMP pathways.[179,180] GPR30 is expressed in the immortalized normal prostate stroma cell line WPWY-1 but does not seem to mediate the growth response induced by high-dose E2.[181] A recent study showed positive staining of GPR30 in both plasma membrane and cytoplasm in the normal and cancerous prostate, and its predominant expression in the luminal epithelium.[182] Activation of GPR30 by a nonestrogenic, synthetic, GPR30-specific ligand G-1 inhibited PCa cell growth in vitro by activating Erk1/2 and upregulating p21-mediated G2-M arrest and attenuated the growth of human PCa xenografts in nude mice.[183] These new findings suggest that GPR30 is a novel estrogen mediator in the prostate and that a specific GPR30 ligand such as G-1 may have therapeutic potential for PCa.

Estrogen-related receptors (ERRs) are orphan nuclear receptors that are highly homologous to ERs, especially in the DNA-binding and ligand-binding domains.[184] However, they do not bind natural estrogens and may have yet-to-be discovered endogenous ligands. There are at least 3 ERRs, namely ERR-α, ERR-β,[185] and ERR-γ.[186,187] They regulate gene expression through transactivation via cis-elements such as the estrogen response element (ERE), steroidogenic factor-1 response element (SFRE), and estrogen-related receptor response element (ERRE).[187–191] Similar to ERs, different ERRs have distinct differential expression patterns in normal and cancerous prostate tissues/cells.[184] Although they do not bind natural estrogens, ERRβ and ERRγ do bind DES, tamoxifen, 4-hydroxytamoxifen, flavones, and isoflavone phytoestrogens,[192–194] and therefore should be considered in devising estrogen-based or antiestrogen-based therapies for PCa.

PREVENTION OF AND THERAPY FOR PCa WITH SERMs, AROMATASE INHIBITORS, PHYTOESTROGENS, AND OTHER ESTROGEN-BASED/ANTIESTROGEN-BASED TREATMENTS

The first effective drug therapy for PCa was found about 70 years ago. DES, a xenoestrogen, was applied for the treatment of metastatic PCa[195] but was found to have cardiovascular toxicity and other serious adverse effects.[33,196,197] Other ER-based treatments for PCa include antiestrogens, SERMs, and aromatase inhibitors. SERMs are estrogenic compounds that act as either ER agonists or antagonists according to the presence of different coregulators in a cell-specific/tissue-specific manner. Consequently, the ERs can be either stimulated or inhibited in the cell/tissue.[198] However, clinical trials have shown that different generations of SERMs, such as tamoxifen, toremifene, raloxifene, and fulvestrant, have limited efficacy as alternatives to DES.[33,199–205] Their lack of efficacy could be caused by their original design for targeting the transactivation of ERα on an ERE and/or blocking the traditional genomic action of estrogen. With the growing knowledge of the wide range of genomic and nongenomic actions of estrogen and the variable expression of ERβ and its isoforms in the prostate and PCa, as well as of the significance of the noncanonical ER, GPR30, the future design of estrogen/antiestrogen therapies and chemopreventive agents will have to take into account the complex nature of estrogen action in the development and progression of PCa.

Many specificities or off-target effects of estrogenic/antiestrogenic drugs are caused by their broad spectrum of activities not restricted to their estrogenicity. Traditionally, estrogen-induced PCa regression is believed to be mediated by its action on the hypothalamic-pituitary axis, thereby inhibiting testosterone synthesis.[206] However, it is now known that many estrogens/antiestrogens/phytoestrogens/SERMs, including DES, 2-methoxy-E2, genistein, resveratrol, licochalcone, raloxifene, toremifene, fulvestrant, and estramustine, have antitumor effects independent of this pathway.[207–223] The ability of these compounds to suppress PCa cell growth has been attributed to a broad range of actions, including direct cytotoxicity,[221] interruption of cell-cycle progression,[208,219,224] induction of apoptosis,[209,219,222,223] depolymerization of microtubules,[207] inhibition of DNA synthesis,[211] inhibition of topoisomerase II,[215] blockade of tyrosine kinase,[215,216] disruption of apoptotic regulators,[220] and activation of death-domain receptors.[212,217] Some of these estrogenic/antiestrogenic compounds are also potent inhibitors of angiogenesis and metastasis, through their actions in upregulating expression of genes related to antiangiogenesis or antimetastasis,[213] activating the cell adhesion–signaling molecule focal adhesion kinase,[214] and reduction in metastatic spreading via the lymphatic system.[218]

As a recent development in the treatment of PCa, the application of estrogen patches has grown in popularity.[225–227] The advantages include reduction in cardiovascular toxicity and the maintenance of adequate hormonal levels for a convenient time period,[228] as well as the additional advantage of alleviating hot flashes and improving bone density after endocrine treatment of PCa.[229,230] Estrogen patches have recently been tested in a phase II clinical trial as a first-line hormonal therapy in patients with locally advanced or metastatic PCa. Preliminary results produced the levels of testosterone and a prostate-specific antigen response similar to those of castration.[226]

Aside from treating PCa, the potential of SERMs for preventing PCa is promising. The rationale stems from several lines of investigation. SERMs were shown to decrease testosterone levels by suppressing the hypothalamic-pituitary axis.[231] Furthermore, age-related increases in PCa prevalence parallel increases in serum estrogen levels, and the incidence of PCa is low in countries with diets rich in phytoestrogens.[232] A multicentered, double-blind, randomized study involving 514 men with high-grade PIN and no cancer reported a significant reduction in PCa incidence in patients treated daily with 20 mg of toremifene for 6 to 12 months compared with placebo.[233] These promising results have prompted the initiation of a large phase III study to examine the potential for toremifene as a chemopreventive agent.

Phytoestrogens are another important class of estrogen-based chemopreventive agents. The most common phytoestrogens, soy isoflavones such as genistein, equol, and daidzein, which are abundant in soy beans and its products, have been found to have estrogenic or antiestrogenic activity.[234–237] They have been some of the most popular agents in studies of the potential of PCa chemoprevention and therapy because of the low incidence of PCa, along with the high levels of phytochemicals, in the diets of Asian populations.[238] Although there is an abundance of in vitro and in vivo experimental data about the antitumor properties of phytoestrogens, the value of their protective or therapeutic effects in cohort studies still remains controversial.[239–246] Nevertheless, phase I clinical trials evaluating the use of phytoestrogen supplementation in patients with PCa have generally seen beneficial effects without any toxicity.[210,247–250]

SUMMARY

Traditionally, androgens have been considered to be the major sex hormones regulating the normal and malignant growth of the prostate. However, recent epidemiologic findings and experimental data suggest that estrogens and their mimics can be responsible for the pathogenesis of PCa. The carcinogenicity of estrogens in the prostate during adulthood is believed to be mediated by the combined effects of the hormone-induced unscheduled cell proliferation and epigenetic silencing of antitumor genes, along with the bioactivation of estrogens to genotoxic carcinogens. Thus, individuals or ethnic groups with polymorphisms in genes encoding ERs and/or estrogen-metabolizing enzymes can modify the risk for PCa caused by altered responsiveness to the hormone and exposure to its carcinogenic metabolites during a lifetime. The age-dependent hormonal shift from androgen to estrogen could also be an important contributing factor to increased estrogen bioavailability. Although PCa has a long latency and starts to develop in men around middle age, recent data strongly suggest that PCa risk could be determined even as early as during prenatal and perinatal life stages by a process known as estrogen imprinting. Thus, primary PCa prevention should probably begin in early life. Among the various cellular mediators, ERβ seems to be a key determinant in the pathogenesis, progression, and metastasis of PCa. Therapeutic approaches targeting its activation/inactivation may have important ramifications in the prevention and treatment of PCa. Epigenetic mechanisms such as DNA methylation play important roles in regulating the expression of the 2 ER subtypes. A change in the methylation status of proximal promoters of these genes constitutes an on/off switch for reversible gene regulation. Moreover, the differential expression of different ER-spliced variants (isoforms) could explain some conflicting observations related to estrogen action in the initiation and progression of PCa. Apart from the canonical genomic action of ERα and ERβ, the therapeutic potential of ER and its variants that function in multiple nongenomic pathways, such as membrane ERα, mitochondrial ER, ERRs, and GPR30, may further contribute to the pathogenesis of PCa. Various estrogenic/antiestrogenic/SERM-like compounds have demonstrable efficacies in causing PCa regression through the use of pathways independent of the hypothalamic-pituitary axis. As the treatment of advanced PCa with transdermal estrogen has gained in popularity, several SERMs, including toremifene, have shown promise as chemopreventive or therapeutic agents in clinical trials. Although data from clinical trials are not conclusive, phytoestrogen supplements, including dietary soy, continue to be used by patients as complementary alternative medicine for PCa. With a greater understanding of the molecular mechanism underlying estrogen carcinogenicity in the prostate, the applicability of estrogen/antiestrogen-based prevention and treatment therapies, as first-line or adjuvant therapies, will be used more in the clinic. Thus, the devising of a new generation of estrogenic/antiestrogenic therapies with higher specificity against PCa and fewer off-target effects is timely.

ACKNOWLEDGMENTS

We thank Nancy K. Voynow for her professional editorial assistance and Dr Xiang Zhang for helpful critiques of the manuscript.

REFERENCES

1. Bostwick DG, Burke HB, Djakiew D, et al. Human prostate cancer risk factors. Cancer 2004;101(Suppl 10):2371–490.
2. Ho SM. Estrogens and anti-estrogens: key mediators of prostate carcinogenesis and new therapeutic candidates. J Cell Biochem 2004;91(3):491–503.
3. Ho SM, Leung YK, Chung I. Estrogens and antiestrogens as etiological factors and therapeutics for prostate cancer. Ann N Y Acad Sci 2006;1089:177–93.
4. Abdelrahaman E, Raghavan S, Baker L, et al. Racial difference in circulating sex hormone-binding globulin levels in prepubertal boys. Metabolism 2005;54(1): 91–6.
5. Hui SL, DiMeglio LA, Longcope C, et al. Difference in bone mass between black and white American children: attributable to body build, sex hormone levels, or bone turnover? J Clin Endocrinol Metab 2003;88(2):642–9.
6. Richards RJ, Svec F, Bao W, et al. Steroid hormones during puberty: racial (black-white) differences in androstenedione and estradiol–the Bogalusa Heart Study. J Clin Endocrinol Metab 1992;75(2):624–31.
7. Rohrmann S, Nelson WG, Rifai N, et al. Serum estrogen, but not testosterone, levels differ between black and white men in a nationally representative sample of Americans. J Clin Endocrinol Metab 2007;92(7):2519–25.
8. Ross R, Bernstein L, Judd H, et al. Serum testosterone levels in healthy young black and white men. J Natl Cancer Inst 1986;76(1):45–8.
9. de Jong FH, Oishi K, Hayes RB, et al. Peripheral hormone levels in controls and patients with prostatic cancer or benign prostatic hyperplasia: results from the Dutch-Japanese case-control study. Cancer Res 1991;51(13):3445–50.
10. Orwoll ES, Nielson CM, Labrie F, et al. Evidence for geographical and racial variation in serum sex steroid levels in older men. J Clin Endocrinol Metab 2010; 95(10):E151–60.
11. Ellem SJ, Risbridger GP. Aromatase and regulating the estrogen:androgen ratio in the prostate gland. J Steroid Biochem Mol Biol 2010;118(4–5):246–51.
12. Feldman HA, Longcope C, Derby CA, et al. Age trends in the level of serum testosterone and other hormones in middle-aged men: longitudinal results from the Massachusetts male aging study. J Clin Endocrinol Metab 2002; 87(2):589–98.
13. Gray A, Berlin JA, McKinlay JB, et al. An examination of research design effects on the association of testosterone and male aging: results of a meta-analysis. J Clin Epidemiol 1991;44(7):671–84.
14. Gray A, Feldman HA, McKinlay JB, et al. Age, disease, and changing sex hormone levels in middle-aged men: results of the Massachusetts Male Aging Study. J Clin Endocrinol Metab 1991;73(5):1016–25.
15. Griffiths K. Estrogens and prostatic disease. International Prostate Health Council Study Group. Prostate 2000;45(2):87–100.
16. Roberts RO, Jacobson DJ, Rhodes T, et al. Serum sex hormones and measures of benign prostatic hyperplasia. Prostate 2004;61(2):124–31.
17. Vermeulen A, Rubens R, Verdonck L. Testosterone secretion and metabolism in male senescence. J Clin Endocrinol Metab 1972;34(4):730–5.

18. Gapstur SM, Gann PH, Kopp P, et al. Serum androgen concentrations in young men: a longitudinal analysis of associations with age, obesity, and race. The CARDIA Male Hormone Study. Cancer Epidemiol Biomarkers Prev 2002;11(10 Pt 1):1041-7.

19. Krieg JM, Vermeulen A. The decline of androgen levels in elderly men and its clinical and therapeutic implications. Endocr Rev 2005;26(6):833-76.

20. Moretti C, Frajese GV, Guccione L, et al. Androgens and body composition in the aging male. J Endocrinol Invest 2005;28(Suppl 3):56-64.

21. Starka L, Pospisilova H, Hill M. Free testosterone and free dihydrotestosterone throughout the life span of men. J Steroid Biochem Mol Biol 2009;116(1-2): 118-20.

22. Krieg M, Nass R, Tunn S. Effect of aging on endogenous level of 5 alpha-dihydrotestosterone, testosterone, estradiol, and estrone in epithelium and stroma of normal and hyperplastic human prostate. J Clin Endocrinol Metab 1993;77(2):375-81.

23. Farnsworth WE. Roles of estrogen and SHBG in prostate physiology. Prostate 1996;28(1):17-23.

24. Ellem SJ, Schmitt JF, Pedersen JS, et al. Local aromatase expression in human prostate is altered in malignancy. J Clin Endocrinol Metab 2004;89(5):2434-41.

25. Ellem SJ, Risbridger GP. Aromatase and prostate cancer. Minerva Endocrinol 2006;31(1):1-12.

26. McPherson SJ, Wang H, Jones ME, et al. Elevated androgens and prolactin in aromatase-deficient mice cause enlargement, but not malignancy, of the prostate gland. Endocrinology 2001;142(6):2458-67.

27. Bain J. Testosterone and the aging male: to treat or not to treat? Maturitas 2010; 66(1):16-22.

28. Prins GS, Korach KS. The role of estrogens and estrogen receptors in normal prostate growth and disease. Steroids 2008;73(3):233-44.

29. Singh PB, Matanhelia SS, Martin FL. A potential paradox in prostate adenocarcinoma progression: oestrogen as the initiating driver. Eur J Cancer 2008;44(7): 928-36.

30. Bosland MC. Use of animal models in defining efficacy of chemoprevention agents against prostate cancer. Eur Urol 1999;35(5-6):459-63.

31. Ho SM, Lane K, Lee K. Neoplastic transformation of the prostate. In: Naz RK, editor. Prostate: basic and clinical aspects. New York: CRC Press; 1997. p. 74-114.

32. Ricke WA, Wang Y, Cunha GR. Steroid hormones and carcinogenesis of the prostate: the role of estrogens. Differentiation 2007;75(9):871-82.

33. Taplin ME, Ho SM. Clinical review 134: the endocrinology of prostate cancer. J Clin Endocrinol Metab 2001;86(8):3467-77.

34. Adams JY, Leav I, Lau KM, et al. Expression of estrogen receptor beta in the fetal, neonatal, and prepubertal human prostate. Prostate 2002;52(1):69-81.

35. Ho SM, Leav I, Merk FB, et al. Induction of atypical hyperplasia, apoptosis, and type II estrogen-binding sites in the ventral prostates of Noble rats treated with testosterone and pharmacologic doses of estradiol-17 beta. Lab Invest 1995; 73(3):356-65.

36. Leav I, Ho SM, Ofner P, et al. Biochemical alterations in sex hormone-induced hyperplasia and dysplasia of the dorsolateral prostates of Noble rats. J Natl Cancer Inst 1988;80(13):1045-53.

37. Leav I, Merk FB, Kwan PW, et al. Androgen-supported estrogen-enhanced epithelial proliferation in the prostates of intact Noble rats. Prostate 1989;15(1):23-40.

38. Yatkin E, Bernoulli J, Talvitie EM, et al. Inflammation and epithelial alterations in rat prostate: impact of the androgen to oestrogen ratio. Int J Androl 2009;32(4): 399–410.
39. Hsu A, Bruno RS, Lohr CV, et al. Dietary soy and tea mitigate chronic inflammation and prostate cancer via NFkappaB pathway in the Noble rat model. J Nutr Biochem 2011;22(5):502–10.
40. Ricke WA, Ishii K, Ricke EA, et al. Steroid hormones stimulate human prostate cancer progression and metastasis. Int J Cancer 2006;118(9):2123–31.
41. Kaplan PJ, Leav I, Greenwood J, et al. Involvement of transforming growth factor alpha (TGFalpha) and epidermal growth factor receptor (EGFR) in sex hormone-induced prostatic dysplasia and the growth of an androgen-independent transplantable carcinoma of the prostate. Carcinogenesis 1996; 17(12):2571–9.
42. Wong YC, Xie W, Tsao SW. Structural changes and alteration in expression of TGF-beta1 and its receptors in prostatic intraepithelial neoplasia (PIN) in the ventral prostate of noble rats. Prostate 2000;45(4):289–98.
43. Wang YZ, Wong YC. Sex hormone-induced prostatic carcinogenesis in the noble rat: the role of insulin-like growth factor-I (IGF-I) and vascular endothelial growth factor (VEGF) in the development of prostate cancer. Prostate 1998;35(3):165–77.
44. Lau KM, Leav I, Ho SM. Rat estrogen receptor-alpha and -beta, and progesterone receptor mRNA expression in various prostatic lobes and microdissected normal and dysplastic epithelial tissues of the Noble rats. Endocrinology 1998; 139(1):424–7.
45. Leav I, Merk FB, Lee KF, et al. Prolactin receptor expression in the developing human prostate and in hyperplastic, dysplastic, and neoplastic lesions. Am J Pathol 1999;154(3):863–70.
46. Leav I, Galluzzi CM, Ziar J, et al. Mitogen-activated protein kinase and mitogen-activated kinase phosphatase-1 expression in the Noble rat model of sex hormone-induced prostatic dysplasia and carcinoma. Lab Invest 1996;75(3): 361–70.
47. Ling MT, Wang X, Ouyang XS, et al. Activation of MAPK signaling pathway is essential for Id-1 induced serum independent prostate cancer cell growth. Oncogene 2002;21(55):8498–505.
48. Ghatak S, Oliveria P, Kaplan P, et al. Expression and regulation of metallothionein mRNA levels in the prostates of noble rats: lack of expression in the ventral prostate and regulation by sex hormones in the dorsolateral prostate. Prostate 1996;29(2):91–100.
49. Ho SM, Leav I, Ghatak S, et al. Lack of association between enhanced TRPM-2/clusterin expression and increased apoptotic activity in sex-hormone-induced prostatic dysplasia of the Noble rat. Am J Pathol 1998;153(1):131–9.
50. Ouyang XS, Wang X, Lee DT, et al. Up-regulation of TRPM-2, MMP-7 and ID-1 during sex hormone-induced prostate carcinogenesis in the Noble rat. Carcinogenesis 2001;22(6):965–73.
51. Ghatak S, Ho SM. Age-related changes in the activities of antioxidant enzymes and lipid peroxidation status in ventral and dorsolateral prostate lobes of noble rats. Biochem Biophys Res Commun 1996;222(2):362–7.
52. Ho SM, Roy D. Sex hormone-induced nuclear DNA damage and lipid peroxidation in the dorsolateral prostates of Noble rats. Cancer Lett 1994;84(2):155–62.
53. Tam NN, Ghatak S, Ho SM. Sex hormone-induced alterations in the activities of antioxidant enzymes and lipid peroxidation status in the prostate of Noble rats. Prostate 2003;55(1):1–8.

54. Tam NN, Szeto CY, Sartor MA, et al. Gene expression profiling identifies lobe-specific and common disruptions of multiple gene networks in testosterone-supported, 17beta-estradiol- or diethylstilbestrol-induced prostate dysplasia in Noble rats. Neoplasia 2008;10(1):20–40.

55. Thompson CJ, Tam NN, Joyce JM, et al. Gene expression profiling of testosterone and estradiol-17 beta-induced prostatic dysplasia in Noble rats and response to the antiestrogen ICI 182,780. Endocrinology 2002;143(6):2093–105.

56. Chan FL, Ho SM. Comparative study of glycoconjugates of the rat prostatic lobes by lectin histochemistry. Prostate 1999;38(1):1–16.

57. Chan FL, Choi HL, Ho SM. Analysis of glycoconjugate patterns of normal and hormone-induced dysplastic Noble rat prostates, and an androgen-independent Noble rat prostate tumor, by lectin histochemistry and protein blotting. Prostate 2001;46(1):21–32.

58. Li SC, Chen GF, Chan PS, et al. Altered expression of extracellular matrix and proteinases in Noble rat prostate gland after long-term treatment with sex steroids. Prostate 2001;49(1):58–71.

59. Bernoulli J, Yatkin E, Konkol Y, et al. Prostatic inflammation and obstructive voiding in the adult Noble rat: impact of the testosterone to estradiol ratio in serum. Prostate 2008;68(12):1296–306.

60. Tam NN, Leav I, Ho SM. Sex hormones induce direct epithelial and inflammation-mediated oxidative/nitrosative stress that favors prostatic carcinogenesis in the noble rat. Am J Pathol 2007;171(4):1334–41.

61. Yatkin E, Bernoulli J, Lammintausta R, et al. Fispemifene [Z-2-{2-[4-(4-chloro-1,2-diphenylbut-1-enyl)-phenoxy]ethoxy}-ethanol], a novel selective estrogen receptor modulator, attenuates glandular inflammation in an animal model of chronic nonbacterial prostatitis. J Pharmacol Exp Ther 2008;327(1):58–67.

62. Bernoulli J, Yatkin E, Laakso A, et al. Histopathological evidence for an association of inflammation with ductal pin-like lesions but not with ductal adenocarcinoma in the prostate of the noble rat. Prostate 2008;68(7):728–39.

63. Cavalieri EL, Rogan EG. A unified mechanism in the initiation of cancer. Ann N Y Acad Sci 2002;959:341–54.

64. Cavalieri E, Frenkel K, Liehr JG, et al. Estrogens as endogenous genotoxic agents–DNA adducts and mutations. J Natl Cancer Inst Monogr 2000;27:75–93.

65. Yager JD, Liehr JG. Molecular mechanisms of estrogen carcinogenesis. Annu Rev Pharmacol Toxicol 1996;36:203–32.

66. Yager JD. Endogenous estrogens as carcinogens through metabolic activation. J Natl Cancer Inst Monogr 2000;27:67–73.

67. Jefcoate CR, Liehr JG, Santen RJ, et al. Tissue-specific synthesis and oxidative metabolism of estrogens. J Natl Cancer Inst Monogr 2000;27:95–112.

68. Lakhani NJ, Sarkar MA, Venitz J, et al. 2-Methoxyestradiol, a promising anticancer agent. Pharmacotherapy 2003;23(2):165–72.

69. Sato F, Fukuhara H, Basilion JP. Effects of hormone deprivation and 2-methoxyestradiol combination therapy on hormone-dependent prostate cancer in vivo. Neoplasia 2005;7(9):838–46.

70. Reiner T, de Las PA, Gomez LA, et al. Low dose combinations of 2-methoxyestradiol and docetaxel block prostate cancer cells in mitosis and increase apoptosis. Cancer Lett 2009;276(1):21–31.

71. Ghosh R, Ganapathy M, Alworth WL, et al. Combination of 2-methoxyestradiol (2-ME2) and eugenol for apoptosis induction synergistically in androgen independent prostate cancer cells. J Steroid Biochem Mol Biol 2009;113(1–2):25–35.

72. Nock NL, Cicek MS, Li L, et al. Polymorphisms in estrogen bioactivation, detox-ification and oxidative DNA base excision repair genes and prostate cancer risk. Carcinogenesis 2006;27(9):1842–8.

73. Acevedo C, Opazo JL, Huidobro C, et al. Positive correlation between single or combined genotypes of CYP1A1 and GSTM1 in relation to prostate cancer in Chilean people. Prostate 2003;57(2):111–7.

74. Caceres DD, Iturrieta J, Acevedo C, et al. Relationship among metabolizing genes, smoking and alcohol used as modifier factors on prostate cancer risk: exploring some gene-gene and gene-environment interactions. Eur J Epidemiol 2005;20(1):79–88.

75. Quinones LA, Irarrazabal CE, Rojas CR, et al. Joint effect among p53, CYP1A1, GSTM1 polymorphism combinations and smoking on prostate cancer risk: an exploratory genotype-environment interaction study. Asian J Androl 2006;8(3): 349–55.

76. Silig Y, Pinarbasi H, Gunes S, et al. Polymorphisms of CYP1A1, GSTM1, GSTT1, and prostate cancer risk in Turkish population. Cancer Invest 2006;24(1):41–5.

77. Sobti RC, Onsory K, Al-Badran AI, et al. CYP17, SRD5A2, CYP1B1, and CYP2D6 gene polymorphisms with prostate cancer risk in North Indian popula-tion. DNA Cell Biol 2006;25(5):287–94.

78. Suzuki M, Mamun MR, Hara K, et al. The Val158Met polymorphism of the catechol-O-methyltransferase gene is associated with the PSA-progression-free survival in prostate cancer patients treated with estramustine phosphate. Eur Urol 2005;48(5):752–9.

79. Tanaka Y, Sasaki M, Shiina H, et al. Catechol-O-methyltransferase gene poly-morphisms in benign prostatic hyperplasia and sporadic prostate cancer. Cancer Epidemiol Biomarkers Prev 2006;15(2):238–44.

80. Tang YM, Green BL, Chen GF, et al. Human CYP1B1 Leu432Val gene polymor-phism: ethnic distribution in African-Americans, Caucasians and Chinese; oes-tradiol hydroxylase activity; and distribution in prostate cancer cases and controls. Pharmacogenetics 2000;10(9):761–6.

81. Leung YK, Lau KM, Mobley J, et al. Overexpression of cytochrome P450 1A1 and its novel spliced variant in ovarian cancer cells: alternative subcellular enzyme compartmentation may contribute to carcinogenesis. Cancer Res 2005;65(9):3726–34.

82. Hiramatsu M, Maehara I, Ozaki M, et al. Aromatase in hyperplasia and carci-noma of the human prostate. Prostate 1997;31(2):118–24.

83. Ito K, Fukabori Y, Shibata Y, et al. Effects of a new steroidal aromatase inhibitor, TZA-2237, and/or chlormadinone acetate on hormone-induced and spontaneous canine benign prostatic hyperplasia. Eur J Endocrinol 2000;143(4):543–54.

84. Radlmaier A, Eickenberg HU, Fletcher MS, et al. Estrogen reduction by aroma-tase inhibition for benign prostatic hyperplasia: results of a double-blind, placebo-controlled, randomized clinical trial using two doses of the aromatase-inhibitor atamestane. Atamestane Study Group. Prostate 1996;29(4):199–208.

85. Suzuki K, Okazaki H, Ono Y, et al. Effect of dual inhibition of 5-alpha-reductase and aromatase on spontaneously developed canine prostatic hypertrophy. Prostate 1998;37(2):70–6.

86. Brodie A, Njar V, Macedo LF, et al. The Coffey Lecture: steroidogenic enzyme inhibitors and hormone dependent cancer. Urol Oncol 2009;27(1):53–63.

87. Djurendic E, Daljev J, Sakac M, et al. Synthesis of some epoxy and/or N-oxy 17-picolyl and 17-picolinylidene-androst-5-ene derivatives and evaluation of their biological activity. Steroids 2008;73(1):129–38.

88. Kruit WH, Stoter G, Klijn JG. Effect of combination therapy with aminoglutethimide and hydrocortisone on prostate-specific antigen response in metastatic prostate cancer refractory to standard endocrine therapy. Anticancer Drugs 2004;15(9):843–7.

89. Sanderson T, Renaud M, Scholten D, et al. Effects of lactone derivatives on aromatase (CYP19) activity in H295R human adrenocortical and (anti)androgenicity in transfected LNCaP human prostate cancer cells. Eur J Pharmacol 2008; 593(1–3):92–8.

90. Suzuki K, Nakazato H, Matsui H, et al. Association of the genetic polymorphism of the CYP19 intron 4[TTTA]n repeat with familial prostate cancer risk in a Japanese population. Anticancer Res 2003;23(6D):4941–6.

91. Suzuki K, Nakazato H, Matsui H, et al. Genetic polymorphisms of estrogen receptor alpha, CYP19, catechol-O-methyltransferase are associated with familial prostate carcinoma risk in a Japanese population. Cancer 2003;98(7):1411–6.

92. Li X, Nokkala E, Yan W, et al. Altered structure and function of reproductive organs in transgenic male mice overexpressing human aromatase. Endocrinology 2001;142(6):2435–42.

93. Rajfer J, Coffey DS. Sex steroid imprinting of the immature prostate. Long-term effects. Invest Urol 1978;16(3):186–90.

94. Arai Y, Suzuki Y, Nishizuka Y. Hyperplastic and metaplastic lesions in the reproductive tract of male rats induced by neonatal treatment with diethylstilbestrol. Virchows Arch A Pathol Anat Histol 1977;376(1):21–8.

95. Arai Y, Mori T, Suzuki Y, et al. Long-term effects of perinatal exposure to sex steroids and diethylstilbestrol on the reproductive system of male mammals. Int Rev Cytol 1983;84:235–68.

96. Prins GS. Neonatal estrogen exposure induces lobe-specific alterations in adult rat prostate androgen receptor expression. Endocrinology 1992;130(6):3703–14.

97. Vorherr H, Messer RH, Vorherr UF, et al. Teratogenesis and carcinogenesis in rat offspring after transplacental and transmammary exposure to diethylstilbestrol. Biochem Pharmacol 1979;28(12):1865–77.

98. McLachlan JA, Newbold RR, Bullock B. Reproductive tract lesions in male mice exposed prenatally to diethylstilbestrol. Science 1975;190(4218):991–2.

99. McLachlan JA. Prenatal exposure to diethylstilbestrol in mice: toxicological studies. J Toxicol Environ Health 1977;2(3):527–37.

100. Pylkkanen L, Santti R, Newbold R, et al. Regional differences in the prostate of the neonatally estrogenized mouse. Prostate 1991;18(2):117–29.

101. Prins GS, Sklarew RJ, Pertschuk LP. Image analysis of androgen receptor immunostaining in prostate cancer accurately predicts response to hormonal therapy. J Urol 1998;159(3):641–9.

102. Prins GS, Birch L, Couse JF, et al. Estrogen imprinting of the developing prostate gland is mediated through stromal estrogen receptor alpha: studies with alphaERKO and betaERKO mice. Cancer Res 2001;61(16):6089–97.

103. vom Saal FS, Timms BG, Montano MM, et al. Prostate enlargement in mice due to fetal exposure to low doses of estradiol or diethylstilbestrol and opposite effects at high doses. Proc Natl Acad Sci U S A 1997;94(5):2056–61.

104. Ho SM, Tang WY, Belmonte de FJ, et al. Developmental exposure to estradiol and bisphenol A increases susceptibility to prostate carcinogenesis and epigenetically regulates phosphodiesterase type 4 variant 4. Cancer Res 2006; 66(11):5624–32.

105. Henderson BE, Feigelson HS. Hormonal carcinogenesis. Carcinogenesis 2000; 21(3):427–33.

106. Potischman N, Troisi R, Thadhani R, et al. Pregnancy hormone concentrations across ethnic groups: implications for later cancer risk. Cancer Epidemiol Biomarkers Prev 2005;14(6):1514–20.

107. Ekbom A, Hsieh CC, Lipworth L, et al. Perinatal characteristics in relation to incidence of and mortality from prostate cancer. BMJ 1996;313(7053):337–41.

108. Ekbom A, Wuu J, Adami HO, et al. Duration of gestation and prostate cancer risk in offspring. Cancer Epidemiol Biomarkers Prev 2000;9(2):221–3.

109. Schrager S, Potter BE. Diethylstilbestrol exposure. Am Fam Physician 2004; 69(10):2395–400.

110. Chapin RE, Adams J, Boekelheide K, et al. NTP-CERHR expert panel report on the reproductive and developmental toxicity of bisphenol A. Birth Defects Res B Dev Reprod Toxicol 2008;83(3):157–395.

111. Ikezuki Y, Tsutsumi O, Takai Y, et al. Determination of bisphenol A concentrations in human biological fluids reveals significant early prenatal exposure. Hum Reprod 2002;17(11):2839–41.

112. Kuroda N, Kinoshita Y, Sun Y, et al. Measurement of bisphenol A levels in human blood serum and ascitic fluid by HPLC using a fluorescent labeling reagent. J Pharm Biomed Anal 2003;30(6):1743–9.

113. Ranjit N, Siefert K, Padmanabhan V. Bisphenol-A and disparities in birth outcomes: a review and directions for future research. J Perinatol 2010;30(1):2–9.

114. Schonfelder G, Wittfoht W, Hopp H, et al. Parent bisphenol A accumulation in the human maternal-fetal-placental unit. Environ Health Perspect 2002;110(11): A703–7.

115. Tsurusaki T, Aoki D, Kanetake H, et al. Zone-dependent expression of estrogen receptors alpha and beta in human benign prostatic hyperplasia. J Clin Endocrinol Metab 2003;88(3):1333–40.

116. Yamada H, Furuta I, Kato EH, et al. Maternal serum and amniotic fluid bisphenol A concentrations in the early second trimester. Reprod Toxicol 2002;16(6):735–9.

117. Braniste V, Jouault A, Gaultier E, et al. Impact of oral bisphenol A at reference doses on intestinal barrier function and sex differences after perinatal exposure in rats. Proc Natl Acad Sci U S A 2010;107(1):448–53.

118. Prins GS, Tang WY, Belmonte J, et al. Developmental exposure to bisphenol A increases prostate cancer susceptibility in adult rats: epigenetic mode of action is implicated. Fertil Steril 2008;89(Suppl 2):e41.

119. Rubin BS, Soto AM, Bisphenol A. Perinatal exposure and body weight. Mol Cell Endocrinol 2009;304(1–2):55–62.

120. Badger TM, Gilchrist JM, Pivik RT, et al. The health implications of soy infant formula. Am J Clin Nutr 2009;89(5):1668S–72S.

121. Joeckel RJ, Phillips SK. Overview of infant and pediatric formulas. Nutr Clin Pract 2009;24(3):356–62.

122. Tuohy PG. Soy infant formula and phytoestrogens. J Paediatr Child Health 2003; 39(6):401–5.

123. Hamilton-Reeves JM, Rebello SA, Thomas W, et al. Effects of soy protein isolate consumption on prostate cancer biomarkers in men with HGPIN, ASAP, and low-grade prostate cancer. Nutr Cancer 2008;60(1):7–13.

124. Ide H, Tokiwa S, Sakamaki K, et al. Combined inhibitory effects of soy isoflavones and curcumin on the production of prostate-specific antigen. Prostate 2010;70(10):1127–33.

125. Kwan W, Duncan G, Van PC, et al. A phase II trial of a soy beverage for subjects without clinical disease with rising prostate-specific antigen after radical radiation for prostate cancer. Nutr Cancer 2010;62(2):198–207.

126. Pendleton JM, Tan WW, Anai S, et al. Phase II trial of isoflavone in prostate-specific antigen recurrent prostate cancer after previous local therapy. BMC Cancer 2008;8:132.
127. Vaishampayan U, Hussain M, Banerjee M, et al. Lycopene and soy isoflavones in the treatment of prostate cancer. Nutr Cancer 2007;59(1):1–7.
128. Risbridger GP, Ellem SJ, McPherson SJ. Estrogen action on the prostate gland: a critical mix of endocrine and paracrine signaling. J Mol Endocrinol 2007;39(3): 183–8.
129. Warner M, Gustafsson JA. The role of estrogen receptor beta (ERbeta) in malignant diseases–a new potential target for antiproliferative drugs in prevention and treatment of cancer. Biochem Biophys Res Commun 2010;396(1):63–6.
130. Katzenellenbogen BS, Sun J, Harrington WR, et al. Structure-function relationships in estrogen receptors and the characterization of novel selective estrogen receptor modulators with unique pharmacological profiles. Ann N Y Acad Sci 2001;949:6–15.
131. Dondi D, Piccolella M, Biserni A, et al. Estrogen receptor beta and the progression of prostate cancer: role of 5alpha-androstane-3beta,17beta-diol. Endocr Relat Cancer 2010;17(3):731–42.
132. Leung YK, Mak P, Hassan S, et al. Estrogen receptor (ER)-beta isoforms: a key to understanding ER-beta signaling. Proc Natl Acad Sci U S A 2006;103(35): 13162–7.
133. McPherson SJ, Hussain S, Balanathan P, et al. Estrogen receptor-beta activated apoptosis in benign hyperplasia and cancer of the prostate is androgen independent and TNFalpha mediated. Proc Natl Acad Sci U S A 2010;107(7):3123–8.
134. Osborne CK, Schiff R, Fuqua SA, et al. Estrogen receptor: current understanding of its activation and modulation. Clin Cancer Res 2001;7(Suppl 12): 4338s–42s.
135. Tremblay GB, Giguere V. Coregulators of estrogen receptor action. Crit Rev Eukaryot Gene Expr 2002;12(1):1–22.
136. Barone I, Brusco L, Fuqua SA. Estrogen receptor mutations and changes in downstream gene expression and signaling. Clin Cancer Res 2010;16(10): 2702–8.
137. Leung YK, Lam HM, Wu S, et al. Estrogen receptor beta2 and beta5 are associated with poor prognosis in prostate cancer, and promote cancer cell migration and invasion. Endocr Relat Cancer 2010;17(3):675–89.
138. Fixemer T, Remberger K, Bonkhoff H. Differential expression of the estrogen receptor beta (ERbeta) in human prostate tissue, premalignant changes, and in primary, metastatic, and recurrent prostatic adenocarcinoma. Prostate 2003;54(2):79–87.
139. Horvath LG, Henshall SM, Lee CS, et al. Frequent loss of estrogen receptor-beta expression in prostate cancer. Cancer Res 2001;61(14):5331–5.
140. Latil A, Bieche I, Vidaud D, et al. Evaluation of androgen, estrogen (ER alpha and ER beta), and progesterone receptor expression in human prostate cancer by real-time quantitative reverse transcription-polymerase chain reaction assays. Cancer Res 2001;61(5):1919–26.
141. Leav I, Lau KM, Adams JY, et al. Comparative studies of the estrogen receptors beta and alpha and the androgen receptor in normal human prostate glands, dysplasia, and in primary and metastatic carcinoma. Am J Pathol 2001; 159(1):79–92.
142. Royuela M, de Miguel MP, Bethencourt FR, et al. Estrogen receptors alpha and beta in the normal, hyperplastic and carcinomatous human prostate. J Endocrinol 2001;168(3):447–54.

143. Torlakovic E, Lilleby W, Torlakovic G, et al. Prostate carcinoma expression of estrogen receptor-beta as detected by PPG5/10 antibody has positive association with primary Gleason grade and Gleason score. Hum Pathol 2002;33(6):646–51.
144. Weihua Z, Warner M, Gustafsson JA. Estrogen receptor beta in the prostate. Mol Cell Endocrinol 2002;193(1–2):1–5.
145. Pasquali D, Staibano S, Prezioso D, et al. Estrogen receptor beta expression in human prostate tissue. Mol Cell Endocrinol 2001;178(1–2):47–50.
146. Pasquali D, Rossi V, Esposito D, et al. Loss of estrogen receptor beta expression in malignant human prostate cells in primary cultures and in prostate cancer tissues. J Clin Endocrinol Metab 2001;86(5):2051–5.
147. Zhu X, Leav I, Leung YK, et al. Dynamic regulation of estrogen receptor-beta expression by DNA methylation during prostate cancer development and metastasis. Am J Pathol 2004;164(6):2003–12.
148. Zhang X, Leung YK, Ho SM. AP-2 regulates the transcription of estrogen receptor (ER)-beta by acting through a methylation hotspot of the 0N promoter in prostate cancer cells. Oncogene 2007;26(52):7346–54.
149. Lai JS, Brown LG, True LD, et al. Metastases of prostate cancer express estrogen receptor-beta. Urology 2004;64(4):814–20.
150. Mak P, Leav I, Pursell B, et al. ERbeta impedes prostate cancer EMT by desta-bilizing HIF-1alpha and inhibiting VEGF-mediated snail nuclear localization: implications for Gleason grading. Cancer Cell 2010;17(4):319–32.
151. Nanni S, Benvenuti V, Grasselli A, et al. Endothelial NOS, estrogen receptor beta, and HIFs cooperate in the activation of a prognostic transcriptional pattern in aggressive human prostate cancer. J Clin Invest 2009;119(5):1093–108.
152. Leung YK, Lee MT, Wang J, et al. Post-transcriptional regulation of estrogen receptor beta isoforms in prostate cancer. In: ENDO 2010 92th Annual Meeting. San Diego (CA), June 19–22, 2010.
153. Lee MT, Leung YK, Chung I, et al. Regulation of ERbeta1 transcriptional activity by acetylation. In: ENDO 2010 92th Annual Meeting. San Diego (CA), June 19–22, 2010.
154. Mak P, Leung YK, Tang WY, et al. Apigenin suppresses cancer cell growth through ERbeta. Neoplasia 2006;8(11):896–904.
155. Krege JH, Hodgin JB, Couse JF, et al. Generation and reproductive phenotypes of mice lacking estrogen receptor beta. Proc Natl Acad Sci U S A 1998;95(26):15677–82.
156. Jiang J, Chang HL, Sugimoto Y, et al. Effects of age on growth and ERbeta mRNA expression of canine prostatic cells. Anticancer Res 2005;25(6B):4081–90.
157. Chang WY, Prins GS. Estrogen receptor-beta: implications for the prostate gland. Prostate 1999;40(2):115–24.
158. Risbridger GP, Bianco JJ, Ellem SJ, et al. Oestrogens and prostate cancer. Endocr Relat Cancer 2003;10(2):187–91.
159. Haqq C, Li R, Khodabakhsh D, et al. Ethnic and racial differences in prostate stromal estrogen receptor alpha. Prostate 2005;65(2):101–9.
160. Tanaka Y, Sasaki M, Kaneuchi M, et al. Polymorphisms of estrogen receptor alpha in prostate cancer. Mol Carcinog 2003;37(4):202–8.
161. Chae YK, Huang HY, Strickland P, et al. Genetic polymorphisms of estrogen receptors alpha and beta and the risk of developing prostate cancer. PLoS One 2009;4(8):e6523.
162. Nicolaiew N, Cancel-Tassin G, Azzouzi AR, et al. Association between estrogen and androgen receptor genes and prostate cancer risk. Eur J Endocrinol 2009;160(1):101–6.

163. McIntyre MH, Kantoff PW, Stampfer MJ, et al. Prostate cancer risk and ESR1 TA, ESR2 CA repeat polymorphisms. Cancer Epidemiol Biomarkers Prev 2007; 16(11):2233–6.

164. Chen YC, Kraft P, Bretsky P, et al. Sequence variants of estrogen receptor beta and risk of prostate cancer in the National Cancer Institute Breast and Prostate Cancer Cohort Consortium. Cancer Epidemiol Biomarkers Prev 2007;16(10): 1973–81.

165. Hedelin M, Balter KA, Chang ET, et al. Dietary intake of phytoestrogens, estrogen receptor-beta polymorphisms and the risk of prostate cancer. Prostate 2006;66(14):1512–20.

166. Thellenberg-Karlsson C, Lindstrom S, Malmer B, et al. Estrogen receptor beta polymorphism is associated with prostate cancer risk. Clin Cancer Res 2006; 12(6):1936–41.

167. Shapiro E, Huang H, Masch RJ, et al. Immunolocalization of estrogen receptor alpha and beta in human fetal prostate. J Urol 2005;174(5):2051–3.

168. Kampa M, Pelekanou V, Castanas E. Membrane-initiated steroid action in breast and prostate cancer. Steroids 2008;73(9–10):953–60.

169. Losel R, Wehling M. Nongenomic actions of steroid hormones. Nat Rev Mol Cell Biol 2003;4(1):46–56.

170. Zhalilo LI, Novominskaia IM. Tissue respiratory activity with a varying potassium ion content in the incubation medium. Fiziol Zh 1976;22(3):410–2 [in Ukrainian].

171. Hammes SR, Levin ER. Extranuclear steroid receptors: nature and actions. Endocr Rev 2007;28(7):726–41.

172. Zhang Z, Maier B, Santen RJ, et al. Membrane association of estrogen receptor alpha mediates estrogen effect on MAPK activation. Biochem Biophys Res Commun 2002;294(5):926–33.

173. Song RX, Zhang Z, Santen RJ. Estrogen rapid action via protein complex formation involving ERalpha and Src. Trends Endocrinol Metab 2005;16(8):347–53.

174. O'Lone R, Knorr K, Jaffe IZ, et al. Estrogen receptors alpha and beta mediate distinct pathways of vascular gene expression, including genes involved in mitochondrial electron transport and generation of reactive oxygen species. Mol Endocrinol 2007;21(6):1281–96.

175. Chen JQ, Russo PA, Cooke C, et al. ERbeta shifts from mitochondria to nucleus during estrogen-induced neoplastic transformation of human breast epithelial cells and is involved in estrogen-induced synthesis of mitochondrial respiratory chain proteins. Biochim Biophys Acta 2007;1773(12):1732–46.

176. Revankar CM, Cimino DF, Sklar LA, et al. A transmembrane intracellular estrogen receptor mediates rapid cell signaling. Science 2005;307(5715): 1625–30.

177. Langer G, Bader B, Meoli L, et al. A critical review of fundamental controversies in the field of GPR30 research. Steroids 2010;75(8–9):603–10.

178. Thomas P, Dressing G, Pang Y, et al. Progestin, estrogen and androgen G-protein coupled receptors in fish gonads. Steroids 2006;71(4):310–6.

179. Maggiolini M, Picard D. The unfolding stories of GPR30, a new membrane-bound estrogen receptor. J Endocrinol 2010;204(2):105–14.

180. Park II, Zhang Q, Liu V, et al. 17Beta-estradiol at low concentrations acts through distinct pathways in normal versus benign prostatic hyperplasia-derived prostate stromal cells. Endocrinology 2009;150(10):4594–605.

181. Zhang Z, Duan L, Du X, et al. The proliferative effect of estradiol on human prostate stromal cells is mediated through activation of ERK. Prostate 2008;68(5): 508–16.

182. Lam HM, Ouyang B, Ho SM. Activation of the G-coupled protein receptor 30 (GPR30) by the non-estrogenic ligand G-1 inhibits prostate cancer cell growth and regulation of its expression via an epigenetic mechanism. In: ENDO 2009 91st Annual Meeting. Washington, DC, June 10–13, 2009.

183. Chan QK, Lam HM, Ng CF, et al. Activation of GPR30 inhibits the growth of prostate cancer cells through sustained activation of Erk1/2, c-jun/c-fos-dependent upregulation of p21, and induction of G(2) cell-cycle arrest. Cell Death Differ 2010;17(9):1511–23.

184. Cheung CP, Yu S, Wong KB, et al. Expression and functional study of estrogen receptor-related receptors in human prostatic cells and tissues. J Clin Endocrinol Metab 2005;90(3):1830–44.

185. Giguere V, Yang N, Segui P, et al. Identification of a new class of steroid hormone receptors. Nature 1988;331(6151):91–4.

186. Chen F, Zhang Q, McDonald T, et al. Identification of two hERR2-related novel nuclear receptors utilizing bioinformatics and inverse PCR. Gene 1999;228(1–2):101–9.

187. Heard DJ, Norby PL, Holloway J, et al. Human ERRgamma, a third member of the estrogen receptor-related receptor (ERR) subfamily of orphan nuclear receptors: tissue-specific isoforms are expressed during development and in the adult. Mol Endocrinol 2000;14(3):382–92.

188. Hong H, Yang L, Stallcup MR. Hormone-independent transcriptional activation and coactivator binding by novel orphan nuclear receptor ERR3. J Biol Chem 1999;274(32):22618–26.

189. Vanacker JM, Pettersson K, Gustafsson JA, et al. Transcriptional targets shared by estrogen receptor- related receptors (ERRs) and estrogen receptor (ER) alpha, but not by ERbeta. EMBO J 1999;18(15):4270–9.

190. Xie W, Hong H, Yang NN, et al. Constitutive activation of transcription and binding of coactivator by estrogen-related receptors 1 and 2. Mol Endocrinol 1999;13(12):2151–62.

191. Zhang Z, Teng CT. Estrogen receptor-related receptor alpha 1 interacts with coactivator and constitutively activates the estrogen response elements of the human lactoferrin gene. J Biol Chem 2000;275(27):20837–46.

192. Suetsugi M, Su L, Karlsberg K, et al. Flavone and isoflavone phytoestrogens are agonists of estrogen-related receptors. Mol Cancer Res 2003;1(13):981–91.

193. Coward P, Lee D, Hull MV, et al. 4-Hydroxytamoxifen binds to and deactivates the estrogen-related receptor gamma. Proc Natl Acad Sci U S A 2001;98(15):8880–4.

194. Tremblay GB, Bergeron D, Giguere V. 4-Hydroxytamoxifen is an isoform-specific inhibitor of orphan estrogen-receptor-related (ERR) nuclear receptors beta and gamma. Endocrinology 2001;142(10):4572–5.

195. Huggins C, Hodges CV. Studies on prostatic cancer. I. The effect of castration, of estrogen and androgen injection on serum phosphatases in metastatic carcinoma of the prostate. CA Cancer J Clin 1072;22(4):232–40.

196. Cox RL, Crawford ED. Estrogens in the treatment of prostate cancer. J Urol 1995;154(6):1991–8.

197. Denis LJ, Griffiths K. Endocrine treatment in prostate cancer. Semin Surg Oncol 2000;18(1):52–74.

198. Shiau AK, Barstad D, Loria PM, et al. The structural basis of estrogen receptor/coactivator recognition and the antagonism of this interaction by tamoxifen. Cell 1998;95(7):927–37.

199. Bergan RC, Reed E, Myers CE, et al. A phase II study of high-dose tamoxifen in patients with hormone-refractory prostate cancer. Clin Cancer Res 1999;5(9):2366–73.

200. Chadha MK, Ashraf U, Lawrence D, et al. Phase II study of fulvestrant (Faslodex) in castration resistant prostate cancer. Prostate 2008;68(13):1461–6.
201. Hamilton M, Dahut W, Brawley O, et al. A phase I/II study of high-dose tamoxifen in combination with vinblastine in patients with androgen-independent prostate cancer. Acta Oncol 2003;42(3):195–201.
202. Lissoni P, Vigano P, Vaghi M, et al. A phase II study of tamoxifen in hormone-resistant metastatic prostate cancer: possible relation with prolactin secretion. Anticancer Res 2005;25(5):3597–9.
203. Shazer RL, Jain A, Galkin AV, et al. Raloxifene, an oestrogen-receptor-beta-targeted therapy, inhibits androgen-independent prostate cancer growth: results from preclinical studies and a pilot phase II clinical trial. BJU Int 2006;97(4):691–7.
204. Smith MR, Morton RA, Barnette KG, et al. Toremifene to reduce fracture risk in men receiving androgen deprivation therapy for prostate cancer. J Urol 2010; 184(4):1316–21.
205. Stein S, Zoltick B, Peacock T, et al. Phase II trial of toremifene in androgen-independent prostate cancer: a Penn cancer clinical trials group trial. Am J Clin Oncol 2001;24(3):283–5.
206. el-Rayes BF, Hussain MH. Hormonal therapy for prostate cancer: past, present and future. Expert Rev Anticancer Ther 2002;2(1):37–47.
207. Dahllof B, Billstrom A, Cabral F, et al. Estramustine depolymerizes microtubules by binding to tubulin. Cancer Res 1993;53(19):4573–81.
208. Fu Y, Hsieh TC, Guo J, et al. Licochalcone-A, a novel flavonoid isolated from licorice root (Glycyrrhiza glabra), causes G2 and late-G1 arrests in androgen-independent PC-3 prostate cancer cells. Biochem Biophys Res Commun 2004;322(1):263–70.
209. Kim HT, Kim BC, Kim IY, et al. Raloxifene, a mixed estrogen agonist/antagonist, induces apoptosis through cleavage of BAD in TSU-PR1 human cancer cells. J Biol Chem 2002;277(36):32510–5.
210. Kumar NB, Cantor A, Allen K, et al. The specific role of isoflavones in reducing prostate cancer risk. Prostate 2004;59(2):141–7.
211. Kuwajerwala N, Cifuentes E, Gautam S, et al. Resveratrol induces prostate cancer cell entry into s phase and inhibits DNA synthesis. Cancer Res 2002; 62(9):2488–92.
212. LaVallee TM, Zhan XH, Johnson MS, et al. 2-Methoxyestradiol up-regulates death receptor 5 and induces apoptosis through activation of the extrinsic pathway. Cancer Res 2003;63(2):468–75.
213. Li Y, Sarkar FH. Gene expression profiles of genistein-treated PC3 prostate cancer cells. J Nutr 2002;132(12):3623–31.
214. Liu Y, Kyle E, Lieberman R, et al. Focal adhesion kinase (FAK) phosphorylation is not required for genistein-induced FAK-beta-1-integrin complex formation. Clin Exp Metastasis 2000;18(3):203–12.
215. Matsukawa Y, Marui N, Sakai T, et al. Genistein arrests cell cycle progression at G2-M. Cancer Res 1993;53(6):1328–31.
216. Misra RR, Hursting SD, Perkins SN, et al. Genotoxicity and carcinogenicity studies of soy isoflavones. Int J Toxicol 2002;21(4):277–85.
217. Mor G, Kohen F, Garcia-Velasco J, et al. Regulation of fas ligand expression in breast cancer cells by estrogen: functional differences between estradiol and tamoxifen. J Steroid Biochem Mol Biol 2000;73(5):185–94.
218. Neubauer BL, Best KL, Counts DF, et al. Raloxifene (LY156758) produces anti-metastatic responses and extends survival in the PAIII rat prostatic adenocarcinoma model. Prostate 1995;27(4):220–9.

219. Qadan LR, Perez-Stable CM, Anderson C, et al. 2-Methoxyestradiol induces G2/M arrest and apoptosis in prostate cancer. Biochem Biophys Res Commun 2001;285(5):1259–66.
220. Rafi MM, Rosen RT, Vassil A, et al. Modulation of bcl-2 and cytotoxicity by licochalcone-A, a novel estrogenic flavonoid. Anticancer Res 2000;20(4):2653–8.
221. Schulz P, Bauer HW, Brade WP, et al. Evaluation of the cytotoxic activity of diethylstilbestrol and its mono- and diphosphate towards prostatic carcinoma cells. Cancer Res 1988;48(10):2867–70.
222. Shimada K, Nakamura M, Ishida E, et al. Requirement of c-jun for testosterone-induced sensitization to N-(4-hydroxyphenyl)retinamide-induced apoptosis. Mol Carcinog 2003;36(3):115–22.
223. Yo YT, Shieh GS, Hsu KF, et al. Licorice and licochalcone-A induce autophagy in LNCaP prostate cancer cells by suppression of Bcl-2 expression and the mTOR pathway. J Agric Food Chem 2009;57(18):8266–73.
224. Kumar AP, Garcia GE, Slaga TJ. 2-Methoxyestradiol blocks cell-cycle progression at G(2)/M phase and inhibits growth of human prostate cancer cells. Mol Carcinog 2001;31(3):111–24.
225. Bland LB, Garzotto M, DeLoughery TG, et al. Phase II study of transdermal estradiol in androgen-independent prostate carcinoma. Cancer 2005;103(4):717–23.
226. Langley RE, Godsland IF, Kynaston H, et al. Early hormonal data from a multicentre phase II trial using transdermal oestrogen patches as first-line hormonal therapy in patients with locally advanced or metastatic prostate cancer. BJU Int 2008;102(4):442–5.
227. Ockrim JL, Lalani EN, Laniado ME, et al. Transdermal estradiol therapy for advanced prostate cancer–forward to the past? J Urol 2003;169(5):1735–7.
228. Ockrim JL, Lalani E, Kakkar AK, et al. Transdermal estradiol therapy for prostate cancer reduces thrombophilic activation and protects against thromboembolism. J Urol 2005;174(2):527–33.
229. Gerber GS, Zagaja GP, Ray PS, et al. Transdermal estrogen in the treatment of hot flushes in men with prostate cancer. Urology 2000;55(1):97–101.
230. Ockrim JL, Lalani EN, Banks LM, et al. Transdermal estradiol improves bone density when used as single agent therapy for prostate cancer. J Urol 2004;172(6 Pt 1):2203–7.
231. Taneja SS, Smith MR, Dalton JT, et al. Toremifene–a promising therapy for the prevention of prostate cancer and complications of androgen deprivation therapy. Expert Opin Investig Drugs 2006;15(3):293–305.
232. Denis L, Morton MS, Griffiths K. Diet and its preventive role in prostatic disease. Eur Urol 1999;35(5–6):377–87.
233. Price D, Stein B, Sieber P, et al. Toremifene for the prevention of prostate cancer in men with high grade prostatic intraepitholial neoplasia: results of a double-blind, placebo controlled, phase IIB clinical trial. J Urol 2006;176(3):965–70.
234. Jian L. Soy, isoflavones, and prostate cancer. Mol Nutr Food Res 2009;53(2):217–26.
235. Lampe JW. Emerging research on equol and cancer. J Nutr 2010;140(7):1369S–72S.
236. Markiewicz L, Garey J, Adlercreutz H, et al. In vitro bioassays of non-steroidal phytoestrogens. J Steroid Biochem Mol Biol 1993;45(5):399–405.
237. Milligan SR, Balasubramanian AV, Kalita JC. Relative potency of xenobiotic estrogens in an acute in vivo mammalian assay. Environ Health Perspect 1998;106(1):23–6.

238. Sonn GA, Aronson W, Litwin MS. Impact of diet on prostate cancer: a review. Prostate Cancer Prostatic Dis 2005;8(4):304–10.
239. Ganry O. Phytoestrogens and prostate cancer risk. Prev Med 2005;41(1):1–6.
240. Hebert JR, Hurley TG, Olendzki BC, et al. Nutritional and socioeconomic factors in relation to prostate cancer mortality: a cross-national study. J Natl Cancer Inst 1998;90(21):1637–47.
241. Hussain M, Banerjee M, Sarkar FH, et al. Soy isoflavones in the treatment of prostate cancer. Nutr Cancer 2003;47(2):111–7.
242. Lee MM, Gomez SL, Chang JS, et al. Soy and isoflavone consumption in relation to prostate cancer risk in China. Cancer Epidemiol Biomarkers Prev 2003;12(7): 665–8.
243. Ozasa K, Nakao M, Watanabe Y, et al. Serum phytoestrogens and prostate cancer risk in a nested case-control study among Japanese men. Cancer Sci 2004;95(1):65–71.
244. Stattin P, Adlercreutz H, Tenkanen L, et al. Circulating enterolactone and prostate cancer risk: a Nordic nested case-control study. Int J Cancer 2002;99(1): 124–9.
245. Strom SS, Yamamura Y, Duphorne CM, et al. Phytoestrogen intake and prostate cancer: a case-control study using a new database. Nutr Cancer 1999;33(1): 20–5.
246. Travis RC, Spencer EA, Allen NE, et al. Plasma phyto-oestrogens and prostate cancer in the European Prospective Investigation into Cancer and Nutrition. Br J Cancer 2009;100(11):1817–23.
247. Dalais FS, Meliala A, Wattanapenpaiboon N, et al. Effects of a diet rich in phytoestrogens on prostate-specific antigen and sex hormones in men diagnosed with prostate cancer. Urology 2004;64(3):510–5.
248. Jarred RA, Keikha M, Dowling C, et al. Induction of apoptosis in low to moderate-grade human prostate carcinoma by red clover-derived dietary isoflavones. Cancer Epidemiol Biomarkers Prev 2002;11(12):1689–96.
249. Miltyk W, Craciunescu CN, Fischer L, et al. Lack of significant genotoxicity of purified soy isoflavones (genistein, daidzein, and glycitein) in 20 patients with prostate cancer. Am J Clin Nutr 2003;77(4):875–82.
250. Takimoto CH, Glover K, Huang X, et al. Phase I pharmacokinetic and pharmacodynamic analysis of unconjugated soy isoflavones administered to individuals with cancer. Cancer Epidemiol Biomarkers Prev 2003;12(11 Pt 1):1213–21.

The Timing and Extent of Androgen Deprivation Therapy for Prostate Cancer: Weighing the Clinical Evidence

Serge Ginzburg, MD, Peter C. Albertsen, MD, MS*

KEYWORDS

- Prostate cancer • Androgen deprivation therapy • Orchiectomy
- Gonadotropin-releasing hormone agonist
- Gonadotropin-releasing hormone antagonist

Estimates from the American Cancer Society suggest that in 2010 more than 217,000 American men were diagnosed with prostate cancer and 32,000 men died of this disease. The lifetime risk of being diagnosed with prostate cancer is now 15.4% for Caucasians and 18.3% for African Americans.[1] As a consequence of widespread screening for prostate-specific antigen (PSA), most of these men will have disease localized to the prostate and will be offered one of four alternative therapies: surgery, radiation therapy (external beam or brachytherapy), androgen deprivation therapy (ADT), or active surveillance.[2] This article reviews the evidence supporting the efficacy of ADT among men with localized and advanced disease.

HISTORY OF ADT

In 1941, Huggins and Hodges[3] published a landmark paper describing significant clinical improvement in men with advanced prostate cancer who underwent surgical castration. Twenty-one consecutive men with advanced prostate cancer, 15 of whom had radiographically demonstrable bone metastases, were treated with bilateral orchiectomy. Fifteen showed significant objective and subjective clinical improvement. As a consequence of these findings, ADT rapidly became the standard of care

The authors have nothing to disclose.
Division of Urology, University of Connecticut Health Center, 263 Farmington Avenue, Farmington, CT 06030, USA
* Corresponding author.
E-mail address: Albertsen@nso.uchc.edu

Endocrinol Metab Clin N Am 40 (2011) 615–623
doi:10.1016/j.ecl.2011.05.005
0889-8529/11/$ – see front matter © 2011 Elsevier Inc. All rights reserved.

for most men presenting with prostate cancer, although clinicians often disagreed whether the treatment was curative or simply palliative.

In 1959, the Veterans Administration Cooperative Urological Research Group (VACURG) was established to coordinate large-scale randomized prospective clinical trials to study the treatment of urologic disorders, with a major focus on prostate cancer.[4] The results of these trials defined the use of androgen deprivation for decades. Androgen deprivation used in these studies consisted of either surgical castration via bilateral orchiectomy or medical suppression using the estrogen diethylstilbestrol (DES) in various doses.

VACURG Study 1 evaluated the use of high-dose DES versus placebo after radical prostatectomy.[5] Results suggested that men with localized disease who were randomized to the placebo arm had a longer survival, but results were not statistically significant because the trials failed to accrue sufficient numbers of patients. Patients with locally advanced and metastatic disease were randomized to receive placebo, orchiectomy, high-dose DES, or orchiectomy plus high-dose DES. Men with locally advanced disease taking DES had slightly longer cancer-specific survival compared with men assigned to orchiectomy plus DES, but neither group showed superior survival when compared with men assigned to the placebo arm. Among men with metastatic disease, no statistical difference was seen in cancer-specific survival. These results discouraged physicians from using androgen deprivation in men with localized disease or asymptomatic advanced disease because the cumulative risks of cardiovascular toxicity outweighed any benefit of improved survival.

The recognition that estrogens caused an increase in deaths from cardiovascular disease led to the second VACURG study to explore various dosing levels. Most men had an excellent response to 1.0 mg of DES, but a dose of 3.0 mg was needed to suppress testosterone in all men.[6] The third VACURG trial evaluated other estrogen compounds, including a conjugated estrogen (Premarin) and progestational agent (Provera). Both of these compounds showed comparable efficacy to DES.

The VACURG established the role of ADT in the management of prostate cancer for the next 2 decades and concluded that (1) high-dose DES led to significant cardiovascular toxicity, (2) orchiectomy plus DES was no better than either orchiectomy or DES alone, and (3) similar cancer control was achieved with DES dosages between 1 and 5 mg, but cardiovascular toxicity increased as the dose was increased.[7]

The continued search for safer methods of ADT led to the discovery and evaluation of luteinizing hormone–releasing hormone (LHRH) agonists and nonsteroidal antiandrogens in the treatment of prostate cancer. In 1983, Labrie and colleagues[8] reported on 37 previously untreated and 21 previously treated men with advanced prostate cancer. They proposed that greater cancer control could be achieved through blocking androgens produced by adrenal synthesis in addition to the 90% to 95% of circulating androgens produced by the testes. He reported that combined androgen therapy with leuprolide and flutamide resulted in a 97% objective response rate in 30 men with previously untreated advanced prostate cancer compared with a 55% response rate in men previously treated with high-dose DES. He advocated total androgen blockade as the initial form of ADT and suggested that this therapy should be initiated early in the course of this disease. The use of a nonsteroidal antiandrogen provided the added benefit of suppressing the flare phenomenon triggered by the rise in androgen production after the initiation of LHRH agonist therapy.

Controversy surrounding the validity of these claims led to a randomized trial organized by the Southwest Oncology Group (SWOG) evaluating the efficacy of combined androgen deprivation in the management of men with metastatic prostate cancer.[9] Men were randomized to receive either leuprolide plus flutamide (n = 303) or leuprolide plus placebo (n = 300). Men receiving combined ADT had an increased median progression-free survival of 16.5 months compared with 13.9 months for men receiving leuprolide alone (*P* = .039), and a median overall survival of 35.6 months compared with 28.3 months (*P* = .035). The report suggested that men with minimal disease had the most significant gain in cause-specific survival, prompting many clinicians to initiate combined antiandrogen therapy much earlier in the course of this disease.

Unfortunately, these findings were not confirmed in a subsequent study designed by SWOG to test whether combined androgen blockade resulted in improved survival in men with minimally advanced disease and better performance status. Eisenberger and colleagues[10] evaluated immediate bilateral orchiectomy with or without flutamide in men with newly diagnosed, previously untreated metastatic prostate cancer. This larger trial consisted of 1387 men and reported a significantly better biochemical response among men receiving flutamide, as measured by the decline of serum PSA levels, but the overall and progression-free survival outcomes were statistically equivalent. Equally important was the observation that men receiving antiandrogen therapy had a lower quality of life, which argued against the early initiation of ADT.

CONTEMPORARY USE OF ADT AMONG MEN WITH LOCALIZED DISEASE
Primary ADT

Little evidence-based support exists for the use of ADT as primary treatment among men with localized prostate cancer. Despite this fact, Cooperberg and colleagues[11] have reported a substantial increase in the use of ADT as primary therapy for men with localized disease. Citing data from CaPSURE, a large longitudinal observational database of 35 academic and community-based urology practices across the United States, they have shown that between 1989 and 2001, the use of ADT more than tripled from 4.6% to 14.2% among men with low-risk disease. A significant rise has also occurred among men with intermediate- and high-risk disease, from 8.9% to 19.7% and 32.8% to 48.2%, respectively.

Several epidemiologic studies have shown no benefit from ADT in this setting.[12,13] Lu-Yao and colleagues[12] reported results from a population-based study using Medicare claims data linked to the Surveillance, Epidemiology and End Results (SEER) database evaluating prostate cancer–specific and overall survival in men older than 65 years with localized disease who were diagnosed between 1992 and 2002 and who received no prior definitive therapy. An instrumental variable analysis was used to address potential biases. When compared with conservative management, primary ADT was associated with lower 10-year prostate cancer–specific survival (80.1% vs 82.6%; hazard ratio [HR], 1.17; 95% CI, 1.03–1.33) and no increase in 10-year overall survival (30.2% vs 30.3%; HR 1.00; 95% CI, 0.90–1.05). A subset analysis of men with poorly differentiated prostate cancer, however, showed a small improvement in prostate cancer–specific survival but not overall survival.

Neoadjuvant ADT

Several researchers have studied the role of neoadjuvant ADT before radical prostatectomy. Soloway and colleagues[14] reported on 282 men with clinical T2b disease randomized to 3 months of leuprolide with radical prostatectomy versus radical prostatectomy alone. They found that positive surgical margins were less frequent among men undergoing ADT, but after 5 years of follow-up no difference was seen in the rate of PSA recurrence. Aus and colleagues[15] conducted a similar study in Europe with nearly identical results. Neoadjuvant ADT seems to have no role for men undergoing radical prostatectomy.

In contrast to these studies, strong evidence exists for the role of neoadjuvant ADT for men with high-risk, advanced (T3), localized disease undergoing external beam radiation therapy (EBRT).[16,17] Widmark and colleagues[18] recently showed the synergy between EBRT and ADT. This multicenter trial enrolled 875 men with locally advanced disease randomized to ADT alone or ADT plus EBRT. ADT was delivered in the form of combined androgen suppression for 3 months followed by ADT. With a median follow-up of 7.6 years, 10-year prostate cancer–specific and overall mortality rates were 23.9% versus 11.9% and 39.4% versus 29.6%, respectively, in favor of men receiving both EBRT and ADT. The PSA recurrence rate at 10 years was 74.7% versus 25.9%.

D'Amico and colleagues[16] reported on outcomes of 206 men with high-risk clinically localized disease randomized to 70 Gy of three-dimensional conformal radiation therapy with or without 6 months of ADT. ADT was delivered in the form of an LHRH agonist and an antiandrogen. After a 4.5-year median follow-up, men receiving neoadjuvant ADT had higher overall survival rates (88% vs 78%; $P = .04$). Men receiving neoadjuvant ADT also showed a higher salvage-free survival rate (82% vs 57%; HR, 2.17; 95% CI, 1.28–3.69; $P = .004$), a lower prostate cancer–specific mortality rate, and a similar non–prostate cancer mortality rate.

Bolla and colleagues[19,20] have provided the most comprehensive support for neoadjuvant therapy in men receiving EBRT. In a series of trials, they have shown a statistically significant survival advantage for men receiving EBRT combined with ADT. A recent randomized trial attempted to define the appropriate duration of therapy by comparing 6 months of therapy against 3 years of ADT after definitive radiation therapy.[21] ADT consisted of 6 months of combined androgen suppression with an LHRH agonist and an antiandrogen followed by an additional 2.5 years of an LHRH agonist alone. After 5 years of follow-up, the overall mortality was 19.0% and 15.2% in favor of longer-term ADT (HR, 1.42; upper 95.71% confidence limit 1.79; $P = .65$ for noninferiority). Prostate cancer–specific mortality was also improved in the 3-year arm (4.7% vs 3.2%; $P = .002$). All of these studies enrolled men with advanced, localized disease (T3). Whether men with low-risk localized disease (T1c) will experience similar benefits is unclear.

Adjuvant ADT

Some support also seems to exist for the use of ADT in the setting of node-positive disease after radical prostatectomy.[22,23] Messing and colleagues[23] randomized 98 patients with positive lymph node metastasis found at radical prostatectomy with lymphadenectomy to immediate continuous ADT versus observation. ADT consisted of goserelin or orchiectomy. At a median follow-up of 11.9 years, improvements in median overall and progression-free survival were 2.6 years ($P = .04$) and 11.5 years ($P<.0001$), respectively, in favor of immediate ADT. Median disease-specific survival was not reached in the immediate ADT arm but was significantly improved (HR, 4.09; 95%CI, 1.76–9.49; $P = .0004$). Unfortunately, this study never achieved its planned accrual and is believed by many to be underpowered.

A recent SEER database review attempted to answer the same question, but arrived at a different conclusion. Wong and colleagues[24] identified 731 men with node-positive disease, among whom 209 received ADT within 3 months of the radical prostatectomy. No statistical difference in overall survival was observed. The role of adjuvant therapy among men with early-stage T4 disease remains uncertain.

ADT AMONG MEN WITH ADVANCED DISEASE

Evidence supporting the role of ADT among men with advanced prostate cancer is well documented. Historically, men have survived an average of 4 years after initiation of ADT when therapy was begun after the appearance of symptomatic disease or bone metastases.[25] During the past decade, several researchers have explored the role of nonsteroidal antiandrogens as primary therapy for men with locally advanced prostate cancer. Wirth and colleagues[26] randomized 309 men with T3 node-negative disease after radical prostatectomy to observation versus flutamide. At a 6.1-year median follow-up, biochemical recurrence-free survival was improved in the flutamide group, but overall survival was unaffected and men receiving antiandrogen therapy showed considerable toxicity.

Wirth and colleagues[27,28] explored the role of bicalutamide, 150 mg daily, among men with locally advanced disease. In this European randomized, double-blind, placebo-controlled trial with a 7.4-year median follow-up, men with locally advanced prostate cancer receiving bicalutamide as either primary therapy or adjuvant therapy to either EBRT or prostatectomy showed increased progression-free survival compared with men receiving placebo.[28] An overall survival advantage was only shown among men undergoing radiation therapy (HR, 0.65; 95% CI, 0.44–0.95; $P = .03$).

A similar trial conducted in North America did not confirm these findings.[29] With a 7.7-year median follow-up, no differences in primary end points were observed between men enrolled in the treatment arm and those in the placebo arm in men with either localized or locally advanced disease. Men enrolled in the North American trial had a much lower risk profile than men enrolled in the European trial, which could explain the different findings. Although of great interest in Europe, the U.S. Food and Drug Administration (FDA) has not approved the use of nonsteroidal antiandrogens as primary therapy for locally advanced prostate cancer in the United States. The 2010 National Comprehensive Cancer Network Clinical Practice Guidelines in Oncology for Prostate Cancer state that antiandrogen monotherapy is less effective than medical or surgical castration and is not recommended.[30]

HOW SHOULD ADT BE ADMINISTERED?

In contemporary practice, few clinicians withhold ADT until patients show clinical symptoms of metastatic disease. Most men are started on ADT much earlier in the course of their disease compared with the men enrolled in the VACURG trials. PSA progression after prostatectomy or definitive radiation therapy is a frequent trigger. As a consequence, men now receive ADT for considerably longer periods, and toxicities of therapy have become more apparent.[28,31,32] Typical side effects include vasomotor flushing, loss of libido, sexual dysfunction, fatigue, gynecomastia, mastodynia, anemia, osteoporosis, osteopenia, and, more recently, metabolic syndrome (obesity, insulin resistance, and lipid alterations) contributing to cardiovascular risks.[31,33,34] Other adverse effects, such as depression, anxiety, malaise, fatigue, and memory difficulties, have also been attributed to chronic ADT. Geriatricians coined the term "androgen deprivation syndrome" to describe these symptoms. Clinicians should carefully consider the impact of chronic treatment before initiating ADT.

ADT can be achieved either through surgical or medical castration. The accepted castrate level of testosterone is less than 50 ng/dL.[30] Although hypophysectomy and bilateral adrenalectomy are of historic interest, bilateral simple or subcapsular orchiectomy is a cost-effective therapy with minimal complications compared with hormonal ablation.[35] Surgical castration is extremely effective in controlling prostate cancer, but is underused, most likely because of its psychological impact.[36] In the CaPSURE database, only 5% of patients elected orchiectomy for ADT.[37]

Medical ADT historically consisted of DES, but this has been abandoned in favor of therapies suppressing LHRH. DES exerted its antiandrogenic effect through negative feedback to the hypothalamus and anterior pituitary gland, thereby downregulating the luteinizing hormone.[38,39] This drug was associated with significant thromboembolic and cardiovascular side effects.

Discovered in 1971, gonadotropin-releasing hormone (GnRH) agonists (leuprolide, goserelin, triptorelin, histrelin) are now the most commonly used drugs in ADT.[40] GnRH is naturally secreted in a pulsatile mode. When present continuously, GnRH agonists act on the anterior pituitary gland through decreasing the release of luteinizing hormone via a downregulation of GnRH receptors.[41] This mode of androgen suppression is associated with an initial androgen surge for up to 3 weeks, which, if unopposed, may be undesirable in men with advanced metastatic disease.[42]

GnRH antagonists (degarelix, abarelix) also exert their action on the anterior pituitary gland through directly inhibiting GnRH receptors.[43] Degarelix was recently approved by the FDA, and unlike GnRH agonists, produces an immediate decline in testosterone levels. Abarelix is no longer available in the United States because of a 3.7% risk of anaphylaxis.[41]

Inhibitors of steroid synthesis (ketoconazole) act at the level of adrenal gland through inhibition of the cytochrome P450 enzyme, thereby decreasing androgen synthesis from steroid precursors.[41] Steroid supplementation is required to prevent adrenal insufficiency. Nonsteroidal androgen receptor antagonists (flutamide, bicalutamide, nilutamide) act at the level of the prostate gland through competitively binding the androgen receptor ligand-binding domain.[41] The steroidal antiandrogen, cyproterone acetate (CPA), has direct androgen receptor–blocking effects and causes a centrally mediated reduction in testicular androgens.[44]

Traditionally, ADT has been continued without interruption until a patient succumbs to a competing medical hazard or develops androgen resistant disease. Several investigators have explored the role of intermittent ADT in an attempt to minimize both the side effects associated with treatment and reduce the cost of treatment.[45] In this scenario, patients are often given ADT until the serum PSA level becomes undetectable. Therapy is then discontinued and resumed only after PSA levels begin to rise again.

Calais da Silva and colleagues[46] recently reported on a phase III trial of intermittent versus continuous ADT for locally advanced or metastatic disease. After a 3-month induction of CPA and an LHRH agonist, 80% of eligible men had a PSA less than 4 ng/dL and were then randomized to intermittent versus continuous ADT with same regimen. Symptomatic men in the intermittent androgen deprivation therapy arm were started back on ADT when their PSA was greater than 10 ng/dl, asymptomatic men when their PSA was greater than 20 ng/dl, and any man with a rise in PSA that was greater than 20% of the nadir PSA if the initial nadir was less than 80% of the initial PSA value. At a follow-up of 4.2 years, no significant difference in disease progression or overall survival was reported. A greater number of cancer-specific deaths reported among men receiving intermittent ADT (106 vs 84) was balanced by an increase in the number of cardiovascular deaths among men receiving continuous ADT (52 vs 41). Side-effects were significantly lower among men receiving intermittent ADT. The median time off therapy was 52 weeks.

Basic criteria for the administration of intermittent ADT, including patient profile and stage of disease, PSA values for treatment suspension and reinitiation, type of ADT, and length of each cycle, remain undefined.[47] Although promising, intermittent ADT remains an experimental approach to treatment.

SUMMARY

ADT is an effective means of palliating symptoms of prostate cancer, but is associated with significant toxicities that increase with duration of treatment. Medical and surgical castration are equally efficacious. Primary ADT in men with localized disease is not indicated because it provides no survival advantage. Neoadjuvant androgen deprivation, when combined with external beam radiation therapy, improves survival for men with locally advanced disease. Immediate adjuvant androgen deprivation does not seem to benefit men undergoing radical prostatectomy except possibly those with lymph-node positive disease. No evidence supports combined androgen blockade or monotherapy with nonsteroidal antiandrogens among men with locally advanced prostate cancer. ADT with orchiectomy or gonadotropin-releasing hormone agonists or antagonists is current standard of care.

ADT still raises controversies among clinicians. Physicians disagree about when to initiate ADT after biochemical recurrence. They also disagree about whether therapy should be administered continuously or intermittently. More controlled randomized studies are needed to guide clinicians in the appropriate use of ADT in contemporary practice.

REFERENCES

1. Jemal A, Siegel R, Xu J, et al. Cancer Statistics, 2010. CA Cancer J Clin 2010;60: 277–300.
2. Cooperberg MR, Broering JM, Litwin MS, et al. The contemporary management of prostate cancer in the United States: lessons from the cancer of the prostate strategic urologic research endeavor (CaPSURE), a national disease registry. J Urol 2004;171(4):1393–401.
3. Huggins C, Hodges CV. Studies on prostatic cancer II: the effects of castration on advanced carcinoma of the prostate gland. Arch Surg 1941;43:209–23.
4. Byar DP. Proceedings: the Veterans Administration Cooperative Urological Research Group's studies of cancer of the prostate. Cancer 1973;32(5):1126–30.
5. Treatment and survival of patients with cancer of the prostate. The Veterans Administration Co-operative Urological Research Group. Surg Gynecol Obstet 1967;124(5):1011–7.
6. Bailar JC III, Byar DP. Estrogen treatment for cancer of the prostate. Early results with 3 doses of diethylstilbestrol and placebo. Cancer 1970;26(2):257–61.
7. Byar DP, Corle DK. Hormone therapy for prostate cancer: results of the Veterans Administration Cooperative Urological Research Group studies. NCI Monogr 1988;(7):165–70.
8. Labrie F, Dupont A, Belanger A, et al. New approach in the treatment of prostate cancer: complete instead of partial withdrawal of androgens. Prostate 1983;4(6): 579–94.
9. Crawford ED, Eisenberger MA, McLeod DG, et al. A controlled trial of leuprolide with and without flutamide in prostatic carcinoma. N Engl J Med 1989;321(7): 419–24 [Erratum appears in N Engl J Med 1989;321(20):1420].
10. Eisenberger MA, Blumenstein BA, Crawford ED, et al. Bilateral orchiectomy with or without flutamide for metastatic prostate cancer. N Engl J Med 1998;339(15): 1036–42.
11. Cooperberg MR, Grossfeld GD, Lubeck DP, et al. National practice patterns and time trends in androgen ablation for localized prostate cancer. J Natl Cancer Inst 2003;95(13):981–9.

12. Lu-Yao GL, Albertsen PC, Moore DF, et al. Survival following primary androgen deprivation therapy among men with localized prostate cancer. JAMA 2008; 300(2):173–81 [Erratum appears in JAMA 2009;301(1):38].

13. Wong YN, Freedland SJ, Egleston B, et al. The role of primary androgen deprivation therapy in localized prostate cancer. Eur Urol 2009;56(4):609–16.

14. Soloway MS, Pareek K, Sharifi R, et al. Neoadjuvant androgen ablation before radical prostatectomy in cT2bNxMo prostate cancer: 5-year results. J Urol 2002;167(1):112–6.

15. Aus G, Abrahamsson PA, Ahlgren G, et al. Three-month neoadjuvant hormonal therapy before radical prostatectomy: a 7-year follow-up of a randomized controlled trial. BJU Int 2002;90(6):561–6.

16. D'Amico AV, Manola J, Loffredo M, et al. 6-month androgen suppression plus radiation therapy vs radiation therapy alone for patients with clinically localized prostate cancer: a randomized controlled trial. JAMA 2004;292(7):821–7.

17. D'Amico AV, Loffredo M, Renshaw AA, et al. Six-month androgen suppression plus radiation therapy compared with radiation therapy alone for men with prostate cancer and a rapidly increasing pretreatment prostate-specific antigen level. J Clin Oncol 2006;24(25):4190–5.

18. Widmark A, Klepp O, Solberg A, et al. Endocrine treatment, with or without radiotherapy, in locally advanced prostate cancer (SPCG-7/SFUO-3): an open randomised phase III trial. Lancet 2009;373(9660):301–8.

19. Bolla M, Gonzalez D, Warde P, et al. Improved survival in patients with locally advanced prostate cancer treated with radiotherapy and goserelin. N Engl J Med 1997;337(5):295–300.

20. Bolla M, Collette L, Blank L, et al. Long-term results with immediate androgen suppression and external irradiation in patients with locally advanced prostate cancer (an EORTC study): a phase III randomised trial. Lancet 2002;360(9327): 103–6.

21. Bolla M, de Reijke TM, Van Tienhoven G, et al. Duration of androgen suppression in the treatment of prostate cancer. N Engl J Med 2009;360(24):2516–27.

22. Messing EM, Manola J, Sarosdy M, et al. Immediate hormonal therapy compared with observation after radical prostatectomy and pelvic lymphadenectomy in men with node-positive prostate cancer. N Engl J Med 1999;341(24):1781–8.

23. Messing EM, Manola J, Yao J, et al. Immediate versus deferred androgen deprivation treatment in patients with node-positive prostate cancer after radical prostatectomy and pelvic lymphadenectomy. Lancet Oncol 2006;7(6):472–9.

24. Wong YN, Freedland S, Egleston B, et al. Role of androgen deprivation therapy for node-positive prostate cancer. J Clin Oncol 2009;27(1):100–5.

25. Krupski TL, Smith MR, Lee WC, et al. Natural history of bone complications in men with prostate carcinoma initiating androgen deprivation therapy. Cancer 2004;101(3):541–9.

26. Wirth MP, Weissbach L, Marx FJ, et al. Prospective randomized trial comparing flutamide as adjuvant treatment versus observation after radical prostatectomy for locally advanced, lymph node-negative prostate cancer. Eur Urol 2004; 45(3):267–70 [discussion: 270].

27. Wirth MP, See WA, McLeod DG, et al. Bicalutamide 150 mg in addition to standard care in patients with localized or locally advanced prostate cancer: results from the second analysis of the early prostate cancer program at median follow-up of 5.4 years. J Urol 2004;172(5 Pt 1):1865–70.

28. McLeod DG, Iversen P, See WA, et al. Bicalutamide 150 mg plus standard care vs standard care alone for early prostate cancer. BJU Int 2006;97(2):247–54.

29. McLeod DG, See WA, Klimberg I, et al. The bicalutamide 150 mg early prostate cancer program: findings of the North American trial at 7.7-year median follow-up. J Urol 2006;176(1):75–80.
30. Mohler J, Bahnson RR, Boston B, et al. NCCN clinical practice guidelines in oncology: prostate cancer. J Natl Compr Canc Netw 2010;8(2):162–200.
31. Saylor PJ, Smith MR. Metabolic complications of androgen deprivation therapy for prostate cancer. J Urol 2009;181(5):1998–2006 [discussion: 2007–8].
32. Schwandt A, Garcia JA. Complications of androgen deprivation therapy in prostate cancer. Curr Opin Urol 2009;19(3):322–6.
33. Basaria S, Lieb J 2nd, Tang AM, et al. Long-term effects of androgen deprivation therapy in prostate cancer patients. Clin Endocrinol (Oxf) 2002;56(6):779–86.
34. Hakimian P, Blute M Jr, Kashanian J, et al. Metabolic and cardiovascular effects of androgen deprivation therapy. BJU Int 2008;102(11):1509–14.
35. Tyrrell CJ, Kaisary AV, Iversen P, et al. A randomised comparison of 'Casodex' (bicalutamide) 150 mg monotherapy versus castration in the treatment of metastatic and locally advanced prostate cancer. Eur Urol 1998;33(5):447–56.
36. Potosky AL, Knopf K, Clegg LX, et al. Quality-of-life outcomes after primary androgen deprivation therapy: results from the Prostate Cancer Outcomes Study. J Clin Oncol 2001;19(17):3750–7.
37. Kawakami J, Cowan JE, Elkin EP, et al. Androgen-deprivation therapy as primary treatment for localized prostate cancer: data from Cancer of the Prostate Strategic Urologic Research Endeavor (CaPSURE). Cancer 2006;106(8):1708–14.
38. Scherr DS, Pitts WR Jr. The nonsteroidal effects of diethylstilbestrol: the rationale for androgen deprivation therapy without estrogen deprivation in the treatment of prostate cancer. J Urol 2003;170(5):1703–8.
39. Cox RL, Crawford ED. Estrogens in the treatment of prostate cancer. J Urol 1995;154(6):1991–8.
40. Gonzalez-Barcena D, Kastin AJ, Schalch DS, et al. Synthetic LH-releasing hormone (LH-RH) administered to normal men by different routes. J Clin Endocrinol Metab 1973;37(3):481–4.
41. Sharifi N, Gulley JL, Dahut WL. Androgen deprivation therapy for prostate cancer. JAMA 2005;294(2):238–44.
42. Limonta P, Montagnani M, Moretti M, et al. LHRH analogues as anticancer agents: pituitary and extrapituitary sites of action. Expert Opin Investig Drugs 2001;10:709–20.
43. Klotz L, Boccon-Gibod L, Shore ND, et al. The efficacy and safety of degarelix: a 12-month, comparative, randomized, open-label, parallel-group phase III study in patients with prostate cancer. BJU Int 2008;102(11):1531–8.
44. Barradell LB, Faulds D. Cyproterone. A review of its pharmacology and therapeutic efficacy in prostate cancer. Drugs Aging 1994;5(1):59–80.
45. Hellerstedt B. Hormonal therapy options for patients with a rising prostate-specific antigen level after primary treatment for prostate cancer. Urology 2003;62(Suppl 1):79–86.
46. Calais da Silva FE, Bono AV, Whelan P, et al. Intermittent androgen deprivation for locally advanced and metastatic prostate cancer: results from a randomised phase 3 study of the South European Uroncological Group. Eur Urol 2009;55(6):1269–77.
47. Abrahamsson PA. Potential benefits of intermittent androgen suppression therapy in the treatment of prostate cancer: a systematic review of the literature. Eur Urol 2010;57(1):49–59.

New Hormonal Therapies for Castration-Resistant Prostate Cancer

Elahe A. Mostaghel, MD, PhD[a], Stephen Plymate, MD[b],*

KEYWORDS

- Prostate cancer • Hormone refractory • Castration resistant
- Androgen ablation • Steroidogenesis • Intracrine • Abiraterone

Androgen deprivation therapy (ADT) remains the primary treatment modality for patients with metastatic prostate cancer, but is uniformly marked by progression to castration-resistant disease over a period of 18 to 20 months with an ensuing median survival of 1 to 2 years. The development of castration-resistant prostate cancer (CRPC) has been the subject of intensive investigation, and continued activation of androgen receptor (AR) signaling despite castration appears to remain a critical driving force in tumor progression.[1] Accumulating data emphasize that "androgen-independent" or "hormone-refractory" tumors retain a clinically relevant degree of hormone sensitivity and highlight the continued importance of AR axis activation in advanced tumors.[2] Accordingly, therapeutic strategies designed to more effectively ablate tumoral androgen activity are required to improve clinical efficacy and prevent disease progression. This article reviews AR-dependent mechanisms underlying CRPC progression and the status of novel hormonal therapies targeting the AR axis that are currently in clinical and preclinical development.

The authors have nothing to disclose.
This work was supported by the Prostate Cancer Foundation (Career Development Award to E.A.M.), Grant K23 CA122820 from the National Institutes of Health (E.A.M.), Grant CI 40 08 from the Damon Runyon Cancer Research Foundation (Damon Runyon-Genentech Clinical Investigator Award to E.A.M.), the Pacific Northwest Prostate Cancer SPORE P50 CA097186 (S.R.P.), and Veterans Affairs Research Service (S.R.P.).
^a Clinical Research Division, Fred Hutchinson Cancer Research Center, 1100 Fairview Avenue N, D4-100, Seattle, WA, USA
^b Department of Medicine, School of Medicine, University of Washington and VAPSHCS/GRECC, 325 9th Avenue, Box 359625, Seattle, WA 98104, USA
* Corresponding author.
E-mail address: splymate@u.washington.edu

Endocrinol Metab Clin N Am 40 (2011) 625–642
doi:10.1016/j.ecl.2011.05.013
0889-8529/11/$ – see front matter © 2011 Elsevier Inc. All rights reserved.

LIGAND-DEPENDENT MECHANISMS MEDIATING AR TRANSACTIVATION IN CRPC

Recent evidence suggests that castration-resistant tumors are not, in fact, androgen independent but develop in a setting of continued AR-mediated signaling potentiated by residual tumoral androgens. The authors and others have demonstrated that castration-resistant tumors are characterized by elevated tumor androgens and by steroid enzyme alterations, which may potentiate de novo androgen synthesis or the use of circulating adrenal androgens.[3–5] These observations suggest that tissue-based alterations in steroid metabolism facilitate the development of CRPC and underscore these metabolic pathways as critical targets of therapy.

Persistence of Intratumoral Androgens Despite Castration

The efficacy of ADT is routinely based on achieving castrate levels of serum testosterone of 20 ng/dL or less. However, tissue androgen measurements in men with either locally recurrent or metastatic CRPC clearly demonstrate that castration does not eliminate androgens from the prostate tumor microenvironment, and that residual androgen levels are well within the range capable of mediating continued AR signaling and AR-mediated gene expression.[6–9] Compared with untreated tissue, prostatic dihydrotestosterone (DHT) levels were decreased approximately 80% in castrate patients with locally recurrent prostate cancer, while testosterone levels were actually equivalent to prostate tissue from untreated men.[7] Moreover, the authors have demonstrated that testosterone levels in metastatic tumors obtained via rapid autopsy from men with CRPC are approximately threefold higher than levels within primary prostate tumors from untreated (eugonadal) patients.[5]

Adrenal androgens have also been detected at significant levels in the prostate tissue of castrate men. Prostatic levels of dehydroepiandrosterone (DHEA), dehydroepiandrosterone sulfate (DHEA-S), and androstenedione (AED) were decreased by about 50% in castrate patients with recurrent prostate cancer, and far exceeded the values of testosterone and DHT in the recurrent tumor tissue.[7] A separate study found no decrease in prostatic levels of 5-androstenediol (a primary metabolite of DHEA and a direct precursor of testosterone, **Fig. 1**) after castration,[10] which is of particular significance, as this androgen has been shown to bind the wild-type AR without being inhibited by flutamide or bicalutamide.[11]

Source of Intratumoral Androgens Despite Castration

Alterations in key enzymes involved in sterol biosynthesis and androgen metabolism have been identified in prostate tumor samples from castrate patients, and the dependence of CRPC on intratumoral androgen metabolism has been modeled in vitro and in vivo.[12–14] These data suggest that the uptake and conversion of adrenal androgens as well as the de novo synthesis of androgens (from progestins, cholesterol, or earlier precursors) may contribute to the residual tissue androgens present after castration.

In the classical pathway of androgen synthesis, C21 steroids generated from cholesterol, such as pregnenolone and progesterone, are first converted to the C19 steroids DHEA and AED via the sequential hydroxylase and lyase activity of CYP17A. These adrenal steroids are then acted on by HSD3B, HSD17B3, and SRD5A to generate testosterone and DHT. In steroidogenic tissues in which both CYP17A and SRD5A are expressed, an alternative route to DHT is possible wherein C21 steroids are first acted on by HSD3B and SRD5A followed by CYP17A and HSD17B3.[15] This "backdoor pathway," wherein steroid flux to DHT bypasses the conventional intermediates of AED and testosterone, has also been postulated to be operative in prostate tumors (see **Fig. 1**).[14]

The enhanced expression of transcripts encoding key enzymes in the cholesterol biosynthetic pathway has been demonstrated in castration-resistant prostate tumors, including expression of squalene epoxidase (SQLE), the rate-limiting enzyme in choles-terol synthesis.[3] The authors and others have reported the altered expression of genes encoding many steroidogenic enzymes including the upregulated expression of FASN, CYP17A1, HSD3B1, HSD17B3, CYP19A1, and UBT2B17 in CRPC metastases, suggesting that castration-resistant tumors have the ability to use progesterone as androgenic precursors.[4,5] Differential expression of several 17β-hydroxysteroid dehy-drogenase family members (HSD17B) has been observed in prostate cancer, suggest-ing a shift in tumoral androgen metabolism toward the formation of testosterone and DHT with increased expression of reductive enzymes catalyzing conversion to active androgens (HSD17B3 and HSD17B5—also known as aldo-keto reductase AKR1C3), and decreased expression of oxidative enzymes catalyzing the reverse reaction (HSD17B2) (reviewed in Ref.[16]). Differential expression of AKR1C1 and AKR1C2, which mediate the catabolism of DHT, has also been observed in prostate tumors, including a selective loss of AKR1C2 and AKR1C1 in primary prostate tumors accompanied by a reduced capacity to catabolize DHT and an increased level of tumoral DHT.

Thus, alterations in several critical enzymes responsible for DHT synthesis and catabolism provide mechanistic support for the role of intracrine androgen production in maintaining the tumor androgen microenvironment in CRPC, and underscore these metabolic pathways as critical therapeutic targets.

AR-BASED ALTERATIONS MEDIATING AR TRANSACTIVATION IN CRPC

Numerous molecular alterations mediating AR signaling at low or absent androgen levels have been described in CRPC, demonstrating that AR activation in CRPC may occur via both ligand-dependent and ligand-independent mechanisms. This section reviews AR-based alterations that promote CRPC progression by facilitating AR transactivation at low or absent androgen levels.

Overexpression/Amplification of Wild-Type AR

AR overexpression is a well-recognized feature of CRPC and is believed to be a critical driver of CRPC progression. In preclinical prostate cancer models, Chen and colleagues[1] identified AR as the most common gene upregulated following androgen deprivation. AR overexpression supported in vitro proliferation of transfected cells at fivefold lower androgen levels than untransfected cells, and it was both necessary and sufficient to induce tumor formation when placed in castrate SCID mice as compared with untransfected controls. Of importance, AR overexpression not only mediated sensitivity to low ligand concentrations but converted antiandrogens such as bicalu-tamide and flutamide from antagonists to agonists via alteration of coactivators recruited to the AR promoter. Though rarely identified in primary prostate tumors, AR gene amplification leading to AR overexpression is present in approximately 30% of clinical CRPC specimens.[17] Additional mechanisms that mediate increased AR transcription and/or AR stability are likely operative, as increased AR expression is frequently observed in the absence of AR amplification. Recent data suggest that dimerization of AR with ligand-independent AR splice variants (discussed later) may increase AR levels by preventing AR protein degradation.[18]

AR Mutations

Mutations in the AR have been identified following castration or ADT in approximately 20% to 40% of CRPC tumors, and are rarely found in hormone-naïve prostate

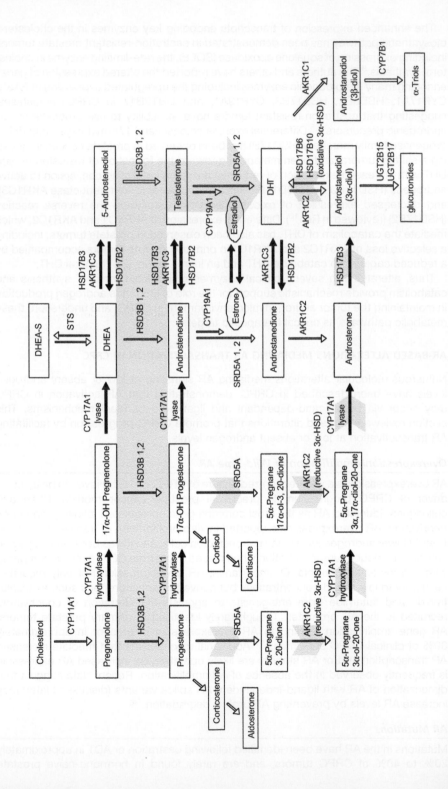

tumors.[19] Multiple mutations are frequently isolated from the same tumor, demonstrating the high degree of heterogeneity present in prostate cancers.[20] Several hundred AR mutations have been described following androgen ablation, but more than 90% are nonsense or missense in nature and result in a nonfunctional AR. Several important AR mutations occur in the ligand-binding domain (LBD), and it is notable that none have been identified in this region in the absence of castration. The most common mutation occurs at or around amino acid 877. The Thr877Ala mutation was originally described in the LNCaP human prostate cancer cell line, and permits binding of an expanded repertoire of steroid ligands such as progestins and estradiol as well as the antiandrogen flutamide, converting its activity as an antiandrogen to an agonist.[21] Gain-of-function mutations also occur in both the N- and C-termini, which can alter the N/C interaction involved in cofactor recruitment. Although AR mutations are associated with castration resistance, none of them occur with a frequency that would suggest they are responsible for the development of castration resistance. However, the potential agonist activity of steroidal antiandrogens in the setting of AR amplification and/or AR mutation has spurred the development of AR antagonists without agonist properties.

Alterations in AR Coregulators

Literally several hundred AR coregulators have been described that influence AR activation via multiple mechanisms, including recruitment of transcriptional machinery, modulation of chromatin-remodeling enzymes, and initiation of RNA polymerase activity.[22] Several AR coactivators are increased in CRPC, including TIF-1, MAGE-II, SRB-1, NFKB, and ARA70, whereas corepressors such as SMRT are downregulated. Whether alterations in the balance between AR and its coregulators can activate AR in the absence of ligand in CRPC is not clear. However, altered coregulator expression may sensitize the AR for activation under low androgen conditions, as well as convert AR antagonists into agonists via corepressor downregulation and/or corepressor dismissal from the AR complex.[23] Inhibition of AR coregulators has been proposed as a target for suppressing AR activity in CRPC.[24]

Activation of AR by Peptide Ligands

Several studies have demonstrated that peptide molecules may transactivate the AR in the absence of ligand, including insulin-like growth factors (IGF-I and IGF-II), epidermal growth factor (EGF), keratinocyte growth factor (KGF), and cytokines

◄────────────────────────

Fig. 1. The classical and backdoor pathways of androgen biosynthesis. In the classical pathway (*solid gray arrow*), C21 precursors (pregnenolone and progesterone) are converted to the C19 adrenal androgens DHEA and androstenedione (AED) by the sequential hydroxylase and lyase activity of CYP17A1. Circulating adrenal androgens (including the sulfated form of DHEA, DHEA-S), enter the prostate and can be converted to testosterone by a series of reactions involving the activity of HSD3B, HSD17B, and AKR1C enzymes. Testosterone is then converted to the potent androgen DHT by the activity of SRD5A. In the backdoor pathway to DHT synthesis (*short gray arrows*), C21 precursors are first acted on by SRD5A and the reductive 3a-HSD activity of the AKR1C family member, AKR1C2, followed by conversion to C19 androgens via the lyase activity of CYP17A. DHT is subsequently generated by the action of HSD17B3 and an oxidative 3a-HSD enzyme, including HSD17B6 (also called RL-HSD) or HSD17B10 (as well as RODH4, RODH5 and NT 3a-HSD, not shown). (*Adapted from* Mostaghel EA, Nelson PS. Intracrine androgen metabolism in prostate cancer progression: mechanisms of castration resistance and therapeutic implications. Best Pract Res Clin Endocrinol Metab 2008;22:243; with permission.)

such as interleukin-6 (IL-6) (reviewed in Ref.[25]). The impact of these factors in vivo is not known, although the authors have shown that inhibition of IGF-I receptor by the IGF-I receptor inhibitory antibody A12 affects AR translocation and transactivation in vivo.[26] Probably the most convincing of these potential AR peptide ligands is IL-6, which has been shown to bind the LBD and transactivate the AR, as determined by ARE-luciferase reporter constructs or by increased expression of androgen-regulated genes. In addition, nuclear translocation of AR by IL-6 has also been described. However, the clinical relevance of IL-6 in prostate cancer is not clear. Although IL-6 is significantly elevated in the serum and bone metastases of patients with advanced prostate cancer, a recent clinical trial in which men with CRPC were treated with an IL-6 inhibitory antibody showed no evidence of benefit.[27]

AR Splice Variants

The authors and others have recently described the generation of posttranscriptional AR splice variants following castration. Approximately 25 variants have been identified in human tissues and human prostate cell lines.[18,28–32] Some of these variants have no function, whereas others appear to enhance the effect of the full-length wild-type receptor. Most significant among these splice variants are those in which the AR LBD is lost, resulting in ligand-independent constitutive AR activation (**Fig. 2**). Mechanisms responsible for generation of the AR splice rearrangements have not been determined, but the consistency with which ARV7/AR3 and AR^v567es are found in human tumors from castrate men suggests that production of these variants may occur in response to castration, and it is notable that the variants most prevalent in

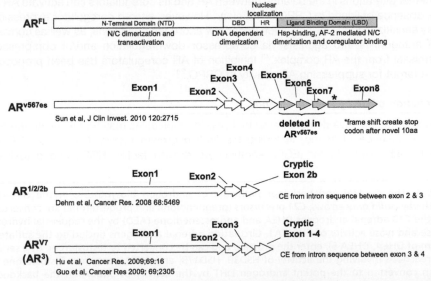

Fig. 2. Androgen receptor splice variants. Domains of the full-length androgen receptor (AR^FL) include the N-terminal domain (NTD), the DNA-binding domain (DBD), the hinge region (HR), and the C-terminal ligand-binding domain (LBD), involved in mediating the indicated functions. The major AR splice variants identified in human prostate cancer cell lines and specimens include the exon-skipping variant, AR^v567es, in which exons 5, 6, and 7 of the LBD are deleted, as well as the indicated truncated AR variants in which exons 2 or 3 become spliced to cryptic exon (CE) sequences. AR^V7 and AR^3 were published separately but later shown to encode the same protein product. (*Data from* Refs.[18,28–30])

human tissues are those most consistently found following androgen deprivation in vitro. The authors have found that the generation of AR^{v567es} is especially sensitive to suppression of intratumoral androgens,[18,32] suggesting that growth of these tumors is dependent on AR variants in the presence of castrate levels of androgen.

While AR variants lacking the LBD are transcriptionally active when placed in AR-negative cell lines, the expression of AR variants has generally been reported to occur in conjunction with ongoing expression of full-length AR. Of interest, Sun and colleagues have demonstrated that in the absence of ligand, the AR^{v567es} AR variant forms a heterodimer with full-length AR, causing it to be translocated to the nucleus, and that in the presence of ligand AR^{v567es} enhances the activity of wtAR. These data suggest that AR variants can activate an AR transcriptional program by themselves, but that they can also potentiate the activity of full-length AR under low ligand conditions by essentially functioning as AR ligands themselves. In this respect, Watson and colleagues[32] recently demonstrated that in the presence of both truncated and full-length AR variants, targeting the full-length AR with the antiandrogen MDV3100 suppressed AR activity and cell growth as efficiently as when only full-length AR was present, suggesting activity of the AR splice variants is mediated through the full-length AR.

NOVEL AGENTS TARGETING INTRATUMORAL ANDROGENS

Because many castration-resistant tumors are not truly androgen independent, therapeutic strategies that more effectively target residual tumoral androgens are necessary. Androgen metabolism within primary prostate tumors is characterized by steroid enzyme alterations, which may potentiate the intracrine conversion of adrenal androgens to testosterone and DHT and/or inhibit the conversion of DHT to inactive metabolites. Enzymes mediating the metabolism of adrenal androgens to testosterone, DHT, and subsequent metabolites are also increased in studies of castration-resistant metastatic tumors, further enhancing the potential use of adrenal androgens in the castrate microenvironment.[4,5] These observations suggest that tissue-based alterations in steroid metabolism may facilitate prostatic tumor development, and underscore these metabolic pathways as critical therapeutic targets.

CYP17A Inhibitors

CYP17A is a single enzyme that catalyzes sequential steps in the conversion of C21 progesterone precursors to the C19 adrenal androgens, DHEA and AED. While ketoconazole (a weak inhibitor of CYP11A and CYP17A) has been used for suppression of residual adrenal androgens in men with CRPC, limited efficacy and significant treatment-related side effects have prompted the development of more potent inhibitors of androgen biosynthesis. Several CYP17A inhibitors have been reported, including a series of novel agents exhibiting both CYP17A inhibition and antiandrogen activity.[33]

Abiraterone

Abiraterone, a pregnenolone derivative, is a selective irreversible inhibitor of both the 17α-hydroxylase and C17,20-lyase activity of CYP17, and has shown promising efficacy in reducing circulating androgen levels and achieving prostate-specific antibody (PSA) responses in men with CRPC. In eugonadal men, abiraterone suppressed testosterone levels by greater than 50% accompanied by a corresponding increase in luteinizing hormone (LH) levels, while in castrate men abiraterone further suppressed serum testosterone levels by 75% or more.[34] Phase 1/2 studies have demonstrated PSA responses and clinical activity in chemotherapy-naïve and post–docetaxel-treated CRPC patients (including patients who have progressed on ketoconazole), and phase 3 studies in these areas are under way.

In men with chemotherapy-naïve metastatic CRPC, phase 1/2 studies have demonstrated durable PSA declines of at least 50% in approximately two-thirds of patients treated with abiraterone, with partial radiographic responses (by RECIST [Response Evaluation Criteria in Solid Tumors] criteria) in 37.5% and a median time to progression of 32 weeks.[35,36] PSA responses of at least 50% were observed in 47% of patients with prior ketoconazole treatment compared with 64% of patients without.[37] Abiraterone generally suppressed DHEA levels by approximately 75% and suppressed DHEA-S, AED, and testosterone levels to essentially undetectable.[36,37] As observed in studies of ketoconazole, patients achieving PSA declines of 50% or more had higher baseline levels of DHEA-S, DHEA, and AED and, in contrast to progression on ketoconazole, increases in testosterone, AED, or DHEA levels were not observed on progression with abiraterone.[35,38]

In a phase 2 study of post–docetaxel-treated CRPC patients, PSA declines of at least 50% were observed in 51% of patients treated with abiraterone alone, with a median time to progression of 24 weeks.[39] In a second study of abiraterone in the postchemotherapy setting, in which 41% of patients had received prior ketoconazole, abiraterone (in combination with prednisone, 5 mg twice daily) achieved PSA declines of a t least 50% in 45% of ketoconazole-naïve patients and in 26% of ketoconazole-treated patients, with a median time to progression of 28 and 14 weeks, respectively.[40] These findings, together with those in the chemotherapy-naïve setting, demonstrate that abiraterone maintains a reasonable degree of clinical efficacy in CRPC patients previously treated with docetaxel and/or ketoconazole. Two phase 3 randomized, placebo-controlled studies of abiraterone in combination with prednisone versus prednisone alone have been ongoing, one in the chemotherapy-naïve setting and one in CRPC patients after docetaxel treatment, both with a primary end point of overall survival. Early results of the phase 3 COU-AA-301 study in the postchemotherapy setting were recently released, demonstrating an overall survival of 14.8 months compared with 10.9 months in the placebo-treated group (hazard ratio 0.646, $P<.0001$), representing a 35% reduction in risk of death with abiraterone treatment.[41]

Abiraterone was associated with expected increases in the C21 steroids upstream of CYP17A (including a 10-fold increase in deoxycorticosterone and 40-fold increase in corticosterone), accounting for the treatment-related side effects. These effects were generally mild and primarily related to symptoms of mineralocorticoid excess (including grade 1 and 2 hypertension, hypokalemia, edema, and fatigue), and responded to treatment with eplerenone or low-dose glucocorticoids (spironolactone should be avoided as it may act as an AR agonist). Decreases in serum cortisol (twofold) with concomitant elevations in corticotropin (fivefold) were also observed. It is interesting that 4 of 15 patients progressing on abiraterone responded to the addition of dexamethasone, which decreased corticotropin and deoxycorticosterone levels to below baseline,[36] consistent with prior reports that steroids upstream of CYP17, including progestins and corticosteroids, can stimulate the AR. At present, use of abiraterone in combination with low-dose prednisone or dexamethasone is recommended to prevent the treatment-related increase in corticotropin and attendant side effects.

TAK-700

TAK-700 (Millennium—Takeda Oncology Company, Cambridge, MA, USA) is a novel nonsteroidal CYP17 inhibitor with high selectivity against the C17,20-lyase over 17α-hydroxylase activity of CYP17. In a phase 1/2 dose-escalation study in men with metastatic CRPC, 11 of 20 patient receiving 300 mg or more twice daily showed PSA declines of greater than 50% and 4 had reductions of greater than 90%. Median testosterone and DHEA-S levels at 4 weeks decreased from 4.9 to 0.6 ng/dL and 53.8 µg/dL to undetectable, respectively. The most common adverse effects included fatigue, nausea, constipation, and anorexia, without a significant incidence of hypertension, consistent with the agent's selective inhibition of 17,20-lyase over 17α-hydroxylase activity.[42] The phase 2 portion, including an arm evaluating the concomitant use of prednisone, is ongoing.

VN-124

VN/124-1, a novel heteroaryl steroid, is a potent CYP17 and AR inhibitor currently being evaluated in a phase 1/2 study under the trade name TOK-001 (Tokai Pharmaceuticals, Cambridge, MA, USA). VN/124-1 exhibits threefold and fourfold stronger inhibition of CYP17 activity than abiraterone and ketoconazole, respectively, and is also a potent inhibitor of the AR, both as a competitive antagonist (with a binding affinity comparable to bicalutamide) and as a dose-dependent inhibitor of AR protein expression, mediated in part via an increase in AR degradation.[43] Of note, VN/124-1 has similar AR inhibitory activity against the T877A AR mutant. In preclinical studies VN/124-1 was significantly more effective than castration or bicalutamide in suppressing growth of the androgen-sensitive LAPC4 xenograft. Moreover, VN/124-1 maintained its potent downregulation of the AR in vivo, leading to a 10-fold reduction in tumor AR levels compared with castration or bicalutamide-treated tumors (both of which demonstrated a 2–3-fold increase in AR expression). Of interest, this agent had also been demonstrated to inhibit the growth of AR-negative prostate cancer cells via induction of the endoplasmic reticulum stress response.[44] Phase 1 studies evaluating this agent in CRPC are in development.

Other Steroidogenic Enzyme Inhibitors

Inhibitors of SRD5A

SRD5A1 and SRD5A2 catalyze the intraprostatic conversion of testosterone to the more potent androgen DHT. SRD5A2 is the primary isoform expressed in benign prostate tissue, while a relative increase in SRD5A1 expression and activity is observed in prostate cancer. Finasteride (a specific inhibitor of SRD5A2) and dutasteride (a dual SRD5A inhibitor) are 4-azasteroids extensively used in the treatment of benign prostatic hyperplasia, and have been explored for the prevention and treatment of prostate cancer. Whereas dutasteride alone has limited activity in men with CRPC, a phase 2 study of ketoconazole, hydrocortisone, and dutasteride (KHAD) demonstrated PSA responses of 50% or greater in 56% of men and a median time to progression of 14.5 months, nearly twice that observed in the phase 2 studies of abiraterone, thus leading the investigators to postulate that intratumoral DHT synthesis may contribute to abiraterone resistance.[45]

Inhibitors of AKR1C3 and HSD17B3

HSD17B3 and AKR1C3 catalyze the final steps in testosterone and DHT biosynthesis: the reduction of the adrenal androgens, AED and androstenedione, to testosterone and DHT. HSD17B3 is primarily expressed in Leydig cells, whereas AKR1C3 mediates production of testosterone and DHT in peripheral tissues. Several studies have demonstrated increased expression of these enzymes in castration-resistant prostate tumors, suggesting they may be important targets for inhibition.[4,5,46] Conversely, the AKR1C family members AKR1C1 and AKR1C2 mediate the catabolism of DHT (to 3b-diol and 3a-diol, respectively), and a selective loss of these enzymes (accompanied by a reduced capacity to metabolize DHT and an increase in tumoral DHT levels) has been reported in prostate tumors.[47] Therefore, agents that selectively target AKR1C3, but not the highly related AKR1C1 and AKR1C2, are under development.

AKR1C family members are inhibited by nonsteroidal anti-inflammatory drugs (NSAIDs) and the cyclooxygenase (COX)-2 selective inhibitor, celecoxib.[48] Indole acetic acids (eg, indomethacin) are among the most potent agents targeting the AKR1C family, and indomethacin analogues that selectively target AKR1C3, but do not inhibit COX-1, COX-2, AKR1C1, and AKR1C2 have been reported.[49] Small molecule inhibitors of HSD17B3 have been developed and tested using in vitro and in vivo systems and have been shown to reduce systemic androgen levels (reviewed in[50]). However, to date no studies in prostate cancer have been reported.

Inhibitors of 3BHSD
3BHSD mediates conversion of δ4 steroids such as DHEA and androstenediol to the δ5 steroids AED and testosterone, respectively. The activity of 3BHSD is required for the de novo biosynthesis of androgens from cholesterol (via either the classical or backdoor pathway) as well as for pathways converting adrenal androgens to testosterone and DHT. The type-1 isoform is expressed in the adrenal, ovary, and testis, and type 2 in peripheral tissues such as the prostate, although transcripts encoding both isoforms have been observed in CRPC metastases. While several studies have demonstrated that DHEA or androstenediol can directly activate wild-type and mutated AR,[10] others have clearly demonstrated a requirement for 3BHSD-mediated conversion to downstream metabolites first,[51] implicating 3BHSD as a therapeutic target for CRPC. Epostane, a competitive inhibitor of 3BHDS1, has already been used in human studies for the medical termination of pregnancy via inhibition of progesterone synthesis and has been shown to inhibit the DHEA-induced proliferation of breast cancer MCF-7 cells,[52] suggesting its study in prostate cancer may be warranted.

Inhibitors of steroid sulfatase
Steroid sulfatase (STS) is the enzyme responsible for hydrolyzing inactive sulfates of estrogen and DHEA to biologically active steroids. Prostate cancer cell lines have demonstrated both STS expression and activity, as demonstrated by hydrolysis of estrone-S and DHEA-S to unconjugated forms, and immunohistochemical expression of STS in prostatic tumors has been reported (reviewed in Ref.[16]). Although not yet tested in prostate cancer, STS inhibitors have been evaluated in patients with breast cancer and may have efficacy in preventing prostatic utilization of the adrenal androgen DHEA, which primarily circulates as the inactive sulfate, DHEA-S. Given the proposed importance of adrenal androgens in maintaining prostate tumor androgen metabolism in anorchid patients, the clinical efficacy of preventing tumoral DHEA-S utilization by STS inhibitors warrants examination.

Apoptone
Apoptone (HE3235; Hollis Eden Pharmaceuticals, San Diego, CA, USA) is a synthetic analogue of 3β-androstanediol, a naturally occurring metabolite of DHT formed in prostate tissue, and has been shown to suppress tumor growth, decrease AR expression and nuclear localization, and suppress levels of intratumoral androgens in castration-resistant prostate cancer xenografts.[53,54] Although its mechanism of activity has not been fully elucidated, HE3235 appears to inhibit conversion of d-cholesterol to d-pregnenolone, without inhibition of CYP17. HE3235 is currently under study in a phase 1/2 clinical trial of men with CRPC, with early results demonstrating promising PSA responses.[55]

LH and LHRH antagonists
Although gonadotropin-releasing hormone (GnRH) analogues are used to achieve medical castration via suppression of the pituitary-testicular axis, variants of the

GnRH and LH-releasing hormone (LHRH) receptor are also present in prostate epithelium.[56] GnRH antagonist therapy may have direct antitumorigenic effects,[57] and LHRH receptors on prostate tumors may serve as targets for LHRH analogues hybridized to cytotoxic moieties.[58] A cytotoxic analogue of LHRH conjugated to doxorubicin has been clinically tested in women with gynecologic tumors expressing LHRH receptors,[59] and studies in prostate cancer may be of interest.

Receptors for LH itself have also been described in prostate cancer specimens. A recent study demonstrated that exposure of both androgen-sensitive (LNCaP) and androgen-independent (22RV1 and C4-2B) prostate cancer cell lines to LH increased the protein expression of steroidogenic enzymes including STAR, CYB5B, CYP11A, and 3BHSD, and a 2.5-fold increase in progesterone synthesis was observed in LH-treated C4-2B cells compared with controls.[60] These data suggest that LH may have a role in the regulation of steroid biosynthesis in prostate cancer cells, and identify the LH receptor as a potential therapeutic target.

NOVEL AGENTS TARGETING THE AR AND DOWNSTREAM AR SIGNALING

The AR, a member of the nuclear receptor superfamily, is a ligand-dependent transcription factor with a 4-domain structure consisting of an N-terminal activation function domain involved in coactivator binding (AF-1), a central DNA-binding domain, a hinge region with a nuclear localization signal, and a C-terminal LBD involved in receptor dimerization as well as ligand-dependent coactivator binding (AF-2). In the absence of ligand, the AR is bound to cytoplasmic chaperones or heat shock proteins (such as HSP90), which maintain receptor conformation and prevent degradation. Ligand binding results in conformational activation, HSP90 dissociation, receptor dimerization, phosphorylation, and nuclear translocation. The dimerized receptor binds to target DNA sequences known as androgen response elements (AREs) in promoter and enhancer regions of androgen-responsive genes, with subsequent recruitment of coregulator proteins that dictate activation or repression of gene expression.

Antiandrogens

AR agonists elicit a structural conformation in the AF-2 domain promoting N-terminal/ C-terminal interactions that stabilize the AR in the agonist conformation, as well as mediating recruitment of coactivator complexes and enhancing stable DNA association. By contrast, AR antagonists prevent the AR from achieving the transcriptionally active conformation required for stable DNA binding. Different antagonists can engage and modulate the AR by distinct mechanisms, including inhibition of chaperone dissociation, alterations in subcellular AR localization, recruitment of nuclear corepressor complexes, and ineffective recruitment of coactivator proteins (reviewed in Ref.[61]). Several mechanisms by which nonsteroidal antiandrogens function as AR agonists have been described, including AR mutations and/or alterations in cofactor recruitment. This aspect has been a critical impetus in the development of novel, more potent AR inhibitors without agonist activity against either wild-type or mutant ARs.

MDV3100

MDV3100 is a second-generation, diarylthiohydantoin-competitive AR antagonist that binds to the AR with fivefold to eightfold greater affinity than bicalutamide and only twofold to threefold lower affinity than DHT. Preclinical studies have demonstrated that, compared with bicalutamide, MDV3100 potently decreases the nuclear translocation of AR, markedly reduces chromatin occupancy at canonical AREs, and is significantly more effective in suppressing the growth of LNCaP tumors.[62] Of importance,

MDV3100 did not elicit agonist activity against LNCaP tumors overexpressing the AR, or against the T877A or W741C AR mutations, situations in which bicalutamide demonstrates agonist activity. Of note, treatment with androgen was able to overcome the AR inhibitory effects of MDV3100 in vitro, suggesting this agent will not have efficacy in the eugonadal setting.

Clinical evaluation of MDV3100 in a phase 1/2 study of 140 men with CRPC has recently been reported. MDV3100 led to PSA declines of greater than 50% in 62% of chemotherapy-naïve patients and 51% of CRPC patients previously treated with docetaxel, with a median time to PSA progression of 41 and 21 weeks, respectively.[63] Two-thirds of patients had partial remissions or stable disease in soft tissue and bone metastases, and all patients who were assessed by [^{18}F]fluorodihydrotestosterone (FDHT) positron emission tomography scans showed declines in FDHT accumulation. Thirty-seven percent of patients with prior ketoconazole treatment achieved a PSA decline of greater than 50% versus 71% of those without. The most common adverse events were fatigue, nausea, dyspnea, anorexia, and back pain. A phase 3, randomized, placebo-controlled trial of MDV3100 in docetaxel-treated men with metastatic CRPC is currently ongoing.

While preclinical studies show that MDV3100 is highly effective in tumors driven by an amplified AR, the observation that ligand can overcome the effect of MDV3100 raises a question as to whether MDV3100 will be equally effective in the setting of a non-amplified AR, particularly if residual tumor androgens are present. AR is amplified in about 20% to 25% of CRPC cases,[17] although AR amplification has been demonstrated in up to 50% of CRPC cases when circulating tumor cells are evaluated,[64] and these may represent cases in which MDV3100 will have most efficacy.

N-terminal AR inhibitors

An alternative approach to targeting the AR LBD is the development of N-terminal domain (NTD) AR inhibitors, as the NTD is essential for both ligand-dependent and ligand-independent AR activation. Agents such as MDV3100 or nonsteroidal antiandrogens do not inhibit ligand-independent transactivation of the AR NTD (mediated by bypass mechanisms such as IL-6 and other peptide growth factors), nor do they directly target constitutively active AR splice variants lacking the LBD. At present the most promising compound that has been published is EPI-001, which is a degradation product of bisphenyl-A that was found by testing a library of products isolated from marine sponges.[65] EPI-001 binds to the amino terminus of the AR and inhibits AR transactivation. EPI-001 does not alter AR nuclear translocation or prevent ligand binding, but disrupts the AR N/C interaction thereby inhibiting cofactor recruitment. When given to castrate mice, EPI-001 decreased the size of human prostate cancer xenografts. No apparent toxicity has been noted in the animals, and it has 85% bioavailability after oral administration. Combined use with LBD and ligand-targeting agents would be of potential benefit by more robustly knocking out AR activity.

Modulators of AR Expression, Stability, and Downstream Signaling

Several agents under investigation for prostate cancer therapy do not target the AR directly, but alter cellular pathways involved in maintaining the expression, stability, and downstream signaling components of the AR axis. While many of these agents are still in development, several have been tested in clinical studies of men with CRPC. The most studied pathways include the heat shock protein (HSP) chaperones, histone deacetylases (HDACs), and mammalian target of rapamycin (mTOR).

HSP inhibitors

HSP90 is an adenosine triphosphate (ATP)-dependent chaperone protein involved in maintaining the stability, localization, and activity of the AR as well as other oncogenic client proteins such as Her2 and Akt. The ansamycin antibiotic, geldenamycin, binds the ATP-binding pocket of HSP90, leading to the degradation of client proteins. In preclinical studies, tanespimycin (17-AA-geldenamycin) inhibited the growth of AR-positive prostate cancer xenografts accompanied by an 80% decrease in AR expression.[66] Phase 1 studies have not shown significant clinical activity in men with CRPC, and agents with improved solubility characteristics are currently being evaluated.

Histone deacetylase inhibitors

Chromatin remodeling determined by the balance of histone acetylation versus deacetylation regulates the transcriptional activity of numerous genes involved in cell survival and differentiation. HDAC inhibitors have been shown to decrease transcription of the AR, to inhibit AR-mediated transcription (by blocking recruitment of RNA polymerase to the promoter of HDAC-dependent AR target genes), and to promote AR degradation (via acetylation-induced inhibition of HSP90 ATP binding).[67] The HDAC inhibitor vorinostat (SAHA) has shown synergistic activity in suppressing prostate cancer cell proliferation in vitro when combined with the AR antagonist bicalutamide.[68] A phase 1 study of vorinostat in combination with docetaxel and a phase 2 study of the single agent vorinostat in the postchemotherapy setting were both associated with minimal clinical response and significant dose-limiting toxicity, suggesting that alternative agents in this class with a more favorable toxicity profile will be required to test the therapeutic efficacy of this approach. A phase 1/2 study of panobinostat (LBH589) in combination with bicalutamide in men with CRPC is ongoing.

mTOR inhibitors

The PI3K/Akt/mTOR pathway is central to several signaling cascades mediating cell growth and survival, and alterations in this pathway (including loss or mutation of the negative regulator PTEN) are present in 30% to 50% of prostate tumors. Moreover, the Akt/mTOR pathway can activate AR in the absence of androgen. Many agents targeting PI3K, Akt, and mTOR have been evaluated in both in vitro and in vivo models of prostate cancer. Clinically the mTOR inhibitors rapamycin and its analogues everolimus (RAD-001) and temsirolimus (CCI-779) have shown the most promise, and multiple phase 1 and phase 2 clinical trials with these agents are currently ongoing.[69]

Src-kinase inhibitors

Src kinases are nonreceptor protein tyrosine kinases involved in signal transduction downstream of multiple cell surface receptors including endothelial growth factor receptor, platelet-derived growth factor receptor, and vascular endothelial growth factor receptor, and have been implicated in the androgen-induced proliferation of CRPC cells. Dasatinib, a dual Abl and Src family kinase inhibitor, has been shown to inhibit AR phosphorylation and activation in vitro,[70] as well as targeting osteoclast and osteoblast activity[71] and has recently been evaluated in a phase 2 study of chemotherapy-naïve men with CRPC. Although progression occurred in 60% and 80% of patients at 12 and 24 weeks, respectively, nearly half of the patients showed a decrease in markers of bone metabolism.[72] A randomized phase 3 study of dasatinib in combination with docetaxel (with skeletal-related events as one end point) is ongoing.

SUMMARY

Hormonal therapy remains the primary treatment modality for patients with advanced prostate cancer, and is associated with significant antitumoral efficacy and clinical benefit. However, many studies demonstrate heterogeneity in the pathologic response to ADT, and the ultimate failure of androgen suppression to control disease progression is well recognized. Data regarding the molecular response of prostate cancer to hormone therapy continues to emerge, providing critical insight into cellular growth and signaling pathways that may be exploited as therapeutic targets. The presence of residual androgens and persistent activation of the AR signaling axis in CRPC suggest that a multitargeted treatment approach to ablate all contributions to AR signaling within the prostate tumor will be required for optimal antitumor efficacy. Such a strategy would include targeting all potential contributors to the prostatic androgen milieu, including testicular, adrenal, and intratumoral sources, as well as novel agents targeting the stability, degradation, and activity of the AR. Although historical studies of combined androgen blockade have yielded small gains in overall survival compared with ADT alone, the introduction of potent steroidogenic inhibitors such as abiraterone and the dual CYP17A/AR inhibitor VN/124-1, in combination with novel AR inhibitors such as MDV3100, hold significant promise for improving the treatment of men with CRPC.

REFERENCES

1. Chen CD, Welsbie DS, Tran C, et al. Molecular determinants of resistance to anti-androgen therapy. Nat Med 2004;10(1):33–9.
2. Scher HI, Sawyers CL. Biology of progressive, castration-resistant prostate cancer: directed therapies targeting the androgen-receptor signaling axis. J Clin Oncol 2005;23(32):8253–61.
3. Holzbeierlein J, Lal P, LaTulippe E, et al. Gene expression analysis of human prostate carcinoma during hormonal therapy identifies androgen-responsive genes and mechanisms of therapy resistance. Am J Pathol 2004;164(1):217–27.
4. Stanbrough M, Bubley GJ, Ross K, et al. Increased expression of genes converting adrenal androgens to testosterone in androgen-independent prostate cancer. Cancer Res 2006;66(5):2815–25.
5. Montgomery RB, Mostaghel EA, Vessella R, et al. Maintenance of intratumoral androgens in metastatic prostate cancer: a mechanism for castration-resistant tumor growth. Cancer Res 2008;68(11):4447–54.
6. Geller J, Liu J, Albert J, et al. Relationship between human prostatic epithelial cell protein synthesis and tissue dihydrotestosterone level. Clin Endocrinol (Oxf) 1987;26(2):155–61.
7. Mohler JL, Gregory CW, Ford OH 3rd, et al. The androgen axis in recurrent prostate cancer. Clin Cancer Res 2004;10(2):440–8.
8. Nishiyama T, Hashimoto Y, Takahashi K. The influence of androgen deprivation therapy on dihydrotestosterone levels in the prostatic tissue of patients with prostate cancer. Clin Cancer Res 2004;10(21):7121–6.
9. Page ST, Lin DW, Mostaghel EA, et al. Persistent intraprostatic androgen concentrations after medical castration in healthy men. J Clin Endocrinol Metab 2006; 91(10):3850–6.
10. Mizokami A, Koh E, Fujita H, et al. The adrenal androgen androstenediol is present in prostate cancer tissue after androgen deprivation therapy and activates mutated androgen receptor. Cancer Res 2004;64(2):765–71.

11. Miyamoto H, Yeh S, Lardy H, et al. Delta5-androstenediol is a natural hormone with androgenic activity in human prostate cancer cells. Proc Natl Acad Sci U S A 1998;95(19):11083-8.

12. Koh E, Kanaya J, Namiki M. Adrenal steroids in human prostatic cancer cell lines. Arch Androl 2001;46(2):117-25.

13. Mizokami A, Koh E, Izumi K, et al. Prostate cancer stromal cells and LNCaP cells coordinately activate the androgen receptor through synthesis of testosterone and dihydrotestosterone from dehydroepiandrosterone. Endocr Relat Cancer 2009;16(4):1139-55.

14. Locke JA, Guns ES, Lubik AA, et al. Androgen levels increase by intratumoral de novo steroidogenesis during progression of castration-resistant prostate cancer. Cancer Res 2008;68(15):6407-15.

15. Auchus RJ. The backdoor pathway to dihydrotestosterone. Trends Endocrinol Metab 2004;15(9):432-8.

16. Mostaghel EA, Nelson PS. Intracrine androgen metabolism in prostate cancer progression: mechanisms of castration resistance and therapeutic implications. Best Pract Res Clin Endocrinol Metab 2008;22(2):243-58.

17. Visakorpi T, Hyytinen E, Koivisto P, et al. In vivo amplification of the androgen receptor gene and progression of human prostate cancer. Nat Genet 1995;9(4):401-6.

18. Sun S, Sprenger CC, Vessella RL, et al. Castration resistance in human prostate cancer is conferred by a frequently occurring androgen receptor splice variant. J Clin Invest 2010;120(8):2715-30.

19. Taplin ME, Balk SP. Androgen receptor: a key molecule in the progression of prostate cancer to hormone independence. J Cell Biochem 2004;91(3):483-90.

20. Steinkamp MP, O'Mahony OA, Brogley M, et al. Treatment-dependent androgen receptor mutations in prostate cancer exploit multiple mechanisms to evade therapy. Cancer Res 2009;69(10):4434-42.

21. Veldscholte J, Berrevoets CA, Ris-Stalpers C, et al. The androgen receptor in LNCaP cells contains a mutation in the ligand binding domain which affects steroid binding characteristics and response to antiandrogens. J Steroid Biochem Mol Biol 1992;41(3-8):665-9.

22. Chmelar R, Buchanan G, Need EF, et al. Androgen receptor coregulators and their involvement in the development and progression of prostate cancer. Int J Cancer 2007;120(4):719-33.

23. Zhu P, Baek SH, Bourk EM, et al. Macrophage/cancer cell interactions mediate hormone resistance by a nuclear receptor derepression pathway. Cell 2006; 124(3):615-29.

24. Rahman MM, Miyamoto H, Lardy H, et al. Inactivation of androgen receptor coregulator ARA55 inhibits androgen receptor activity and agonist effect of antiandrogens in prostate cancer cells. Proc Natl Acad Sci U S A 2003;100(9):5124-9.

25. Culig Z. Androgen receptor cross-talk with cell signalling pathways. Growth Factors 2004;22(3):170-04.

26. Wu JD, Haugk K, Woodke L, et al. Interaction of IGF signaling and the androgen receptor in prostate cancer progression. J Cell Biochem 2006;99(2):392-401.

27. Dorff TB, Goldman B, Pinski JK, et al. Clinical and correlative results of SWOG S0354: a phase II trial of CNTO328 (siltuximab), a monoclonal antibody against interleukin-6, in chemotherapy-pretreated patients with castration-resistant prostate cancer. Clin Cancer Res 2010;16(11):3028-34.

28. Dehm SM, Schmidt LJ, Heemers HV, et al. Splicing of a novel androgen receptor exon generates a constitutively active androgen receptor that mediates prostate cancer therapy resistance. Cancer Res 2008;68(13):5469-77.

29. Hu R, Dunn TA, Wei S, et al. Ligand-independent androgen receptor variants derived from splicing of cryptic exons signify hormone-refractory prostate cancer. Cancer Res 2009;69(1):16–22.

30. Guo Z, Yang X, Sun F, et al. A novel androgen receptor splice variant is up-regulated during prostate cancer progression and promotes androgen depletion-resistant growth. Cancer Res 2009;69(6):2305–13.

31. Marcias G, Erdmann E, Lapouge G, et al. Identification of novel truncated androgen receptor (AR) mutants including unreported pre-mRNA splicing variants in the 22Rv1 hormone-refractory prostate cancer (PCa) cell line. Hum Mutat 2010;31(1):74–80.

32. Watson PA, Chen YF, Balbas MD, et al. Constitutively active androgen receptor splice variants expressed in castration-resistant prostate cancer require full-length androgen receptor. Proc Natl Acad Sci U S A 2010;107(39):16759–65.

33. Handratta VD, Vasaitis TS, Njar VCO, et al. Novel C-17-heteroaryl steroidal CYP17 inhibitors/antiandrogens: synthesis, in vitro biological activity, pharmacokinetics, and antitumor activity in the LAPC4 human prostate cancer xenograft model. J Med Chem 2005;48(8):2972–84.

34. O'Donnell A, Judson I, Dowsett M, et al. Hormonal impact of the 17alpha-hydroxylase/C(17,20)-lyase inhibitor abiraterone acetate (CB7630) in patients with prostate cancer. Br J Cancer 2004;90(12):2317–25.

35. Attard G, Reid AH, A'Hern R, et al. Selective inhibition of CYP17 with abiraterone acetate is highly active in the treatment of castration-resistant prostate cancer. J Clin Oncol 2009;27(23):3742–8.

36. Attard G, Reid AH, Yap TA, et al. Phase I clinical trial of a selective inhibitor of CYP17, abiraterone acetate, confirms that castration-resistant prostate cancer commonly remains hormone driven. J Clin Oncol 2008;26(28):4563–71.

37. Ryan CJ, Smith MR, Fong L, et al. Phase I clinical trial of the CYP17 inhibitor abiraterone acetate demonstrating clinical activity in patients with castration-resistant prostate cancer who received prior ketoconazole therapy. J Clin Oncol 2010; 28(9):1481–8.

38. Ryan CJ, Halabi S, Ou SS, et al. Adrenal androgen levels as predictors of outcome in prostate cancer patients treated with ketoconazole plus antiandrogen withdrawal: results from a cancer and leukemia group B study. Clin Cancer Res 2007;13(7):2030–7.

39. Reid AH, Attard G, Danila DC, et al. Significant and sustained antitumor activity in post-docetaxel, castration-resistant prostate cancer with the CYP17 inhibitor abiraterone acetate. J Clin Oncol 2010;28(9):1489–95.

40. Danila DC, Morris MJ, de Bono JS, et al. Phase II multicenter study of abiraterone acetate plus prednisone therapy in patients with docetaxel-treated castration-resistant prostate cancer. J Clin Oncol 2010;28(9):1496–501.

41. de Bono JS, Logothetis CJ, Molina A, et al. Abiraterone and increased survival in metastatic prostate cancer. N Engl J Med 2011;364(21):1995–2005.

42. Dreicer R, Agus DB, MacVicar GR, et al. Safety, pharmacokinetics, and efficacy of TAK-700 in castration-resistant, metastatic prostate cancer: a phase I/II, open-label study. Paper presented at: 2010 Genitourinary Cancers Symposium. San Francisco (CA), March 7, 2010.

43. Vasaitis T, Belosay A, Schayowitz A, et al. Androgen receptor inactivation contributes to antitumor efficacy of 17{alpha}-hydroxylase/17,20-lyase inhibitor 3beta-hydroxy-17-(1H-benzimidazole-1-yl)androsta-5,16-diene in prostate cancer. Mol Cancer Ther 2008;7(8):2348–57.

44. Bruno RD, Gover TD, Burger AM, et al. 17alpha-Hydroxylase/17,20 lyase inhibitor VN/124-1 inhibits growth of androgen-independent prostate cancer cells via induction of the endoplasmic reticulum stress response. Mol Cancer Ther 2008;7(9):2828–36.
45. Taplin ME, Regan MM, Ko YJ, et al. Phase II study of androgen synthesis inhibition with ketoconazole, hydrocortisone, and dutasteride in asymptomatic castration-resistant prostate cancer. Clin Cancer Res 2009;15(22):7099–105.
46. Bauman D, Steckelbroeck S, Peehl D, et al. Transcript profiling of the androgen signal in normal prostate, benign prostatic hyperplasia and prostate cancer. Endocrinology 2006;147(12):5806–16.
47. Ji Q, Chang L, Stanczyk FZ, et al. Impaired dihydrotestosterone catabolism in human prostate cancer: critical role of AKR1C2 as a pre-receptor regulator of androgen receptor signaling. Cancer Res 2007;67(3):1361–9.
48. Bauman DR, Rudnick SI, Szewczuk LM, et al. Development of nonsteroidal anti-inflammatory drug analogs and steroid carboxylates selective for human aldo-keto reductase isoforms: potential antineoplastic agents that work independently of cyclooxygenase isozymes. Mol Pharmacol 2005;67(1):60–8.
49. Byrns MC, Steckelbroeck S, Penning TM. An indomethacin analogue, N-(4-chlorobenzoyl)-melatonin, is a selective inhibitor of aldo-keto reductase 1C3 (type 2 3alpha-HSD, type 5 17beta-HSD, and prostaglandin F synthase), a potential target for the treatment of hormone dependent and hormone independent malignancies. Biochem Pharmacol 2008;75(2):484–93.
50. Day JM, Tutill HJ, Purohit A, et al. Design and validation of specific inhibitors of 17beta-hydroxysteroid dehydrogenases for therapeutic application in breast and prostate cancer, and in endometriosis. Endocr Relat Cancer 2008;15(3):665–92.
51. Evaul K, Li R, Papari-Zareei M, et al. 3beta-hydroxysteroid dehydrogenase is a possible pharmacological target in the treatment of castration-resistant prostate cancer. Endocrinology 2010;151(8):3514–20.
52. Thomas JL, Bucholtz KM, Kacsoh B. Selective inhibition of human 3beta-hydroxysteroid dehydrogenase type 1 as a potential treatment for breast cancer. J Steroid Biochem Mol Biol 2010;125(1–2):57–65.
53. Koreckij TD, Trauger RJ, Montgomery RB, et al. HE3235 inhibits growth of castration-resistant prostate cancer. Neoplasia 2009;11(11):1216–25.
54. Ahlem C, Kennedy M, Page T, et al. 17alpha-Alkynyl 3alpha, 17beta-androstanediol non-clinical and clinical pharmacology, pharmacokinetics and metabolism. Invest New Drugs 2010. [Epub ahead of print].
55. Montgomery RB, Morris MJ, Ryan CJ, et al. HE3235, a synthetic adrenal hormone, in patients with castration-resistant prostate cancer (CRPC): clinical phase I/II trial results. Paper presented at: 2010 Genitourinary Cancers Symposium. San Francisco (CA), March 7, 2010.
56. Liu SV, Schally AV, Hawes D, et al. Expression of receptors for luteinizing hormone-releasing hormone (LH-RH) in prostate cancers following therapy with LH-RH agonists. Clin Cancer Res 2010;16(18):4675–80.
57. Gnanapragasam V, Darby S, Khan M, et al. Evidence that prostate gonadotropin-releasing hormone receptors mediate an anti-tumourigenic response to analogue therapy in hormone refractory prostate cancer. J Pathol 2005;206(2):205–13.
58. Pinski J, Schally AV, Yano T, et al. Inhibition of growth of experimental prostate cancer in rats by LH-RH analogs linked to cytotoxic radicals. Prostate 1993;23(2):165–78.

59. Emons G, Sindermann H, Engel J, et al. Luteinizing hormone-releasing hormone receptor-targeted chemotherapy using AN-152. Neuroendocrinology 2009;90(1): 15–8.

60. Pinski JK, Xiong S, Wang Q, et al. Effect of luteinizing hormone on the steroid biosynthesis pathway in prostate cancer. Paper presented at: 2010 Genitourinary Cancers Symposium. San Francisco (CA), March 7, 2010.

61. Singh P, Uzgare A, Litvinov I, et al. Combinatorial androgen receptor targeted therapy for prostate cancer. Endocr Relat Cancer 2006;13(3):653–66.

62. Tran C, Ouk S, Clegg NJ, et al. Development of a second-generation antiandrogen for treatment of advanced prostate cancer. Science 2009;324(5928):787–90.

63. Scher HI, Beer TM, Higano CS, et al. Antitumour activity of MDV3100 in castration-resistant prostate cancer: a phase 1-2 study. Lancet 2010;375(9724):1437–46.

64. Leversha MA, Han J, Asgari Z, et al. Fluorescence in situ hybridization analysis of circulating tumor cells in metastatic prostate cancer. Clin Cancer Res 2009;15(6): 2091–7.

65. Andersen RJ, Mawji NR, Wang J, et al. Regression of castrate-recurrent prostate cancer by a small-molecule inhibitor of the amino-terminus domain of the androgen receptor. Cancer Cell 2010;17(6):535–46.

66. Solit DB, Zheng FF, Drobnjak M, et al. 17-Allylamino-17-demethoxygeldanamycin induces the degradation of androgen receptor and HER-2/neu and inhibits the growth of prostate cancer xenografts. Clin Cancer Res 2002;8(5):986–93.

67. Welsbie DS, Xu J, Chen Y, et al. Histone deacetylases are required for androgen receptor function in hormone-sensitive and castrate-resistant prostate cancer. Cancer Res 2009;69(3):958–66.

68. Marrocco DL, Tilley WD, Bianco-Miotto T, et al. Suberoylanilide hydroxamic acid (vorinostat) represses androgen receptor expression and acts synergistically with an androgen receptor antagonist to inhibit prostate cancer cell proliferation. Mol Cancer Ther 2007;6(1):51–60.

69. Morgan TM, Koreckij TD, Corey E. Targeted therapy for advanced prostate cancer: inhibition of the PI3K/Akt/mTOR pathway. Curr Cancer Drug Targets 2009;9(2):237–49.

70. Liu Y, Karaca M, Zhang Z, et al. Dasatinib inhibits site-specific tyrosine phosphorylation of androgen receptor by Ack1 and Src kinases. Oncogene 2010;29(22): 3208–16.

71. Koreckij T, Nguyen H, Brown LG, et al. Dasatinib inhibits the growth of prostate cancer in bone and provides additional protection from osteolysis. Br J Cancer 2009;101(2):263–8.

72. Yu EY, Wilding G, Posadas E, et al. Phase II study of dasatinib in patients with metastatic castration-resistant prostate cancer. Clin Cancer Res 2009;15(23): 7421–8.

Androgens and Prostate Cancer Bone Metastases: Effects on Both the Seed and the Soil

Wei Yang, BA, Alice C. Levine, MD*

KEYWORDS

• Androgens • Androgen receptor • Prostate cancer
• Bone metastases

Metastases that are resistant to therapy represent the major cause of death from cancer and the primary clinical challenge in the field. Prostate cancer (PCa) preferentially metastasizes to bone with a resulting mortality of approximately 70%. The metastases are associated with crippling complications, including severe pain, fractures, spinal cord compression, and bone marrow suppression.[1,2] Unfortunately, there are currently no effective therapies for the prevention or treatment of PCa bone metastases. Androgens are essential for normal prostate development[3] and are necessary, but not sufficient, for the development of prostate cancer.[4] Androgen deprivation therapy (ADT) has long been the mainstay of treatment for PCa bone metastases, providing palliation of symptoms in the majority of patients, followed by relapse and progression.[5–7] In spite of these demonstrated effects of androgens on the early and very late phases of PCa, less is known about androgenic effects at varying stages during the multistep process leading to incurable bone metastases.

To metastasize, PCa cells need to develop a vascular network, escape from the primary tumor, invade surrounding tissues, and enter the circulatory and lymphatic systems.[8] Escape into the circulation does not ensure the establishment of distant metastases because most of the tumor cells that enter the blood stream are rapidly eliminated.[9] The small percentage of circulating PCa cells that eventually establish metastases must home and adhere to distant organs, extravasate, proliferate, vascularize, defend against host immune responses, continue to grow in the new

The authors have nothing to disclose.
Division of Endocrinology, Diabetes and Bone Disease, Department of Medicine, Mount Sinai School of Medicine, One Gustave L. Levy Place, Box 1055, New York, NY 10029, USA
* Corresponding author.
E-mail address: alice.Levine@mountsinai.org

Endocrinol Metab Clin N Am 40 (2011) 643–653
doi:10.1016/j.ecl.2011.05.001
0889-8529/11/$ – see front matter © 2011 Elsevier Inc. All rights reserved.

endo.theclinics.com

microenvironment, and then reinitiate these processes to establish more metastases from metastases. Stephen Paget[2] originally identified the critical role of host-tumor interaction in the successful establishment of tumor cell distant metastases in 1889 when he proposed his now widely accepted seed-and-soil hypothesis, noting "When a plant goes to seed, its seeds are carried in all directions; but they can only grow if they fall on congenial soil."[2] Androgens have proven effects on both the seed (PCa cells) and the favorable soil (bone).

ANDROGENS AND PROSTATE CANCER GROWTH IN THE PRIMARY SITE

The process of cancer metastases begins with growth in the primary site. In the normal prostate, the androgen receptor (AR) is expressed in both stromal and epithelial cells. Growth and survival effects of androgens on noncancerous prostate epithelial cells are mainly caused by paracrine actions of androgens, that is, androgenic stimulation of stromal AR resulting in the enhanced transcription and secretion of paracrine growth factors, andromedins. In contrast, the direct action of androgens on normal prostate epithelial cells is to suppress growth and promote differentiation. In PCa cells, AR signaling is often dysregulated because of AR mutations, amplification, alterations in AR coactivators or corepressors, or increased mitogen-activated protein kinase signaling mediated by oncogenes resulting in ligand-independent activation of AR. These alterations in AR signaling result in direct growth-promoting effects of androgens on PCa cells with a decreased dependence of these cells on stromal andromedins.[10,11]

ANDROGENS AND ANGIOGENESIS

Growing tumors must adapt to conditions of low oxygen and low nutrient availability. Tumor angiogenesis is the proliferation of a network of blood vessels that penetrates into cancerous growths, supplying nutrients and oxygen and removing waste products. Folkman[12] was the first to demonstrate that angiogenesis, the development of new blood vessels, is an essential step in tumor growth. Without angiogenesis, tumor growth at both primary and metastatic sites stops at a volume of 1 to 3 mm^3.

Several growth factors have been demonstrated to induce angiogenesis, but vascular endothelial growth factor (VEGF), originally noted for its permeability effects and also called vascular permeability factor, is unique among angiogenic molecules in that it specifically targets endothelial cells and promotes their proliferation and migration, 2 essential steps in angiogenesis.[13] Although endothelial cells are the specific target of VEGF, the molecule itself is expressed in a variety of cell types in the benign and malignant prostate. In a xenograft model of human PCa, LNCaP tumor cells that were co-inoculated with human prostate fetal fibroblasts subcutaneously into nude mice developed highly vascular tumors with high VEGF expression in stromal cells. Treatment of tumor-bearing animals with VEGF neutralizing antibodies resulted in significant tumor growth suppression.[14] Androgens were subsequently demonstrated to induce VEGF expression in human fetal prostate fibroblasts.[15] Androgens were also shown to stimulate angiogenesis and VEGF in PCa cells and the normal rat ventral prostate.[16,17] Furthermore, androgen withdrawal inhibited the hypoxic induction of VEGF in LNCaP xenografts.[18] Finally, prostate endothelial cells have been shown to express AR and to be androgen sensitive, suggesting a direct action of androgens on the prostatic vasculature.[19] Taken together, these reports demonstrate that androgens enhance PCa angiogenesis via direct effects on prostate endothelial cells and indirect effects on tumor vasculature via stimulation of stromal and epithelial cell VEGF expression.

ANDROGENIC EFFECTS ON TUMOR INVASION

Androgens have been demonstrated to promote PCa invasion via both direct effects on PCa cells and indirect effects on prostatic stroma. The stroma is a major component of the primary prostate environment affecting tumor dynamics.[20] Stromal-derived fibroblasts are involved in cancer progression in addition to structurally supporting epithelial cell growth.[21] In patients with PCa, there is a close association between low AR levels in the stroma adjacent to malignant epithelium with a poor clinical outcome.[22]

The hallmark characteristic of a reactive stroma that supports tumor proliferation is the presence of myofibroblasts, a cellular intermediate between a fibroblast and a smooth muscle cell.[23,24] PCa progression to a highly aggressive malignant state is closely linked to the myofibroblast component of the gland.[25] Crosstalk between androgens and transforming growth factor beta-1 (TGFβ1) signaling in prostate stromal cells affects AR localization, cell proliferation, and myodifferentiation.[20] There is a significant correlation between AR and TGFβ1 levels in the stromal component of prostatic intraepithelial neoplasia.[26] TGFβ1induces nuclear to cytoplasmic distribution of the androgen receptor and inhibits the androgen response in prostate smooth muscle cells.[27,28] In contrast, androgens enhance TGFβ1-mediated proliferation of prostate smooth muscle cells (PSMC1).[29] Moreover, AR signaling in prostate fibroblasts may promote prostate epithelial cell proliferation and mediate a functional exchange between prostate epithelial and stromal cells, thereby contributing to the epithelial to mesenchymal transition (EMT) effect.[30]

EPITHELIAL TO MESENCHYMAL TRANSITION

Cell motility is a critical determinant of PCa metastasis. The disruption of intercellular adhesion in tumors causes the cells to detach from the tumor cell mass. EMT is a conserved embryonic program where polarized immotile epithelial cells transition to motile mesenchymal cells.[31] Embryologically, EMT is mediated by the TGFβ and Wnt signaling systems,[32] both of which drive epithelial cell layers to lose polarity and cell-cell contacts, subsequently triggering remodeling of the cytoskeleton.[33] Specifically, molecules, such as Snail, Twist, Par6, and nuclear factor-κB (NF-κB), have been implicated in coordinating TGFβs participation in the EMT process In embryogenesis and PCa progression.[24] Smad-dependent induction of Snail, Slug, Twist and Smad-independent phosphorylation of Par6 contribute to the dissolution of cell junction complexes. NF-κB has been indirectly linked to tumor metastasis via its ability to regulate the expression of matrix metalloproteinases, interleukin-8, VEGF, and CXCR4.[34] The EMT transition is marked by the loss of epithelial cell markers, such as E-cadherin and β-catenin, and the gain of mesenchymal cell markers, such as N-cadherin and vimentin. The mesenchymal phenotype exhibits enhanced migration and survival in an anchorage-independent environment and ultimately promotes metastasis.[35,36] This process is supported by evidence that in high Gleason grade PCa, expression of syndecan-1, E-cadherin, and β-catenin is significantly decreased.[37] Furthermore, β-catenin is translocated into the nucleus, suggesting its role in gene regulation of MMPs and integrins.[37]

ANDROGENS AND EMT

Androgens suppress E-cadherin expression and induce mesenchymal marker expression in PCa cells.[30] Androgenic stimulation of critical polymerization protein expression in LNCaP cells suggests that they also affect actin polymerization to promote cell motility and migration, possibly facilitating interaction with adherent molecules in the extracellular matrix.[30] The interplay of androgens and TGFβ signaling has been investigated as a determining factor in the EMT process. In PC-3 and LNCaP cells, Smad3, a downstream mediator in the TGFβ pathway, enhances AR transactivation, whereas cotransfection of Smad3 and Smad4 repress AR transactivation.[38–40] Activation of β-catenin by androgen signaling can serve as an alternative mechanism of androgen-induced EMT.[30,41] Furthermore, Zhu and Kyprianou's[30] results suggest that androgens can independently induce EMT, potentially bypassing the effect of TGFβ.

Interestingly, experiments show that overexpression of AR in PCa cells suppresses the androgen-induced EMT phenotype,[30] whereas low AR content sensitizes PCa cells to androgen-induced EMT.[30] Because long-term ADT may downregulate AR expression, this form of therapy may actually facilitate DHT-induced EMT and promote cancer metastasis.[30]

ANDROGENS AND PROSTATE CANCER BONE TARGETING

Once cancer cells escape the prostate and enter the circulation, they must then arrest and adhere to the bone marrow to begin the process of bone metastases. Stromal cell-derived factor 1a (SDF1a or CXCL12) is expressed in bone marrow cells and has an affinity for the chemokine receptor CXCR4 that is expressed in PCa cells.[42,43] Interestingly, androgens have been shown to induce CXCR4 in PCa cells through ERG factor expression in PCa cells that express the TMPRSS2-ERG fusion protein. This finding is highly clinically relevant because TMPRSS2-ERG fusion transcripts (expression driven by androgens) have been shown to be present in a majority of patients with PCa because of chromosomal translocations or deletions involving the TMPRSS2 gene promoter and the ERG gene coding sequence.[44] This finding provides a link between expression of the fusion protein and androgen-driven PCa bone adherence and metastases.

ANDROGENS AND PROSTATE CANCER BONE SEEDING AND INITIAL OSTEOLYTIC LESIONS

PCa cell growth in bone is dependent upon the crosstalk between PCa and bone cells (osteoclasts and osteoblasts). The mineralized bone matrix, the largest storehouse for growth factors in the body, also plays a seminal role in the bone-metastatic process (**Fig. 1**). Bone metastases are classified as osteolytic when a decrease in bone density occurs via increased bone resorption or as osteoblastic when bone formation overcomes bone resorption.[45] Although PCa cells are somewhat unique among the solid tumors in that they often produce osteoblastic lesions in bone, accumulating evidence suggests that there is an initial and ongoing osteolytic phase that is *essential* for both bone targeting and continued PCa growth in bone. Osteoclastic bone resorption releases soluble growth factors from the bone matrix that further stimulate PCa growth in bone. By producing osteoclast-activating soluble factors, PCa cells co-opt these normal osteoclasts and induce them to initiate bone resorption with the subsequent release of stored growth factors from the matrix, thereby aiding both PCa entry into and growth in the bone microenvironment.[46–48]

A variety of osteoclast-activating cytokines and growth factors are secreted by PCa cells. More recently, it has been determined that the major regulation of osteoclast activity, both in normal bone and metastatic disease, is via a tumor necrosis factor ligand, receptor activator of nuclear factor-κB (RANKL), an essential osteoclast differentiation factor normally secreted by osteoblasts in the bone microenvironment.

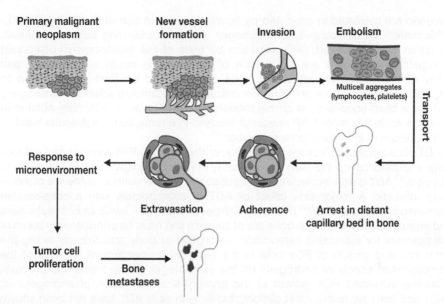

Fig. 1. Stages in PCa bone metastases. (*From* Vinik A. "Chapter 2: carcinoid tumors" (Endotext.org, Section: Carcinoid Bone metastasis - Osteolytic and Osteoblastic). Version of November 22, 2010; with permission.)

RANKL binding to RANK on osteoclasts induces their differentiation and bone resorbing activity. Conversely, osteoprotegerin (OPG) (also secreted by normal osteoblasts as well as tumor cells) acts as a decoy receptor to RANKL and halts osteoclastic activity.[49] Bone-metastatic PCa cells have been shown to express RANKL.[50] PCa cell secretion of RANKL is involved in EMT, migration, and osteomimicry.[51–53] LNCaP human PCa cells express RANKL and induce osteoclastogenesis, an effect that can be blocked with OPG.[46] As mentioned, PCa cells express growth factors and cytokines, notably PTHrP, TGF-β, and interleukin-1, and these factors have been demonstrated to increase RANKL secretion by osteoblasts in the bone microenvironment, thereby facilitating osteoclastic resorption and metastases.[54]

Although androgens have not been shown to directly stimulate RANKL secretion by PCa cells, AR signaling has been demonstrated to inhibit RANKL expression by osteoblasts.[55] AR has also been reported to bind to the transcription factor Runx2 and abrogate its recruitment to DNA.[56] Runx2, a mandatory transcription factor in the differentiation of osteoblasts, postnatal bone metabolism, and control of bone mass, promotes osteoblast-mediated osteoclastogenesis and bone resorption, partially via the stimulation of RANKL.[57] Runx2 is also expressed in PCa cells and may play a role in their tumorigenicity and metastatic potential.[56,58] In an intratibial metastasis model of PCa, high Runx2 levels were associated with large tumors, increased expression of metastasis-related genes, and the promotion of osteolytic activity.[58] Therefore, androgens and AR may indirectly regulate PCa effects on osteolysis via effects on Runx2 activity.

ANDROGENS, ESTROGENS, AND AR: EFFECTS ON BONE CELLS

Sex steroids have profound effects on bone cells. Estrogen withdrawal results in an increased osteoclast number and accelerated bone resorption.[59] These effects of estrogen are mediated in large part by estrogenic modulation of the RANK/RANKL/ OPG system by osteoblasts, with estrogen withdrawal favoring increased RANKL secretion and decreased OPG secretion by cells of the mesenchymal-osteoblast lineage.[60,61] Androgens are the source of estrogens in males and females, and many of the androgenic effects on bone are mediated via their aromatization to estrogen. However, there are also aromatization-independent effects of androgens that have been uncovered in animal models where AR was conditionally ablated in osteoblasts. In this model, AR knockout resulted in a reduction in trabecular number and evidence of increased bone resorption.[62]

ADT via surgical orchiectomy, estrogens, or the use of GnRH agonists and antago-nists ± antiandrogens, has been the mainstay of therapy for advanced PCa for almost 70 years.[63] ADT is now increasingly being used to treat men without evidence of meta-static disease. A major side effect of ADT is osteoporosis with a considerable increased risk of fractures.[64] Because ADT generally lowers levels of both estrogens and androgens, the effects on bone are of concern and must be considered in terms of the potential for increasing osteoclastic resorption of bone and thereby aiding the entry into and growth of PCa cells in the bone microenvironment. In spite of the demonstrated effects of androgens on the early stages of the metastatic process, including increased PCa growth at the primary site, promotion of angiogenesis, EMT, and bone targeting, most clinical studies with early ADT have not been shown to prevent PCa bone metastases or result in a survival advantage, with the exception of high-risk, advanced (T3) localized disease in men receiving external beam radiation therapy.[65] It is possible that the beneficial effects of ADT on PCa progression and bone targeting (decreased PCa growth, angiogenesis, motility, and EMT) are counter-balanced by the direct effect of ADT on the activation of bone resorption, accounting for the disappointing results so far in clinical studies using ADT in the prevention of PCa progression, bone metastases, and survival.

ANDROGENIC EFFECTS ON ESTABLISHED PCa BONE METASTASES

Androgen deprivation is the mainstay of treatment for established PCa bone-metastatic disease and appears to be effective via multiple mechanisms, including induction of apoptosis of AR-expressing PCa cells in bone, inhibition of angiogenesis, and possibly suppression of the osteoblastic reaction often seen in this disorder. These metastases eventually become resistant to ADT, although castration-resistant cells often still express functional AR and may respond to further lowering of intratumoral androgens or more potent androgen receptor blockers.[11,66]

Although the initial bone lesions are often osteolytic, the later stages of PCa growth in bone are characterized by crosstalk between PCa cells, osteoclasts, and osteoblasts.[48] The Wnt signaling pathway plays a central role in osteoblast develop-ment and formation.[67] Wnts promote the lineage commitment of mesenchymal precursor cells and the differentiation of progenitor cell lines into osteoblasts.[67,68] In addition, they stimulate osteoblast maturation and exert direct effects on the formation and turnover of the mature skeleton. Wnts also directly stimulate tumor cell growth and survival via autocrine regulation in several types of human cancer, including PCa.[69]

There is significant crosstalk between the Wnt/β-catenin and AR signaling path-ways. Functional colocalization of AR, β-catenin, and T cell factor (Tcf) in the nucleus has been reported.[70,71] It has also been shown that β-catenin preferentially binds AR over several other steroid hormone receptors.[70] Androgens induce Wnt signaling and differentiation of preosteoblast cells as evidenced by increased nuclear expression of

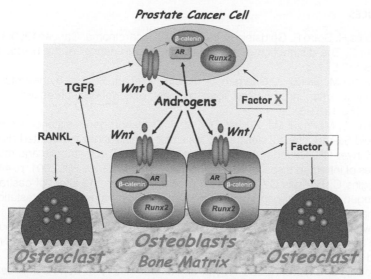

Fig. 2. Androgens/AR interactions with TGF-β and Wnt signaling systems in PCa and bone cells. Androgens modulate Runx2 activity in PCa cells and may thereby promote EMT and PCa metastatic potential. In PCa cells, AR also interacts with β-catenin, an important component of the canonical Wnt signaling system. Androgens stimulate Wnt signaling in osteoblasts leading to increases in Runx2 expression, osteoblast differentiation, and enhanced secretion of both known (RANKL) and, possibly, unknown growth factors that promote osteoclast differentiation. These mature osteoclasts initiate bone resorption with the release of growth factors from the bone matrix, most notably TGF-β, which, in collaboration with androgens/AR, can stimulate further PCa growth and EMT. Thus, the androgenic signaling pathway profoundly influences the vicious cycle of bone metastases at multiple steps in the process.

β-catenin and increased expression of the Runx2 nuclear transcription factor. Further, androgen-induced Wnt signaling in preosteoblasts promoted the growth of MDA-PCa-2b human PCa cells via induction of soluble growth factors from the osteoblast lineage cells.[72] This data provides yet another mechanism whereby androgens/AR, working cooperatively with the Wnt/β-catenin/Runx2 signaling pathway in osteoblasts can further stimulate PCa growth in bone. **Fig. 2** depicts some of the complex, interrelated pathways stimulated by androgens/AR in PCa and bone cells that may contribute to PCa EMT, bone targeting, growth in bone, and the osteoblastic bone reaction commonly seen in PCa bone metastases.

SUMMARY

A complex interplay of factors secreted by PCa cells, local stroma, endothelial cells, and bone cells contribute to the bone metastatic phenotype, morbidity, and mortality associated with the disease. Androgens influence many of these interactions, either directly via AR signaling or indirectly by aromatization to estrogens. The majority of preclinical data indicates a stimulatory effect of androgens on the various stages of the bone-metastatic process. However, ADT also increases osteoclastogenesis and may thereby promote PCa seeding to and growth in bone. Combination therapy with early ADT and antiresorptive agents to prevent the deleterious effects of ADT on bone may prevent PCa bone metastases and improve overall survival.

REFERENCES

1. Abrams H, Spiro R, Goldstein N. Metastases in carcinoma. Cancer 1950;3:74–85.
2. Paget S. The distribution of secondary growths in cancer of the breast. Lancet 1889;133:571–3.
3. Imperato-McGinley J, Guerrero L, Guatier T, et al. Steroid 5α-reductase deficiency in man: an inherited form of male pseudohermaphroditism. Science 1974;186:1213–5.
4. Griffin JE, McPhaul MJ, Russell DW, et al. The androgen resistance syndromes: steroid 5α-reductase 2 deficiency, testicular feminization, and related disorders. In: Scriver CR, Beaudet AL, Sly WS, et al, editors. The metabolic and molecular bases of inherited disease. 8th edition. New York: McGraw-Hill; 2001. p. 4117–46.
5. Huggins C, Hodges CV. Studies on prostatic cancer: the effect of castration, of estrogen and androgen injection on serum phosphatases in metastatic carcinoma of the prostate. Cancer Res 1941;1:293–7.
6. Crawford ED, Eisenberger MA, McLeod DG, et al. A controlled trial of leuprolide with and without flutamide in prostatic carcinoma [Erratum appears in N Engl J Med 1989;321(20):1420]. N Engl J Med 1989;321(7):419–24.
7. Krupski TL, Smith MR, Lee WC, et al. Natural history of bone complications in men with prostate carcinoma initiating androgen deprivation therapy. Cancer 2004;101(3):541–9.
8. Talmadge JE, Fidler IJ. AACR centennial series: the biology of cancer metastasis: historical perspective. Cancer Res 2010;70(14):5649–69.
9. Fidler IJ. Metastasis: quantitative analysis of distribution and fate of tumor emboli labeled with 125I-5-iodo-2'-deoxyuridine. J Natl Cancer Inst 1970;45:773–82.
10. Isaacs JT, Isaacs WB. Androgen receptor outwits prostate cancer drugs. Nat Med 2004;10(1):26–7.
11. Chen CD, Welsbie DS, Tran C, et al. Molecular determinants of resistance to antiandrogen therapy. Nat Med 2004;10(1):33–9.
12. Folkman J. What is the evidence that tumors are angiogenesis dependent? J Natl Cancer Inst 1990;82:4–7.
13. Ferrara N, Houck K, Jakeman L, et al. Molecular and biological properties of the vascular endothelial growth factor family of proteins. Endocr Rev 1992;13:18–32.
14. Kirschenbaum A, Wang JP, Ren M, et al. Inhibition of vascular endothelial cell growth factor suppresses the in vivo growth of human prostate tumors. Urol Oncol 1997;3:3–10.
15. Levine AC, Liu X-H, Greenberg PD, et al. Androgens induce the expression of vascular endothelial growth factor in human fetal prostatic fibroblasts. Endocrinology 1998;139(11):4672–7.
16. Joseph IB, Nelson JB, Denmeade SR, et al. Androgens regulate vascular endothelial growth factor content in normal and malignant prostate tissue. Clin Cancer Res 1997;3:2507–11.
17. Franck-Lissbrandt I, Haggstrom S, Damber JE, et al. Testosterone stimulates angiogenesis and vascular regrowth in the ventral prostate in castrated adult rats. Endocrinology 1998;139:451–6.
18. Shibata Y, Kasiwagi B, Arai S, et al. Direct regulation of prostate blood flow by vascular endothelial growth factor and its participation in the androgenic regulation of prostate blood flow in vivo. Endocrinology 2004;145:4507–12.
19. Godoy A, Watts A, Sotomayor P, et al. Androgen receptor is causally involved in the homeostasis of the human prostate endothelial cell. Endocrinology 2008;149:2959–69.

20. Zhu ML, Kyprianou N. Androgen receptor and growth factor signaling cross-talk in prostate cancer cells. Endocr Relat Cancer 2008;15(4):841–9.
21. Wang X, Yin L, Rao P, et al. Targeted treatment of prostate cancer. J Cell Biochem 2007;102:571–9.
22. Henshall SM, Quinn DI, Lee CS, et al. Altered expression of androgen receptor in the malignant epithelium and adjacent stroma is associated with early relapse in prostate cancer. Cancer Res 2001;61(2):423–7.
23. Gabbiani G, Hirschel BJ, Ryan GB, et al. Granulation tissue as a contractile organ. A study of structure and function. J Exp Med 1972;135:719–34.
24. Rennebeck G, Martelli M, Kyprianou N. Anoikis and survival connections in the tumor microenvironment: is there a role in prostate cancer metastasis? Cancer Res 2005;65(24):11230–5.
25. Tuxhorn JA, McAlhany SJ, Dang TD, et al. Stromal cells promote angiogenesis and growth of human prostate tumors in a differential reactive stroma (DRS) xeno-graft model. Cancer Res 2002;62:3298–307.
26. Cardillo MR, Petrangeli E, Perracchio L, et al. Transforming growth factor-beta expression in prostate neoplasia. Anal Quant Cytol Histol 2000;22:1–10.
27. Gerdes MJ, Dang TD, Larsen M, et al. Transforming growth factor-beta1 induces nuclear to cytoplasmic distribution of androgen receptor and inhibits androgen response in prostate smooth muscle cells. Endocrinology 1998;139: 3569–77.
28. Gerdes MJ, Larsen M, Dang TD, et al. Regulation of rat prostate stromal cell my-odifferentiation by androgen and TGF-beta1. Prostate 2004;58:299–307.
29. Salm SN, Koikawa Y, Ogilvie V, et al. Generation of active TGF-beta by prostatic cell cocultures using novel basal and luminal prostatic epithelial cell lines. J Cell Physiol 2000;184:70–9.
30. Zhu ML, Kyprianou N. Role of androgens and the androgen receptor in epithelial-mesenchymal transition and invasion of prostate cancer cells. FASEB J 2010; 24(3):769–77.
31. Josson S, Matsuoka Y, Chung LW, et al. Tumor-stroma co-evolution in prostate cancer progression and metastasis. Semin Cell Dev Biol 2010;21(1):26–32.
32. Yang J, Weinberg RA. Epithelial-mesenchymal transition: at the crossroads of development and tumor metastasis. Dev Cell 2008;14(6):818–29.
33. Liu YN, Liu Y, Lee HJ, et al. Activated androgen receptor downregulates E-cad-herin gene expression and promotes tumor metastasis. Mol Cell Biol 2008;28(23): 7096–108.
34. Massague J. TGF-β in cancer. Cell 2008;134:215–30.
35. Thiery JP. Epithelial-mesenchymal transitions in tumour progression. Nat Rev Cancer 2002;2:442–54.
36. Huber MA, Kraut N, Beug H. Molecular requirements for epithelial-mesenchymal transition during tumor progression. Curr Opin Cell Biol 2005;17:548–58.
37. Contreras HR, Ledezma RA, Vergara J, et al. The expression of syndecan-1 and -2 is associated with Gleason score and epithelial-mesenchymal transition markers, E-cadherin and β-catenin, in prostate cancer. Urol Oncol 2010;28(5): 534–40.
38. Bruckheimer EM, Kyprianou N. Dihydrotestosterone enhances transforming growth factor-β-induced apoptosis in hormone-sensitive prostate cancer cells. Endocrinology 2001;142:2419–26.
39. Kang HY, Huang KE, Chang SY, et al. Differential modulation of androgen receptor-mediated transactivation by Smad3 and tumor suppressor Smad4. J Biol Chem 2002;277:43749–56.

40. Kang HY, Lin HK, Hu YC, et al. From transforming growth factor-beta signaling to androgen action: identification of Smad3 as an androgen receptor coregulator in prostate cancer cells. Proc Natl Acad Sci U S A 2001;98:3018–23.

41. Derynck R, Akhurst RJ. Differentiation plasticity regulated by TGF-β family proteins in development and disease. Nat Cell Biol 2007;9:1000–4.

42. Wang J, Loberg R, Taichman RS. The pivotal role of CXCL12(SDF-1)CXCR4 axis in bone metastasis. Cancer Metastasis Rev 2006;25:573–87.

43. Taichman RS, Cooper C, Keller ET, et al. Use of the stromal cell-derived factor-1/CXCR4 pathway in prostate cancer metastases to one. Cancer Res 2002;62:1832–7.

44. Cai J, Kandagatia P, Singareddy R, et al. Androgens induce functional CSCR4 through ERG factor expression in RMPRSS2-ERG fusion-positive prostate cancer cells. Transl Oncol 2010;3(3):195–203.

45. Kakonen SM, Mundy GR. Mechanisms of osteolytic bone metastases in breast carcinoma. Cancer 2003;97:834–9.

46. Zhang J, Dai J, Qi Y, et al. Osteoprotegerin inhibits prostate cancer-induced osteoclastogenesis and prevents prostate tumor growth in the bone. J Clin Invest 2001;107:1235–44.

47. Jacobs SC. Spread of prostatic carcinoma to bone. Urology 1983;21:337–44.

48. Guise TA, Mohammed KS, Clines G, et al. Basic mechanisms responsible for osteolytic and osteoblastic bone metastases. Clin Cancer Res 2006;12(Suppl 20): 6213s–6s.

49. Mundy GR. Metastasis to bone: causes, consequences and therapeutic opportunities. Nat Rev Cancer 2002;2(8):584–93.

50. Chen G, Sircar K, Aprikian A, et al. Expression of RANKL/RANK/OPG in primary and metastatic human prostate cancer as markers of disease stage and functional regulation. Cancer 2006;107:289–98.

51. Odero-Marah VA, Wang R, Chu G, et al. Receptor activator of NF-κ B ligand (RANKL) expression is associated with epithelial to mesenchymal transition in human prostate cancer cells. Cell Res 2008;18:858–70.

52. Sabbota AL, Kim HR, Zhe X, et al. Shedding of RANKL by tumor-associated MT1-MMP activates Src-dependent prostate cancer cell migration. Cancer Res 2010; 70(13):5558–66.

53. Graham TR, Agrawal KC, Mageed-Abdel AB. Independent and cooperative roles of tumor necrosis factor-α, nuclear factor-κB, and bone morphogenetic protein-2 in regulation of metastasis and osteomimicry of prostate cancer cells and differentiation and mineralization of MC3T3-E1 osteoblast-like cells. Cancer Sci 2010; 101(1):103–11.

54. Angelucci A, Garofalo S, Speca S, et al. Arachidonic acid modulates the crosstalk between prostate carcinoma and bone stromal cells. Endocr Relat Cancer 2008;15:91–100.

55. Kawano H, Sato T, Yamada T, et al. Suppressive function of androgen receptor in bone resorption. Proc Natl Acad Sci U S A 2003;100:9416–21.

56. Baniwal SK, Khalid O, Sor D, et al. Repression of Runx2 by androgen receptor (AR) in osteoblasts and prostate cancer cells: AR binds Runx2 and abrogates its recruitment to DNA. Mol Endocrinol 2009;23:1203–14.

57. Geoffroy V, Kneissel M, Fournier B, et al. High bone resorption in adult aging transgenic mice overexpressing cbfa/runx2 in cells of the osteoblastic lineage. Mol Cell Biol 2002;22:6222–3.

58. Akech J, Wixted JJ, Bedard K, et al. Runx2 association with progression of prostate cancer in patients: mechanisms mediating bone osteolysis and osteoblastic bone metastatic lesions. Oncogene 2010;29:811–21.

59. Riggs BL, Khosla S, Melton LJ 3rd. Sex steroids and the construction and conservation of the adult skeleton. Endocr Rev 2002;23:279–302.

60. Frenkel B, Hong A, Baniwal SK, et al. Regulation of adult bone turnover by sex steroids. J Cell Physiol 2010;224:305–10.

61. Hofbauer LC, Gori F, Riggs BL, et al. Stimulation of osteoprotegerin ligand and inhibition of osteoprotegerin production by glucocorticoids in human osteoblastic lineage cells: potential paracrine mechanisms of glucocorticoid-induced osteoporosis. Endocrinology 1999;140:4382–9.

62. Notini AJ, McManus JF, Moore A, et al. Osteoblast deletion of exon 3 of the androgen receptor gene results in trabecular bone loss in adult male mice. J Bone Miner Res 2007;22:347–56.

63. Huggins C, Hodges CV. Studies on prostatic cancer II: the effects of castration on advanced carcinoma of the prostate gland. Arch Surg 1941;43:209–23.

64. Smith MR, Lee WC, Brandman J, et al. Gonadotropin-releasing hormone agonists and fracture risk: a claims-based cohort study of men with nonmetastatic prostate cancer. J Clin Oncol 2005;23:7897–903.

65. Widmark A, Klepp O, Solberg A, et al. Endocrine treatment, with or without radiotherapy, in locally advanced prostate cancer (SPCG-7/SFUO-3): an open randomized phase III trial. Lancet 2009;373(9660):301–8.

66. Montgomery RB, Mostaghel EA, Vessella R, et al. Maintenance of intratumoral androgens in metastatic prostate cancer: a mechanism for castration-resistant tumor growth. Cancer Res 2008;68(11):4447–54.

67. Westendorf J, Kahler RA, Schroeder TM. Wnt signaling in osteoblasts and bone diseases. Gene 2004;341:19–39.

68. Gregory CA, Gunn WG, Reyes E, et al. How Wnt signaling affects bone repair by mesenchymal stem cells from the bone marrow. Ann N Y Acad Sci 2005;1049: 97–106.

69. Verras M, Brown J, Li X, et al. Wnt3a growth factor induces androgen receptor-mediated transcription and enhances cell growth in human prostate cancer cells. Cancer Res 2004;64:8860–6.

70. Yang F, Li X, Sharma M, et al. Linking β-catenin to androgen-signaling pathway. J Biol Chem 2002;277:11336–44.

71. Pawlowski JE, Ertel JR, Allen MP, et al. Liganded androgen receptor interaction with β-catenin nuclear co-localization and modulation of transcriptional activity in neuronal cells. J Biol Chem 2002;277:20702–10.

72. Liu XH, Kirschenbaum A, Yao S, et al. Androgen-induced Wnt signaling in preosteoblasts promotes the growth of MDA-PCa-2b human prostate cancer cells. Cancer Res 2007;67(12):5747–53.

Management of Side Effects of Androgen Deprivation Therapy

Mathis Grossmann, MD, PhD, FRACP[a,b],
Jeffrey D. Zajac, MBBS, PhD, FRACP[a,b],*

KEYWORDS

- Androgen deprivation • Prostate cancer • Osteoporosis
- Insulin resistance • Testosterone

Prostate cancer is the most common solid-organ cancer in men, with a lifetime risk of 1 in 9.[1] The contemporary 5-year relative survival rate for men with all stages of prostate cancer combined is estimated to be 98.8%.[2] Because of such high rates in cancer-specific survival, the consideration of treatment-related toxicity assumes major significance. More than 30% of men with prostate cancer die of cardiovascular disease, which constitutes the most common cause of mortality in this patient population.[3,4] Androgen deprivation therapy (ADT) for the treatment of prostate cancer is being used increasingly. Because larger numbers of men are being treated with this therapy, it is becoming clear that substantial side effects can occur with this treatment (**Box 1**). These side effects range from osteoporosis leading to fractures, changes in glucose metabolism leading to an increase in diabetes, and increases in cardiovascular risk factors. Other side effects relate to lifestyle factors, mood, and sexual function. Anemia and a decrease in muscle mass can worsen the general sense of well-being in these patients and increase their risk of falls and consequent fractures. This article reviews the current side effects of ADT and suggests evidence-based approaches to reducing them.

ADT

ADT has long been a mainstay for the treatment of metastatic prostate cancer. It is being used more widely for localized disease and biochemical recurrence. This

Disclosures: The authors have nothing to disclose.
This work was supported by a National Health and Medical Research Council Health Professional Fellowship given to M.G.
[a] Department of Medicine Austin Health/Northern Health, University of Melbourne, Studley Road, Heidelberg, Victoria 3084, Australia
[b] Department of Endocrinology, Austin Health, Studley Road, Heidelberg, Victoria 3084, Australia
* Corresponding author. Department of Medicine, Austin Hospital, Studley Road, Heidelberg, Victoria 3084, Australia.
E-mail address: j.zajac@unimelb.edu.au

Endocrinol Metab Clin N Am 40 (2011) 655–671
doi:10.1016/j.ecl.2011.05.004
0889-8529/11/$ – see front matter © 2011 Published by Elsevier Inc.

| Box 1 |
| Adverse effects associated with ADT |

- Sexual dysfunction
- Hot flushes
- Fatigue
- Anemia
- Neurophysiologic effects (reduced mood, cognition)
- Sarcopenia
- Increased fat mass
- Increased insulin resistance and incident diabetes
- Increase in cardiovascular risk factors
- Osteoporosis and fractures

therapy comes with substantial metabolic and other side effects that need to be balanced against its beneficial effects. This therapy involves depot preparations of gonadotropin-releasing hormone (GnRH) agonists.[5] Compounds approved in the United States include leuprolide, goserelin, and triptorelin. Long-term treatment with GnRH agonists, by overriding the stimulatory effects of physiologically pulsatile endogenous GnRH, downregulates the GnRH receptors in the anterior pituitary gland and leads to castrate levels of testosterone within 3 weeks.[6] ADT, which intentionally reduces serum testosterone levels to castrate range (<5% of the normal value) and serum estrogen levels to less than 20%,[7] can now be considered the most common cause of severe male hypogonadism.

In addition to its palliative role in metastatic disease, ADT has also been shown to improve survival in men with locally advanced or high-risk localized disease who receive radiation therapy or in men with lymph node–positive disease who are treated with radical prostatectomy.[5] Although there has been debate about the duration of ADT, a recent study has shown that, in combination with radiotherapy, 3 years of ADT significantly improves survival in patients with locally advanced prostate cancer compared with 6 months.[8] The use of ADT in North American men with nonmetastatic prostate cancer has increased from 3.7% in 1991 to 31% in 1999 with 600,000 men, with one-third of the estimated 2 million prostate cancer survivors in the US receiving this therapy.[9] There are similar trends in other parts of the world, including Australia, where the use of ADT from 2003 to 2009 has increased by more than 40%.[10] ADT is increasingly being used in situations in which a survival benefit has not been demonstrated. These situations include primary therapy for early-stage (localized) prostate cancer, neoadjuvant therapy for low-risk disease, or biochemical prostate-specific antigen (PSA) recurrence (defined as rising PSA levels in the absence of other signs of disease) after surgery or radiotherapy.[5,6] Because such men have a relatively good prognosis and low cancer-specific mortality, the benefits of ADT in these patients need to be carefully balanced against the toxicity. Observational data and post hoc analyses from randomized trials suggest that men with low- or intermediate-risk prostate cancer treated with ADT may have worse survival compared with those who do not receive this treatment.[11,12] Thus, the current National Comprehensive Cancer Network guidelines recommend ADT only for situations in which a survival benefit has clearly been documented.[13]

ADVERSE EFFECTS

The adverse effects of ADT include fatigue, sexual dysfunction, hot flushes, and anemia.[14] Other recognized consequences include osteoporosis leading to fractures, weight gain, insulin resistance, and diabetes.[6] Skeletal and metabolic complications are of particular concern because of their effect on morbidity and mortality in a population that already has a high background prevalence of these conditions (**Fig. 1**). One in 5 men older than 50 years suffer an osteoporotic fracture during their lifetime,[15] and recent data from the National Health and Nutritional Examination Survey have shown that one-third of men in the United States who are 65 years or older have diabetes.[16]

In the Endocrine Men's Health Clinic, Austin Health, Melbourne, Australia, all men with nonmetastatic prostate cancer started on ADT are routinely reviewed. A survey of the first 100 men referred with nonmetastatic prostate cancer, with a mean age of 69 years (range, 48–92 years), showed that 85% were overweight or obese, 51% had hypertension, 50% were current smokers, 25% had previous cardiovascular events, 21% had known diabetes, and 25% had osteoporosis, defined as T score of hip or spine of −2.5 or less (Grossmann and colleagues, unpublished data, 2010). These observations indicate a high baseline risk of cardiovascular and skeletal events in such men even before ADT is commenced. The authors expect that the data is similar for men in the United States.

A diagnosis of prostate cancer does not alter life expectancy for most men, and the 10-year survival approaches 90% even for those who present with metastatic disease.[17] Given the diverse nature of ADT-associated side effects, management of patients with prostate cancer receiving ADT should consist of an individualized multidisciplinary approach. This approach should include, as appropriate, experts in urology, radiation and medical oncology, endocrinology, geriatric medicine, dietetics, exercise physiotherapy, sex therapy, and psychology. Before the commencement of ADT, all patients should be counseled about ADT-associated side effects, including its association with adverse bone and metabolic health. Adverse effects should be considered in the decision-making process of commencing ADT for prostate cancer, especially in patients with high baseline risk for fractures or cardiovascular events and

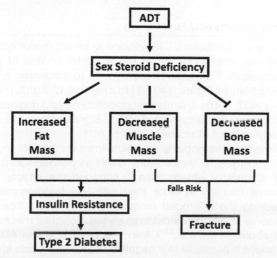

Fig. 1. Adverse effects of ADT.

with low-risk prostate cancer for which the survival benefit of ADT has not been established.

Health-Related Quality of Life, Mood, and Cognition

There has been only one long-term prospective study to assess heath-related quality of life after diagnosis of localized prostate cancer. In this questionnaire-based population-based study, men younger than 70 years were followed up for 3 years after the diagnosis of prostate cancer. Men receiving ADT had poorer adjusted physical and mental health scores than those undergoing radical prostatectomy, external beam radiotherapy, or active surveillance.[18] Poorer quality-of-life scores in men receiving ADT have also been reported in short-term cohort studies, for example, from the Cancer of the Prostate Strategic Urologic Research Endeavor database.[19] These studies are not randomized and may suffer from selection bias and unmeasured confounders. The clinical significance of such differences, therefore, remains unclear. The effect of ADT on mood and cognition is controversial. Observational studies, generally small and with short-term follow-up, reported that 47% to 69% of men receiving ADT had a decline in at least 1 cognitive area, most commonly visuospatial abilities and executive functioning.[20] One study did not suggest any decline in cognition with ADT but rather found an improvement in object recall.[21] A population-based study from the Surveillance, Epidemiology and End Results (SEER)-Medicare database suggested that advanced age, disease stage, and coexisting illness may account for a significant proportion of cognitive and emotional changes. In this study of 50,613 men with prostate cancer, 31% of the men receiving ADT developed at least 1 depressive, cognitive, or constitutional diagnosis compared with 24% of the men who did not. However, after correction for age, disease stage, and comorbidities, these differences were largely eliminated.[22] Given that this study only examined claims-based diagnoses, it is likely that mild to moderate neuropsychological disorders were underreported. Overall, it is important to recognize that men with prostate cancer are generally a high-risk group for emotional and cognitive disturbances. Although there has been little study on the effects of intervention on depression and cognitive decline specific to men with prostate cancer receiving ADT, physicians should be vigilant for early signs of such conditions and manage and refer patients as appropriate.

Fatigue, Sarcopenia, and Physical Functioning

Fatigue is common and multifactorial. In addition to neurophysiologic factors, sarcopenia and anemia may contribute, given the anabolic actions of testosterone on muscle and erythropoiesis.[23] Anemia is usually mild to moderate, with mean hemoglobin level declining from 14.9 g/dL [149 g/L] to a nadir of 12.3 g/dL [123 g/L] 6 months after the initiation of ADT.[24] The anemia is normochromic and normocytic and usually resolves over the months after cessation of ADT.[24] Significant anemia should be investigated appropriately and not attributed solely to ADT.

Loss of muscle mass, or sarcopenia, is a significant contributor to falls, frailty, and loss of functional mobility. Low testosterone level has been associated with frailty in population-based studies of elderly men,[25] although the effects of testosterone therapy on functional mobility in older men with low testosterone levels are not certain.[26] Mice lacking the androgen receptor also have significant reductions in muscle mass and serve as a good model to study the molecular mechanisms by which testosterone is anabolic to muscle.[27] Given that men receiving ADT have castrate levels of testosterone, it is plausible that negative effects on muscle strength and functioning are more pronounced than that of ageing men with borderline testosterone levels, although this has not been formally demonstrated. A recent meta-analysis of mostly short-term (<6 months) studies showed that in men receiving ADT, lean body mass decreased by 2.8%, with more extensive changes seen with a longer duration of treatment.[28] The increased fat mass of 7.7% observed may further contribute to or alternatively be a consequence of decreased mobility. Activity levels, however, were not consistently assessed in these studies.[28] In a cross-sectional study, men receiving ADT had reduced limb strength and physical function compared with men who had prostate cancer and were not given ADT.[29] Several trials have shown that exercise programs may reduce the adverse effects of ADT on fatigue and muscle loss. In a 12-week trial, 57 men with prostate cancer commencing ADT were randomized to a resistance and aerobic exercise program or usual care. The men undergoing the exercise program showed significant increases in lean body mass, better muscle strength, and better 6-meter walk time test results and were less fatigued compared with controls.[30] Similarly, in a 12-week resistance exercise intervention in men commencing ADT, 155 men showed significant improvement in, compared with controls, self-reported fatigue, quality of life, and muscular fitness.[31] Thus, given the safety of an appropriately tailored exercise regimen and the additional possible benefits on insulin resistance, bone density, falls reduction, and mood, all patients should be repeatedly counseled regarding regular exercise. Whether formal review by a physical therapist and/or the administration of a specifically designed exercise program is cost effective is unknown.

Sexual Dysfunction

Sexual dysfunction develops in most men who were potent before the initiation of ADT, usually within months of initiation. In the Prostate Cancer Outcomes Study of the SEER program, the proportion of men reporting no sexual interest increased from 31% to 58% after GnRH agonist treatment, and the proportion of men who achieved no erections increased from 38% to 74%. Less than 20% of the men maintained any sexual activity during ADT.[32] Thus, sexual dysfunction should be expected, and men and their partners should be counseled before the commencement of ADT. In many instances, sexual dysfunction may not be of primary concern, especially in older men. Although controlled data regarding the efficacy of phosphodiesterase type 5 inhibitors is lacking, there is evidence that tissue androgenization is required for optimal response to such agents. Indeed, the commencement of ADT may worsen response to phosphodiesterase type 5 inhibitors.[33] Other options that have even been less well studied include intracavernosal therapy, vacuum devices, and penile implants.

Vasomotor Symptoms

Hot flushes are experienced by 50% to 80% of patients receiving ADT. Up to 27% of the men report hot flushes as being the most troublesome side effect of ADT,[6] and more than 50% of the men with hot flushes report that flushes have a significant adverse effect on their quality of life.[34] Hot flushes commence within weeks of ADT initiation and may persist long term. Common sense recommendations, not tested in prospective trials, are to reduce hot flushes by reducing ambient temperature, sleeping in cool bedrooms, and drinking cold water when the flush starts. Although most hot flushes occur spontaneously, triggers, which may include overheating, spicy food, alcohol, and smoking, should be avoided. The only controlled trial that directly compared different drug options enrolled 919 men at commencement of ADT.[34] A total of 311 men requested treatment and were randomized to medroxyprogesterone acetate (20 mg daily), cyproterone acetate (100 mg daily), or venlafaxine (75 mg daily), with no placebo control. At 4 weeks, the hot flush score decreased by 84% in the medroxyprogesterone group, by 95% in the cyproterone group, and by 47% in the venlafaxine group. Both hormonal treatments were significantly better compared with venlafaxine, but there was no difference between medroxyprogesterone and cyproterone.[34] There were no serious drug-related side effects in this 12-week study. A randomized controlled trial of megestrol acetate (20 mg twice daily) led to a significantly greater reduction in hot flushes than placebo (85% vs 21%).[35] However, PSA levels have been reported to increase with the commencement of megestrol and to decline with its discontinuation, and this drug can, therefore, not be recommended.[34] Antidepressants have not been tested in placebo-controlled trials, and their effectiveness is partly inferred by controlled trials in menopausal women. In a before-after study in men receiving ADT, venlafaxine reduced hot flushes by more than 50% in 10 of 16 men,[36] with similar results for paroxetine.[37] If hot flushes remain bothersome despite simple measures, the authors usually commence low-dose venlafaxine or a selective serotonin reuptake inhibitor and gradually uptitrate as required and tolerated. Given the less favorable side effect profile, the authors use the significantly more effective hormonal therapies with considerable caution and reserve them for truly refractory cases, which in their experience are uncommon.

Gynecomastia and Other Adverse Effects on Body Image

Gynecomastia is caused by a change in the estrogen to testosterone ratio and may cause discomfort and psychologically distressing disturbances in body image. This condition occurs in up to 80% of men receiving antiandrogen monotherapy and is less common (1%–16%) with GnRH agonists.[6] Tamoxifen appears to be more effective than the aromatase inhibitor anastrozole in men receiving antiandrogen monotherapy. In a trial of 88 men with prostate cancer, gynecomastia developed in 73%, 51%, and 10% of men receiving bicalutamide alone, bicalutamide with anastrozole, and bicalutamide with tamoxifen, respectively.[38] Options for treating established gynecomastia include radiotherapy, which may be more effective in reducing pain compared with reduction in breast tissue volume and surgery.[6] Other potentially distressing effects of ADT include decreases in testicular size and penile size, as well as body hair loss.[6] Men should be informed about these changes before the commencement of ADT.

Osteoporosis and Fractures

Fractures are a significant cause of morbidity in men. Lifetime fracture risk for men in the general population aged 50 years or more is 20%, and 30% of all hip fractures occur in men.[15] Mortality after fracture is higher in men compared with women, with age-standardized mortality ratios of 2.2 to 3.2 compared with 1.7 to 2.2 in women.[39] The 3 most common causes of secondary osteoporosis in men are hypogonadism, corticosteroid exposure, and excessive alcohol use.[15] ADT for prostate cancer results in severe sex steroid deficiency. Reduced bone mineral density (BMD) and osteoporosis have been well described in men who are on this therapy.[14,40–42] BMD begins to decline within months after the initiation of ADT[43] in men with prostate cancer, reflecting the rapid decrease in sex steroid levels, which reach a nadir within 2 to 4 weeks. Rates of bone loss reported in prospective studies range between 2% and 8% per year at the lumbar spine and between 1.8% and 6.5% per year at the femoral neck.[14,40–42,44] Although these studies were generally small and lacked adequate controls, the rate of bone loss in patients undergoing ADT seems much more rapid than that in the general population. In community-dwelling aging men, BMD is typically only 0.5% to 1.0% per year, and, in early female menopause, BMD is around 2% per year.[42] Two prospective studies have compared short-term (<12 months) with longer-term ADT. Both studies showed that BMD loss was maximal within the first year of ADT.[43,45] In one study of 152 men, bone loss increased 5- to 10-fold during the first 12 months of ADT use compared with men with prostate cancer who did not receive ADT.[43] Men in the highest tertile of bone turnover markers at 6 months experienced the greatest BMD loss at 12 months.[43] Cross-sectional studies suggest that BMD continues to decline even with long-term ADT, albeit at a lower rate.[41,42] In an observational study of 390 men on continuous ADT, the prevalence of osteoporosis was 43% after 2 years of ADT and 81% after 10 or more years, compared with a prevalence of 35% in hormone-naive patients.[46] A recent prospective study using high-resolution, peripheral, quantitative computed tomography has shown that ADT is associated with marked microarchitectural decay of bone with both cortical and trabecular bone losses.[47] Further studies will determine whether microarchitectural decay predicts fracture risk more accurately than BMD loss measured by conventional dual energy x-ray absorptiometry (DEXA). Mice with global[48] or osteoblast-specific[49] deletion of the androgen receptor also have decreased cortical and trabecular bone masses, confirming an essential role for testosterone in the maintenance of both bone compartments.

Several retrospective population-based studies have shown that men with prostate cancer managed with ADT have an increased risk of fractures.[50–54] In a retrospective cohort study of the SEER-Medicare database of more than 50,000 patients with prostate cancer who survived at least 5 years after the diagnosis of prostate cancer, 19.4% of the men who received ADT had a clinically apparent fracture compared with 12.6% of those who were not on ADT (P<.001).[52,55,56] Despite this compelling evidence of reduced BMD and increased fracture risk in men receiving ADT, the awareness of this issue is poor among health professionals, and osteoporosis remains undertreated in this group.[57,58] A prospective study from Canada found that bone health was discussed with only 1 of 7 patients commencing ADT. Lifestyle measures or calcium/vitamin D supplementation were recommended in less than 20% of patients, despite 60% of patients having osteopenia or osteoporosis at baseline.[57]

ASSESSMENT OF BONE HEALTH

All men undergoing ADT should have a baseline assessment of fracture risk (Box 2). Risk factors for osteoporosis should be ascertained, such as the history of minimal trauma fracture (MTF), cigarette smoking, excess alcohol intake, any use of glucocorticoids, and relevant coexisting medical conditions.[59] The risk of falls should be evaluated. BMD by DEXA should be measured in all patients at the commencement of ADT. In men with osteopenia, posteroanterior and lateral radiographs of the thoracolumbar spine should be performed to identify clinically silent vertebral fractures. DEXA should be repeated 12 months after commencement of ADT. Routine laboratory tests to screen for secondary causes of osteoporosis include measurements of serum calcium, phosphate, creatinine, vitamin D, and thyroid-stimulating hormone concentrations and liver function and a complete blood cell count.[10]

LIFESTYLE MEASURES AND CALCIUM AND VITAMIN D SUPPLEMENTATIONS

Recommended lifestyle measures include smoking cessation and reducing alcohol intake to less than 2 standard drinks per day.[59] Resistance exercise reduces fatigue and improves muscle strength and balance in men with prostate cancer receiving ADT,[31,60] which may in turn decrease the risk of falls. Exercise also increases BMD in older men in some studies.[59] Although there is no such evidence specific for men with prostate cancer, regular physical activity involving weight-bearing exercise and

Box 2
Assessment and management of bone health in men with prostate cancer receiving ADT

- Assessment at commencement of ADT should include a history of MTFs and risk factors for osteoporosis and BMD measurement by DEXA in all men. In men with osteopenia (T score < −1.5), posteroanterior as well as lateral thoracolumbar spine radiographies should be performed to evaluate for vertebral MTF.

- Total daily calcium intake should be 1200 mg to 1500 mg through dietary intake, supplements, or both. Calcium supplements should be avoided in patients with kidney stones, and emerging data about cardiovascular safety should be taken into account.

- Vitamin D supplementation should be prescribed to achieve a target serum vitamin D level of 75 nmol/L.

- In men with a clinical or radiological MTF, treatment with an antiresorptive agent such as a bisphosphonate should be commenced, unless contraindicated.

- Antiresorptive therapy for primary prevention of MTFs should be individualized and considered in men with a baseline BMD T score of −2.0 to −2.5 or less or in those with a 10-year absolute risk of a major osteoporotic fracture of 20% or more or of a hip fracture of 3% or more.

- BMD measurement should be repeated after 12 months of ADT, with subsequent individualized testing frequency.

Data from National Osteoporosis Foundation treatment guidelines. Available at: http://www. nof.org/professionals/clinical-guidelines.

resistance training should be encouraged because it likely confers multiple other health benefits. Epidemiologic studies have shown a possible association between high calcium intake and increased prostate cancer risk.[61] However, this seems not to be the case if daily calcium intake remains 1500 mg or less.[41] In contrast to demonstrated antifracture efficacy in men older than 50 years,[59] it is unknown whether vitamin D supplementation independently improves BMD or reduces the risk of fractures in men with prostate cancer receiving ADT. A retrospective analysis of 87 men with prostate cancer receiving ADT showed an independent association of vitamin D deficiency with spinal fractures (P = .003).[62] In line with the 2008 National Osteoporosis Foundation (NOF) guidelines for men who are 50 years and older, vitamin D supplementation (cholecalciferol 800–1000 IU/d) should be prescribed routinely to achieve vitamin D serum levels of 75 nmol/L. Calcium and vitamin sufficiency, however, are not sufficient to fully prevent bone loss during ADT.[63]

BISPHOSPHONATE THERAPY

Bisphosphonates including intravenous pamidronate,[63,64] intravenous zoledronic acid,[65–68] weekly oral alendronate,[69,70] and weekly or monthly oral risedronate[71,72] prevent ADT-induced loss of BMD in randomized controlled trials. Although placebo-treated patients receiving ADT lost 2% to 8% of BMD per year, patients randomized to bisphosphonates had either stable BMD or increases of up to 8% at the lumbar spine, with lesser but significant increases, around 2%, at the hip.[63–72] To date, there have been no trials of adequate size or duration to determine the effect of bisphosphonate therapy on fracture incidence in men receiving ADT for prostate cancer.

NONBISPHOSPHONATE PHARMACOTHERAPY

In contrast to the lack of current evidence with bisphosphonate therapy in ADT, 2 recent controlled trials have shown that both denosumab and the selective estrogen receptor modulator (SERM) toremifene reduce fracture incidence in men with nonmetastatic prostate cancer receiving ADT.[73,74] However, because neither agent has been compared head to head with bisphosphonates in a prospective trial powered for fracture end points, the superiority of these agents to bisphosphonates remains unproven. The first randomized controlled trial that demonstrated antifracture efficacy in men receiving ADT used denosumab. This study randomized men with mild osteopenia (baseline femoral neck T score of −1.5) and a median prior duration of ADT treatment of 20 months. At 36 months, denosumab increased lumbar spine BMD by 5.6% compared with a decrease of 1% with placebo.[73] Denosumab also reduced the incidence of vertebral fractures (cumulative incidence compared with placebo 0.3% vs 1.9% at 1 year and 1.5% vs 3.9% at 3 years). The number needed to treat to prevent one new vertebral fracture over three years was 42. Denosumab appeared well tolerated without a significant difference in adverse events. Denosumab is undergoing priority review by the Food and Drug Administration (FDA) for the prevention of bone loss in men receiving ADT.

The SERM toremifene significantly increased BMD at the hip and lumbar spine by 1.3% to 1.8% after 6 months.[75] In a recently completed 2-year randomized trial of 1389 men at high risk of fracture because of age greater than 70 years or low BMD, 80-mg toremifene daily decreased the incidence of new vertebral fractures in men receiving ADT by 53% ($P = .034$) compared with placebo and significantly increased BMD at the lumbar spine by 2% and at the hip by 1.6%.[74] In addition, toremifene had small but favorable effects on lipid profile and reduced hot flushes as well as breast tenderness.

RECOMMENDATION FOR PHARMACOTHERAPY

Evidence-based current NOF guidelines for the general male population recommend pharmacologic therapy with a bisphosphonate for primary prevention in men older than 50 years of age with a T score of −2.5 or less or if the 10-year major osteoporotic fracture probability exceeds 20% or if the 10-year hip fracture risk exceeds 3% (www. nof.org/professionals/Clinicians_Guide.htm). In addition, bisphosphonates are recommended for all men who are 50 years or older with a history of MTF. Therefore, all men with prostate cancer who are 50 years or older receiving ADT with a previous history of a clinical or radiological MTF should be commenced on antiresorptive therapy with a bisphosphonate, unless contraindicated (see **Box 2**).

In contrast, there is insufficient evidence specific to men with prostate cancer receiving ADT to make firm evidence-based recommendations as to when pharmacotherapy for primary prevention of osteoporotic fracture should be commenced. To date, there are no FDA-approved medications for fracture prevention in men receiving ADT, although denosumab is under review for this indication. A cutoff BMD T score of −2.0 or less to consider bisphosphonate therapy has been recommended by an expert panel for women with nonmetastatic breast cancer initiating aromatase inhibitors, who experience similar rates of bone loss and increases in fracture risk compared with men initiating ADT.[76] Thus, pharmacotherapy should be considered as primary prevention if the BMD T score of men with prostate cancer while receiving ADT is −2.0 or less to −2.5 or less, depending on clinical fracture risk.[10] In addition, antiresorptive therapy should be selectively considered for older men with multiple osteoporosis risk factors, especially if, based on FRAX (WHO Fracture Risk Assessment Tool), the 10-year absolute risk of a major osteoporotic fracture exceeds 20% or that of a hip fracture exceeds 3%. A recent analysis has concluded that in men starting ADT for localized prostate cancer, BMD testing followed by selective alendronate use for those with osteoporosis (T score <−2.5) is cost effective.[77]

METABOLIC HEALTH IN MEN WITH PROSTATE CANCER RECEIVING ADT

In men, even mildly reduced testosterone levels are associated with increased insulin resistance, type 2 diabetes, and features of the metabolic syndrome, such as obesity, hypertriglyceridemia, and reduced high-density lipoprotein (HDL) cholesterol.[78] Because men receiving ADT have testosterone levels in the castrate range,[7] they may be at even higher risk of developing such complications.

ADT-Induced Changes in Body Composition

Androgens are important determinants of body composition in men. Men with untreated hypogonadism have increased fat mass and decreased lean body mass. In contrast, testosterone therapy increases lean body mass and decreases fat mass in hypogonadal men.[79] Body composition changes, especially increased visceral adipose tissue, are a major factor in the inverse relationship between testosterone levels and insulin sensitivity.[80] Cross-sectional studies have revealed that men undergoing ADT have increased fat mass compared with eugonadal controls with prostate cancer.[29] In longitudinal observational studies, GnRH agonist therapy increased fat mass by about 10% and decreased lean body mass by about 3%, with 80% of these changes occurring within the first 3 months of therapy.[81,82] In a recent meta-analysis of 16 longitudinal studies, ADT increased fat mass by 7.7% and decreased lean body mass by 2.8%.[28] Thus, ADT causes sarcopenic obesity. Increased abdominal fat mass promotes insulin resistance, and reduced lean body mass aggravates insulin resistance by reducing glucose uptake in muscles (see **Fig. 1**).[83] Increased visceral obesity, possibly through the secretion of bone catabolic cytokines, has been associated with reduced BMD and reduced bone strength.[84]

Effects of ADT on Insulin Resistance and Glucose Metabolism

ADT is associated with an increase of 26% to 65% in insulin levels and corresponding increases in the indices of insulin resistance.[82,85] These changes become apparent within 3 months of ADT. In short-term (<6 months) prospective studies, fasting glucose levels did not increase, suggesting that compensatory hyperinsulinemia prevents progression to type 2 diabetes, at least temporarily.[82,86] Multiple population-based studies consistently show a significant association between the use of longer-term (>12 months) ADT and incident diabetes.[9,14] The largest study involved more than 73,000 men who were treated for 9 years.[87] Amongst a third of those men who received ADT, the risk of new diabetes was significantly increased with an adjusted hazard ratio of 1.44 (95% confidence interval [CI], 1.34–1.55).[87] In a cohort study of 19,079 men who are 66 years or older from the Ontario Cancer Registry, men given ADT had an increased risk of diabetes of 1.16 (95% CI, 1.11–1.21), and the number needed to harm for 1 new case of diabetes was 91.[88] The limitations of all such studies include nonrandomization, a reliance on administrative data to obtain information on diabetes incidence, and detection bias because men receiving ADT may have more frequent contact with health care providers.

ADT and Alterations in Lipid Profile

ADT has been associated with alterations in lipid profile in several prospective studies. Lipid changes occur early, during the first 3 to 12 months of therapy. Triglyceride levels increase by more than 25% and total cholesterol by 7% to 10%.[81,89] HDL-cholesterol levels increase by 8% to 20%, whereas changes in low-density lipoprotein cholesterol levels are variable (no change to up to 7% increase).[9,14]

ADT and Cardiovascular Risk

There is strong observational evidence that ADT is associated with insulin resistance, an independent cardiovascular risk factor,[90] and incident diabetes.[91] ADT has been shown to increase arterial stiffness.[85] Five large observational retrospective studies, with a total of almost 200,000 men with prostate cancer, have assessed whether ADT increases the risk of cardiovascular events,[87,88,92–94] already the most common cause of death in the population with prostate cancer.[3,4] The first study of 73,196 men with prostate cancer from the SEER database showed that ADT was associated with modestly increased risks of coronary heart disease (absolute hazard ratio [AHR], 1.16; 95% CI, 1.10–1.21), myocardial infarction (AHR, 1.11; 95% CI, 1.01–1.21), and sudden cardiac death (AHR, 1.16; 95% CI, 1.05–1.27).[87] This finding has been confirmed in a study from the Veterans Administration database, with increased risk of coronary heart disease (AHR, 1.19; 95% CI, 1.10–1.28), myocardial infarction (AHR, 1.28; 95% CI, 1.08–1.52), and sudden cardiac death (AHR, 1.35; 95% CI, 1.18–1.54).[94] The increased risk, however, was relatively modest, with an estimated 1 extra myocardial infarction for every 200 men treated with ADT for a mean of 2.6 years. Similarly, a Swedish National Prostate Cancer Registry study of 31,000 patients with prostate cancer estimated that 10 ischemic heart disease events a year occur for every 1000 men receiving ADT.[93] A study of 23,000 men showed an AHR of 1.20 for serious cardiovascular morbidity even after 1 year of ADT,[92] and a pooled analysis of 3 randomized trials reported a shorter time to fatal myocardial infarction in men treated with 6 months of ADT compared with men who were hormone naive.[95] A systematic review based on more than 80,000 patients with prostate cancer has shown that ADT is associated with an increase in cardiovascular mortality of 17%.[56] A recent science advisory from the American Heart Association, the American Cancer Society, and the American Urological Association has concluded that "there may be a relationship between ADT and cardiovascular events and death."[96] The advisory acknowledged plausibility based on the adverse effect of ADT on cardiovascular risk factors and suggested that future trials of ADT should assess cardiovascular risk factors and monitor cardiovascular events.[96] No published intervention study has assessed insulin resistance, glycemia, or cardiovascular risk in this patient population. There is currently no evidence that routine cardiac stress testing or ultrasound imaging of the carotid artery affects outcomes, especially in asymptomatic patients.

ASSESSMENT AND MANAGEMENT OF METABOLIC AND CARDIOVASCULAR HEALTH

Older men with prostate cancer are at relatively high risk of metabolic syndrome, diabetes, and cardiovascular events. These risks may be further aggravated by ADT. Such risk needs to be weighed against the expected benefits of ADT.[10] Despite the absence of high-level evidence of outcome benefits specific to men with prostate cancer receiving ADT, the authors recommend close monitoring and intervention, especially during the first year of ADT, given that the available data suggest that metabolic complications occur within 3 to 6 months (**Box 3**). Cardiovascular risk factors should be managed according to current clinical practice. Lifestyle intervention should be instituted at the commencement of ADT to prevent weight gain and insulin resistance. Macrovascular targets for men with prediabetes should be the same as those for established diabetes,[97] with blood pressure less than 130/80 mm Hg and lipid targets according to the National Cholesterol Education Program Adult Treatment Panel III. In men with preexisting diabetes, antiglycemic therapy may need intensification to maintain individualized HbA1c targets.

It is incumbent on treating doctors to fully inform patients of the effects, both beneficial and detrimental, of ADT. Not infrequently, physicians treating such patients are

---

Box 3
Assessment and management of metabolic and cardiovascular health in men with prostate cancer receiving ADT

- Before commencing ADT, metabolic risk assessment should include body mass index, waist circumference, blood pressure, fasting blood glucose, oral glucose tolerance test (if fasting glucose between 100–125 mg/dL), and fasting lipid profile.

- During the first year of ADT, metabolic assessment should be repeated at 6 and 12 months, with subsequent testing frequency.

- Intensive lifestyle intervention should be instituted to prevent weight gain and worsening of insulin resistance.

- Management includes reducing cardiovascular risk factors, particularly smoking cessation. Blood pressure should be less than 130/80 mm Hg and lipid targets according to the National Cholesterol Education Program Adult Treatment Panel III treatment guidelines.

Data from the American Diabetes Association. Available at: http://care.diabetesjournals.org/content/34/Supplement_1; the National Cholesterol Education Program Adult Treatment Panel III. Available at: http://www.nhlbi.nih.gov/guidelines/cholesterol/index.htm; and the American Heart Association treatment guidelines. Available at: http://my.americanheart.org/professional/StatementsGuidelines/Statements-Guidelines_UCM_316885_SubHomePage.jsp.

---

referred symptomatic men to whom no specific information about the metabolic and other effects of ADT has been supplied. This situation should be avoided at all costs.

FUTURE DIRECTIONS

The current information is inadequate to assess the risk-benefit ratio of ADT for a large proportion of men with prostate cancer. Controlled trials are required to assess the effect of ADT on survival in men with localized prostate cancer or PSA recurrence. In addition, such trials should be designed to help determine the optimal length of ADT for specific patient populations. The role of using intermittent ADT to minimize adverse effects while maintaining antitumor efficacy needs to be defined. Trials are necessary to better define the harm caused by ADT, especially with respect to fracture and cardiovascular events. Randomized intervention trials using pharmacologic therapy powered for fracture outcomes should be available in the near future to provide more definitive criteria as to when to institute such treatment for primary prevention and to guide the duration of therapy. The effect of ADT on glucose metabolism and cardiovascular events and the value of preventive strategies need to be defined more precisely in prospective studies. Such information is crucial to better quantitate the risk-benefit ratio of ADT for the individual patient with prostate cancer.

REFERENCES

1. Crawford ED. Epidemiology of prostate cancer. Urology 2003;62:3–12.
2. SEER. Surveillance, Epidemiology and End Results (SEER): stat fact sheets: prostate cancer 2008. Available at: http://seercancergov/statfacts/html/prosthtml. Accessed August 26, 2010.
3. Satariano WA, Ragland KE, Van Den Eeden SK. Cause of death in men diagnosed with prostate carcinoma. Cancer 1998;83:1180–8.
4. Lu-Yao G, Stukel TA, Yao SL. Changing patterns in competing causes of death in men with prostate cancer: a population based study. J Urol 2004;171:2285–90.

5. Damber JE, Aus G. Prostate cancer. Lancet 2008;371:1710–21.
6. Sharifi N, Gulley JL, Dahut WL. Androgen deprivation therapy for prostate cancer. JAMA 2005;294:238–44.
7. Leuprolide versus diethylstilbestrol for metastatic prostate cancer. The Leuprolide Study Group. N Engl J Med 1984;311:1281–6.
8. Bolla M, de Reijke TM, Van Tienhoven G, et al. Duration of androgen suppression in the treatment of prostate cancer. N Engl J Med 2009;360:2516–27.
9. Shahani S, Braga-Basaria M, Basaria S. Androgen deprivation therapy in prostate cancer and metabolic risk for atherosclerosis. J Clin Endocrinol Metab 2008;93: 2042–9.
10. Grossmann M, Hamilton EJ, Gilfillan C, et al. Bone and metabolic health in patients with prostate cancer receiving androgen deprivation therapy—management guidelines on behalf of the Endocrine Society of Australia, the Australian and New Zealand Bone and Mineral Society, and the Urological Society of Australia and New Zealand. Med J Aust 2011;194:301–6.
11. Wong YN, Freedland SJ, Egleston B, et al. The role of primary androgen deprivation therapy in localized prostate cancer. Eur Urol 2009;56:609–16.
12. D'Amico AV, Chen MH, Renshaw AA, et al. Androgen suppression and radiation versus radiation alone for prostate cancer: a randomized trial. JAMA 2008;299:289–95.
13. Network NCC. NCCN practice guidelines in oncology. Version 1. Available at: http://www.nccn.org/professionals/physician_gls/f_guidelines.asp. Accessed August 1, 2010.
14. Smith MR. Androgen deprivation therapy for prostate cancer: new concepts and concerns. Curr Opin Endocrinol Diabetes Obes 2007;14:247–54.
15. Khosla S. Update in male osteoporosis. J Clin Endocrinol Metab 2010;95:3–10.
16. Cowie CC, Rust KF, Byrd-Holt DD, et al. Prevalence of diabetes and high risk for diabetes using A1C criteria in the U.S. population in 1988-2006. Diabetes Care 2010;33:562–8.
17. Tangen CM, Faulkner JR, Crawford ED, et al. Ten-year survival in patients with metastatic prostate cancer. Clin Prostate Cancer 2003;2:41–5.
18. Smith DP, King MT, Egger S, et al. Quality of life 3 years after diagnosis of localised prostate cancer: population based cohort study. BMJ 2009;339: b4817.
19. Lubeck DP, Grossfeld GD, Carroll PR. The effect of androgen deprivation therapy on health-related quality of life in men with prostate cancer. Urology 2001;58:94–100.
20. Nelson CJ, Lee JS, Gamboa MC, et al. Cognitive effects of hormone therapy in men with prostate cancer: a review. Cancer 2008;113:1097–106.
21. Salminen E, Portin R, Korpela J, et al. Androgen deprivation and cognition in prostate cancer. Br J Cancer 2003;89:971–6.
22. Shahinian VB, Kuo YF, Freeman JL, et al. Risk of the "androgen deprivation syndrome" in men receiving androgen deprivation for prostate cancer. Arch Intern Med 2006;166:465–71.
23. Handelsman DJ, Zajac JD. 11: androgen deficiency and replacement therapy in men. Med J Aust 2004;180:529–35.
24. Strum SB, McDermed JE, Scholz MC, et al. Anaemia associated with androgen deprivation in patients with prostate cancer receiving combined hormone blockade. Br J Urol 1997;79:933–41.
25. Hyde Z, Flicker L, Almeida OP, et al. Low free testosterone predicts frailty in older men: the health in men study. J Clin Endocrinol Metab 2010;95:3165–72.
26. Basaria S, Coviello AD, Travison TG, et al. Adverse events associated with testosterone administration. N Engl J Med 2010;363:109–22.

27. MacLean HE, Chiu WS, Notini AJ, et al. Impaired skeletal muscle development and function in male, but not female, genomic androgen receptor knockout mice. FASEB J 2008;22:2676–89.
28. Haseen F, Murray LJ, Cardwell CR, et al. The effect of androgen deprivation therapy on body composition in men with prostate cancer: systematic review and meta-analysis. J Cancer Surviv 2010;4:128–39.
29. Basaria S, Lieb J 2nd, Tang AM, et al. Long-term effects of androgen deprivation therapy in prostate cancer patients. Clin Endocrinol (Oxf) 2002;56:779–86.
30. Galvao DA, Taaffe DR, Spry N, et al. Combined resistance and aerobic exercise program reverses muscle loss in men undergoing androgen suppression therapy for prostate cancer without bone metastases: a randomized controlled trial. J Clin Oncol 2010;28:340–7.
31. Segal RJ, Reid RD, Courneya KS, et al. Resistance exercise in men receiving androgen deprivation therapy for prostate cancer. J Clin Oncol 2003;21:1653–9.
32. Potosky AL, Knopf K, Clegg LX, et al. Quality-of-life outcomes after primary androgen deprivation therapy: results from the prostate cancer outcomes study. J Clin Oncol 2001;19:3750–7.
33. Teloken PE, Ohebshalom M, Mohideen N, et al. Analysis of the impact of androgen deprivation therapy on sildenafil citrate response following radiation therapy for prostate cancer. J Urol 2007;178:2521–5.
34. Irani J, Salomon L, Oba R, et al. Efficacy of venlafaxine, medroxyprogesterone acetate, and cyproterone acetate for the treatment of vasomotor hot flushes in men taking gonadotropin-releasing hormone analogues for prostate cancer: a double-blind, randomised trial. Lancet Oncol 2010;11:147–54.
35. Loprinzi CL, Michalak JC, Quella SK, et al. Megestrol acetate for the prevention of hot flashes. N Engl J Med 1994;331:347–52.
36. Quella SK, Loprinzi CL, Sloan J, et al. Pilot evaluation of venlafaxine for the treatment of hot flashes in men undergoing androgen ablation therapy for prostate cancer. J Urol 1999;162:98–102.
37. Loprinzi CL, Barton DL, Carpenter LA, et al. Pilot evaluation of paroxetine for treating hot flashes in men. Mayo Clin Proc 2004;79:1247–51.
38. Boccardo F, Rubagotti A, Battaglia M, et al. Evaluation of tamoxifen and anastrozole in the prevention of gynecomastia and breast pain induced by bicalutamide monotherapy of prostate cancer. J Clin Oncol 2005;23:808–15.
39. Center JR, Nguyen TV, Schneider D, et al. Mortality after all major types of osteoporotic fracture in men and women: an observational study. Lancet 1999;353:878–82.
40. Holmes-Walker DJ, Woo H, Gurney H, et al. Maintaining bone health in patients with prostate cancer. Med J Aust 2006;184:176–9.
41. Greenspan SL. Approach to the prostate cancer patient with bone disease. J Clin Endocrinol Metab 2008;93:2–7.
42. Higano CS. Androgen-deprivation-therapy-induced fractures in men with nonmetastatic prostate cancer: what do we really know? Nat Clin Pract Urol 2008;5:24–34.
43. Greenspan SL, Coates P, Sereika SM, et al. Bone loss after initiation of androgen deprivation therapy in patients with prostate cancer. J Clin Endocrinol Metab 2005;90:6410–7.
44. Diamond TH, Higano CS, Smith MR, et al. Osteoporosis in men with prostate carcinoma receiving androgen-deprivation therapy: recommendations for diagnosis and therapies. Cancer 2004;100:892–9.
45. Morote J, Orsola A, Abascal JM, et al. Bone mineral density changes in patients with prostate cancer during the first 2 years of androgen suppression. J Urol 2006;175:1679–83 [discussion: 1683].

46. Morote J, Morin JP, Orsola A, et al. Prevalence of osteoporosis during long-term androgen deprivation therapy in patients with prostate cancer. Urology 2007;69: 500–4.
47. Hamilton EJ, Ghasem-Zadeh A, Gianatti E, et al. Structural decay of bone micro-architecture in men with prostate cancer treated with androgen deprivation therapy. J Clin Endocrinol Metab 2010;95(12):E456–63.
48. MacLean HE, Moore AJ, Sastra SA, et al. DNA-binding-dependent androgen receptor signaling contributes to gender differences and has physiological actions in males and females. J Endocrinol 2010;206:93–103.
49. Chiang C, Chiu M, Moore AJ, et al. Mineralization and bone resorption are regulated by the androgen receptor in male mice. J Bone Miner Res 2009;24:621–31.
50. Smith MR, Lee WC, Brandman J, et al. Gonadotropin-releasing hormone agonists and fracture risk: a claims-based cohort study of men with nonmetastatic prostate cancer. J Clin Oncol 2005;23:7897–903.
51. Smith MR, Boyce SP, Moyneur E, et al. Risk of clinical fractures after gonadotropin-releasing hormone agonist therapy for prostate cancer. J Urol 2006;175:136–9 [discussion: 139].
52. Shahinian VB, Kuo YF, Freeman JL, et al. Risk of fracture after androgen deprivation for prostate cancer. N Engl J Med 2005;352:154–64.
53. Abrahamsen B, Nielsen MF, Eskildsen P, et al. Fracture risk in Danish men with prostate cancer: a nationwide register study. BJU Int 2007;100:749–54.
54. Oefelein MG, Ricchuiti V, Conrad W, et al. Skeletal fracture associated with androgen suppression induced osteoporosis: the clinical incidence and risk factors for patients with prostate cancer. J Urol 2001;166:1724–8.
55. Alibhai SM, Duong-Hua M, Cheung AM, et al. Fracture types and risk factors in men with prostate cancer on androgen deprivation therapy: a matched cohort study of 19,079 men. J Urol 2010;184:918–24.
56. Taylor LG, Canfield SE, Du XL. Review of major adverse effects of androgen-deprivation therapy in men with prostate cancer. Cancer 2009;115:2388–99.
57. Panju AH, Breunis H, Cheung AM, et al. Management of decreased bone mineral density in men starting androgen-deprivation therapy for prostate cancer. BJU Int 2009;103:753–7.
58. Tanvetyanon T. Physician practices of bone density testing and drug prescribing to prevent or treat osteoporosis during androgen deprivation therapy. Cancer 2005;103:237–41.
59. Ebeling PR. Clinical practice. Osteoporosis in men. N Engl J Med 2008;358:1474–82.
60. Galvao DA, Nosaka K, Taaffe DR, et al. Resistance training and reduction of treatment side effects in prostate cancer patients. Med Sci Sports Exercise 2006;38: 2045–52.
61. Giovannucci E, Rimm EB, Wolk A, et al. Calcium and fructose intake in relation to risk of prostate cancer. Cancer Res 1998;58:442–7.
62. Diamond TH, Bucci J, Kersley JH, et al. Osteoporosis and spinal fractures in men with prostate cancer: risk factors and effects of androgen deprivation therapy. J Urol 2004;172:529–32.
63. Smith MR, McGovern FJ, Zietman AL, et al. Pamidronate to prevent bone loss during androgen-deprivation therapy for prostate cancer. N Engl J Med 2001; 345:948–55.
64. Diamond TH, Winters J, Smith A, et al. The antiosteoporotic efficacy of intravenous pamidronate in men with prostate carcinoma receiving combined androgen blockade: a double blind, randomized, placebo-controlled crossover study. Cancer 2001;92:1444–50.

65. Michaelson MD, Kaufman DS, Lee H, et al. Randomized controlled trial of annual zoledronic acid to prevent gonadotropin-releasing hormone agonist-induced bone loss in men with prostate cancer. J Clin Oncol 2007;25:1038–42.
66. Smith MR, Eastham J, Gleason DM, et al. Randomized controlled trial of zoledronic acid to prevent bone loss in men receiving androgen deprivation therapy for nonmetastatic prostate cancer. J Urol 2003;169:2008–12.
67. Satoh T, Kimura M, Matsumoto K, et al. Single infusion of zoledronic acid to prevent androgen deprivation therapy-induced bone loss in men with hormone-naive prostate carcinoma. Cancer 2009;115:3468–74.
68. Ryan CW, Huo D, Bylow K, et al. Suppression of bone density loss and bone turnover in patients with hormone-sensitive prostate cancer and receiving zoledronic acid. BJU Int 2007;100:70–5.
69. Greenspan SL, Nelson JB, Trump DL, et al. Effect of once-weekly oral alendronate on bone loss in men receiving androgen deprivation therapy for prostate cancer: a randomized trial. Ann Intern Med 2007;146:416–24.
70. Planas J, Trilla E, Raventos C, et al. Alendronate decreases the fracture risk in patients with prostate cancer on androgen-deprivation therapy and with severe osteopenia or osteoporosis. BJU Int 2009;104(11):1637–40.
71. Ishizaka K, Machida T, Kobayashi S, et al. Preventive effect of risedronate on bone loss in men receiving androgen-deprivation therapy for prostate cancer. Int J Urol 2007;14:1071–5.
72. Izumi K, Mizokami A, Sugimoto K, et al. Risedronate recovers bone loss in patients with prostate cancer undergoing androgen-deprivation therapy. Urology 2009;73:1342–6.
73. Smith MR, Egerdie B, Hernandez Toriz N, et al. Denosumab in men receiving androgen-deprivation therapy for prostate cancer. N Engl J Med 2009;361:745–55.
74. Smith MR, Morton RA, Barnette KG, et al. Toremifene to reduce fracture risk in men receiving androgen deprivation therapy for prostate cancer. J Urol 2010; 184(4):1316–21.
75. Smith MR, Malkowicz SB, Chu F, et al. Toremifene increases bone mineral density in men receiving androgen deprivation therapy for prostate cancer: interim analysis of a multicenter phase 3 clinical study. J Urol 2008;179:152–5.
76. Reid DM, Doughty J, Eastell R, et al. Guidance for the management of breast cancer treatment-induced bone loss: a consensus position statement from a UK Expert Group. Cancer Treat Rev 2008;34(Suppl 1):S3–18.
77. Ito K, Elkin EB, Girotra M, et al. Cost-effectiveness of fracture prevention in men who receive androgen deprivation therapy for localized prostate cancer. Ann Intern Med 2010;152:621–9.
78. Grossmann M, Thomas MC, Panagiotopoulos S, et al. Low testosterone levels are common and associated with insulin resistance in men with diabetes. J Clin Endocrinol Metab 2008;93:1834–40.
79. Allan CA, McLachlan RI. Age-related changes in testosterone and the role of replacement therapy in older men. Clin Endocrinol (Oxf) 2004;60:653–70.
80. Grossmann M, Gianatti EJ, Zajac JD. Testosterone and type 2 diabetes. Curr Opin Endocrinol Diabetes Obes 2010;17:247–56.
81. Smith MR, Finkelstein JS, McGovern FJ, et al. Changes in body composition during androgen deprivation therapy for prostate cancer. J Clin Endocrinol Metab 2002;87:599–603.
82. Smith MR, Lee H, Nathan DM. Insulin sensitivity during combined androgen blockade for prostate cancer. J Clin Endocrinol Metab 2006;91:1305–8.

83. Shepherd PR, Kahn BB. Glucose transporters and insulin action—implications for insulin resistance and diabetes mellitus. N Engl J Med 1999;341:248–57.
84. Gilsanz V, Chalfant J, Mo AO, et al. Reciprocal relations of subcutaneous and visceral fat to bone structure and strength. J Clin Endocrinol Metab 2009;94:3387–93.
85. Smith JC, Bennett S, Evans LM, et al. The effects of induced hypogonadism on arterial stiffness, body composition, and metabolic parameters in males with prostate cancer. J Clin Endocrinol Metab 2001;86:4261–7.
86. Dockery F, Bulpitt CJ, Agarwal S, et al. Testosterone suppression in men with prostate cancer leads to an increase in arterial stiffness and hyperinsulinaemia. Clin Sci (Lond) 2003;104:195–201.
87. Keating NL, O'Malley AJ, Smith MR. Diabetes and cardiovascular disease during androgen deprivation therapy for prostate cancer. J Clin Oncol 2006;24:4448–56.
88. Alibhai SM, Duong-Hua M, Sutradhar R, et al. Impact of androgen deprivation therapy on cardiovascular disease and diabetes. J Clin Oncol 2009;27:3452–8.
89. Eri LM, Urdal P, Bechensteen AG. Effects of the luteinizing hormone-releasing hormone agonist leuprolide on lipoproteins, fibrinogen and plasminogen activator inhibitor in patients with benign prostatic hyperplasia. J Urol 1995;154:100–4.
90. Despres JP, Lamarche B, Mauriege P, et al. Hyperinsulinemia as an independent risk factor for ischemic heart disease. N Engl J Med 1996;334:952–7.
91. Faris JE, Smith MR. Metabolic sequelae associated with androgen deprivation therapy for prostate cancer. Curr Opin Endocrinol Diabetes Obes 2010;17:240–6.
92. Saigal CS, Gore JL, Krupski TL, et al. Androgen deprivation therapy increases cardiovascular morbidity in men with prostate cancer. Cancer 2007;110:1493–500.
93. Van Hemelrick M, Garmo H, Bratt H, et al. Increased cardiovascular morbidity and mortality following endocrine treatment for prostate cancer: an analysis in 30,642 men in PCBaSe Sweden. Eur J Cancer Suppl 2009;7:1.
94. Keating NL, O'Malley AJ, Freedland SJ, et al. Diabetes and cardiovascular disease during androgen deprivation therapy: observational study of veterans with prostate cancer. J Natl Cancer Inst 2010;102:39–46.
95. D'Amico AV, Denham JW, Crook J, et al. Influence of androgen suppression therapy for prostate cancer on the frequency and timing of fatal myocardial infarctions. J Clin Oncol 2007;25:2420–5.
96. Levine GN, D'Amico AV, Berger P, et al. Androgen-deprivation therapy in prostate cancer and cardiovascular risk: a science advisory from the American Heart Association, American Cancer Society, and American Urological Association: endorsed by the American Society for Radiation Oncology. Circulation 2010; 121:833–40.
97. Twigg SM, Kamp MC, Davis TM, et al. Prediabetes: a position statement from the Australian Diabetes Society and Australian Diabetes Educators Association. Med J Aust 2007;186:461–5.

Index

Note: Page numbers of article titles are in **boldface** type.

A

Endocrinol Metab Clin N Am 40 (2011) 673–701
doi:10.1016/S0889-8529(11)00084-3
0889-8529/11/$ – see front matter © 2011 Elsevier Inc. All rights reserved.

endo.theclinics.com

Printed and bound by CPI Group (UK) Ltd, Croydon, CR0 4YY

03/10/2024

01040455-0007